Workbook for

McCurnin's Clinical Textbook for Veterinary Technicians

Ninth Edition

Sherry Castle Boyer
President
Castle Media Consultants
Jackson, Mississippi

ELSEVIER

ELSEVIER

3251 Riverport Lane
St. Louis, Missouri 63043

Notices

Knowledge and best practice in this field are constantly changing. As new research and experience broaden
our understanding, changes in research methods, professional practices, or medical treatment may become
necessary.

Practitioners and researchers must always rely on their own experience and knowledge in evaluating and
using any information, methods, compounds, or experiments described herein. In using such information or
methods they should be mindful of their own safety and the safety of others, including parties for whom
they have a professional responsibility.

With respect to any drug or pharmaceutical products identified, readers are advised to check the most
current information provided (i) on procedures featured or (ii) by the manufacturer of each product to be
administered, to verify the recommended dose or formula, the method and duration of administration, and
contraindications. It is the responsibility of practitioners, relying on their own experience and knowledge of
their patients, to make diagnoses, to determine dosages and the best treatment for each individual patient,
and to take all appropriate safety precautions.

To the fullest extent of the law, neither the Publisher nor the authors, contributors, or editors, assume any
liability for any injury and/or damage to persons or property as a matter of products liability, negligence or
otherwise, or from any use or operation of any methods, products, instructions, or ideas contained in the material herein.

Content Strategist: Brandi Graham
Content Development Manager: Ellen Wurm-Cutter
Associate Content Development Specialist: Erin Garner
Publishing Services Manager: Deepthi Unni
Project Manager: Nadhiya Sekar
Design Direction: Muthukumaran Thangaraj

Working together
to grow libraries in
developing countries

www.elsevier.com • www.bookaid.org

Printed in the United States of America

Last digit is the print number: 9 8 7 6 5 4 3 2

Previous Edition Contributors

Paige A. Allen, MS, RVT, AS, BSBA
Instructional Technologist
Veterinary Technology Program
College of Veterinary Medicine
Purdue University
West Lafayette, Indiana

Josh L. Clark, MS, RVT
Instructional Technologist
Veterinary Technology Program
Purdue University
West Lafayette, Indiana

Brenda Arth Johnson, DVM
Professor and Program Coordinator
Veterinary Technology Program
Columbus State Community College
Columbus, Ohio

Erin M. Kelly, DVM
Adjunct Faculty
Veterinary Technology
Columbus State Community College
Columbus, Ohio

Kathianne Komurek, DVM, MA
Program Coordinator
Veterinary Technology
Manor College
Jenkintown, Pennsylvania

Carla Mayers Bletsch, DVM
Assistant Professor
Veterinary Technology
Columbus State Community College
Columbus, Ohio

Terence A. Olive, DVM
Associate Professor
Lead Attending Veterinarian
Veterinary Technology
Columbus State Community College
Columbus, Ohio

Stuart L. Porter, VMD
Professor and Program Coordinator
Veterinary Technology Program
Blue Ridge Community College
Weyers Cave, Virginia

Lori Renda-Francis, PhD, MA, BBA, LVT
Professor/Program Director
Veterinary Technology Department
Macomb Community College
Clinton Township, Michigan

Marianne Tear, MS, LVT
Program Director
Veterinary Technology
Baker College of Clinton Township
Clinton Township, Michigan

John A. Thomas, DVM
Assistant Professor
Veterinary Technology
Cuyahoga Community College
Cleveland, Ohio

Preface

This workbook is intended to accompany the ninth edition of the textbook *McCurnin's Textbook for Veterinary Technicians.* Each chapter in the workbook relates to a corresponding chapter in the textbook and stresses the essential information of the chapter through the use of definitions, short answer (comprehension), photo quizzes, matching, fill-in-the-blank, true or false, multiple choice questions, word searches, and crossword puzzles.

Learning objectives are included at the beginning of each chapter to help you focus on the material that you are expected to learn and understand how these concepts can be applied in the veterinary clinical setting.

The following suggestions will help you use this workbook to identify strengths and weaknesses:

1. Review the contents of each chapter before you attempt to do the exercise. Do not treat the questions individually and then refer to the text for the correct answer. Deal with the chapter's subject matter as a whole, as many of the questions are interrelated. This is a learning exercise meant to help you learn the material presented in the textbook, not an examination for grades.

2. Remember that the same subject matter may be repeated in different question forms in each chapter or other chapters, as the material overlaps. The subjects of the questions are not necessarily in the same order as they appear in the textbook, although the questions in each exercise are grouped to match the order of the main sections in the text.

3. Read each question and study each illustration carefully before answering. You may know the answer or you may arrive at the correct answer by knowing which answers are incorrect.

4. This workbook is designed so that the pages can be easily removed and submitted, if required, and placed in your notebook with the corresponding lecture notes.

The answers to all the exercises appear as an Instructor Resource for *McCurnin's Textbook for Veterinary Technicians* on the Evolve website. For additional study, review questions for each chapter are available in the Student Resources on the Evolve website.

Contents

v

1 Introduction to Veterinary Technology: Its Laws and Ethics

LEARNING OBJECTIVES

When you have completed this chapter, you will be able to:
1. Pronounce, define, and spell all of the Key Terms in this chapter.
2. Describe the events from 1963 to 1990 that led to the development of modern veterinary technology in the United States and Canada.
3. Describe the educational and credentialing requirements established in most states for entry into the profession of veterinary technology.
4. Explain the structure, format, and scheduling of the VTNE.
5. List the six features that characterize the profession.
6. Describe the five steps of the veterinary technician practice model.
7. Describe the scope of practice for veterinary technicians, and list four duties performed only by veterinarians.
8. Describe areas of responsibility for veterinary technicians in clinical practice.
9. List the members of the veterinary health care team and describe their respective roles. In your description of veterinary technician specialists, include a list of the veterinary technician academies recognized by NAVTA.
10. Describe professional appearance, conduct, and communication.
11. Name the organizations represented by the acronyms AVMA, CVMA, CVTEA, NAVTA, AAVSB, and RVTTC and describe their roles in the education and credentialing of veterinary technicians.
12. Describe professional ethics.
13. Differentiate between statutes (laws) and regulations.
14. Describe the role of state boards in the credentialing of veterinary professionals.
15. List possible grounds for disciplinary action by state or provincial boards, list three levels of supervision defined in the NAVTA Model Rules and Regulations, and describe how these levels affect the veterinary technician's scope of practice.
16. Describe steps and possible sanctions carried out during disciplinary action against a licensee.
17. Describe how laws related to labor, medical waste, controlled substances, and animals relate to the profession of veterinary technology.
18. Name and describe laws that are specific to Canada regarding animals.

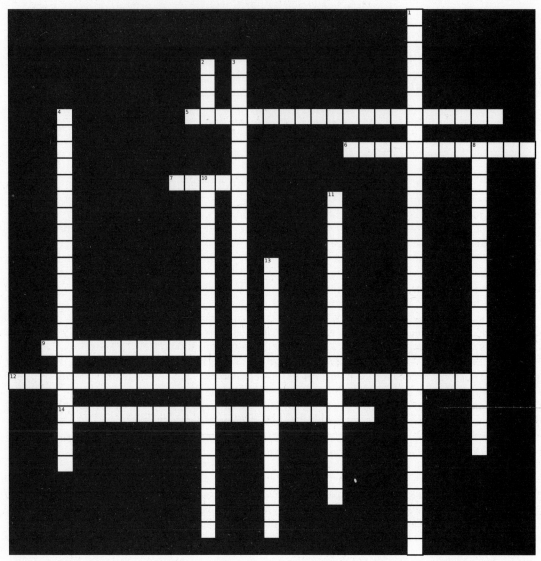

Across

5 The science and art of providing professional support to veterinarians. (two words)
6 A member of the veterinary health care team who may prognose, diagnose, and prescribe.
7 The acronym for a veterinary technician association that has written the code of ethics and the veterinary technician oath.
9 The primary state law or statute written and passed by the legislature to govern the practice of a profession in that state. (two words)
12 A member of the veterinary health care team with a higher level of skill in a particular discipline of veterinary technology. (three words)
14 Conclusions drawn from patient assessment and analysis of the database. (two words)

Down

1 The process carried out by veterinary technicians when assessing, caring for and reevaluating animal patients, which provides a methodology for providing consistently excellent patient care. (four words)
2 In most states, a passing score on this test is required to become an LVT, CVT, or RVT.
3 A member of the veterinary health care team with an AS degree, who completes all patient care duties except those exclusive to the practice of veterinary medicine. (two words)
4 An action planned and implemented by the veterinary technician to address a patient's reaction to illness, risk of future problems, and owner knowledge deficit. (two words)
8 Mandates written by the state board. (three words)
10 A member of the veterinary health care team with a BS in veterinary technology. (two words)
11 A member of the veterinary health care team who may be trained on the job. (two words)
13 The "father" of veterinary technology.

EXERCISE 1.2 MATCHING #1: IMPORTANT EVENTS IN THE HISTORY OF VETERINARY TECHNOLOGY (SEE TIMELINE IN THE FRONT MATTER OF THE TEXTBOOK)

Instructions: Place the 16 listed events in the proper chronological order (least recent to most recent) by placing the appropriate letter in the space provided on the left. Then, in the space on the right, place the year that each event occurred.

Column A

Event	Year
1. _____	_____
2. _____	_____
3. _____	_____
4. _____	_____
5. _____	_____
6. _____	_____
7. _____	_____
8. _____	_____
9. _____	_____
10. _____	_____
11. _____	_____
12. _____	_____
13. _____	_____
14. _____	_____
15. _____	_____
16. _____	_____

Column B

A. The first specialty in veterinary technology is established (the Academy of Veterinary Emergency and Critical Care Technicians).

B. The AVMA Advisory Committee on Animal Technicians urges all state veterinary medical associations to establish advisory committees on animal technicians.

C. A group of eight students graduate from the SUNY at Delhi animal technician program. (This represents the first group of graduates from an animal technician program.)

D. NAVTA adopts a national code of ethics for veterinary technicians.

E. The Committee on Accreditation of Training for Animal Technicians (CATAT) is formed by the AVMA to accredit training programs for animal technicians.

F. Walter Collins, DVM, receives federal funding to develop model curricula for training veterinary technicians.

G. The Canadian Association of Animal Health Technicians (CAAHT) is formed.

H. The first professional journal for veterinary technicians, *Methods: The Journal for Animal Health Technicians,* is published.

I. The first Animal Technician National Exam (predecessor to the VTNE) is given in Maine.

J. The AVMA accredits the first distance-learning program in veterinary technology.

K. The North American Veterinary Technician Association (NAVTA) is organized.

L. The first two programs are accredited by the AVMA (Michigan State University and Nebraska College of Technical Agriculture).

M. Members of the Ontario Association of Veterinary Technicians (OAVT) in Canada pass bylaws establishing it as the first self-regulating group in the profession of veterinary technology.

N. The AVMA House of Delegates approves the use of the term *veterinary technician*, which replaces animal technician.

O. NAVTA creates the Committee on Veterinary Technician Specialties (CVTS) to oversee the development of veterinary technician academies.

P. In December, the premier issue of *The NAVTA Journal* is released.

EXERCISE 1.3 MATCHING #2: ACRONYMS RELATED TO ASSOCIATIONS, AGENCIES, AND COMMITTEES

Instructions: Match each acronym in column A with the corresponding description in column B by writing the appropriate letter in the space provided.

Column A

1. _____ AALAS
2. _____ CVMA
3. _____ AAVSB
4. _____ CAAHTT
5. _____ ACC
6. _____ CALAS
7. _____ IACUC
8. _____ AVTE
9. _____ CVTEA
10. _____ USFWS
11. _____ AVMA

Column B

A. The committee that accredits veterinary technology programs in the United States under the auspices of the AVMA.

B. A Canadian association dedicated to advancing the knowledge, skills, and status of those who work with laboratory animals.

C. The agency that coadministers the Endangered Species Act in the United States.

D. An association dedicated to strengthening the animal health technologist/veterinary technician profession in Canada.

E. An organization that accredits veterinary technology programs in Canada.

F. A committee that works with research and educational institutions in the United States to help ensure compliance with and to enforce the Animal Welfare Act.

G. A professional association in the United States that is dedicated to the humane care and treatment of laboratory animals.

H. A group whose members are primarily instructors, staff, and managers of veterinary technology programs.

I. The organization responsible for appointing members of the Veterinary Technician National Exam Committee (VTNE).

J. A committee that oversees the care and use of animals in education and research in Canada.

K. The organization responsible for accrediting U.S. programs of veterinary technology.

EXERCISE 1.4 MATCHING #3: ACRONYMS RELATED TO CERTIFICATIONS, LAWS, AND OTHER ENTITIES

Instructions: Match each acronym in column A with the corresponding description in column B by writing the appropriate letter in the space provided.

Column A

1. _____ RACE
2. _____ ALAT
3. _____ VTS
4. _____ RMLAT
5. _____ LATG
6. _____ AWA
7. _____ LAT
8. _____ VTNE
9. _____ HPA
10. _____ PES

Column B

A. The second highest level of certification for technicians caring for laboratory animals in the United States.

B. A designation that a veterinary technician has the credentials to qualify as a specialist.

C. The highest level of certification for technicians caring for laboratory animals in the United States.

D. A program administered by the AAVSB to uphold quality standards of continuing education.

E. An entity that works with the AAVSB to develop the Veterinary Technician National Exam.

F. The U.S. law that requires minimum standards of care and treatment be provided for some warm-blooded animals bred for commercial sale, used in research and higher education, transported commercially, and exhibited to the public.

G. A law designed to protect horses from the practice of "soring."

H. The first level of certification for technicians caring for laboratory animals.

I. The highest level of certification for technicians caring for laboratory animals in Canada.

J. A passing score on this test is required to practice in most states and provinces.

EXERCISE 1.5 TRUE OR FALSE: COMPREHENSIVE

Instructions: Read the following statements and write "T" for true or "F" for false in the blanks provided. If the statement is false, correct the statement to make it true.

1. _____ Graduates of accredited Canadian Veterinary Technology programs are eligible for recognition in the United States.

2. _____ Most states and provinces require veterinary technicians to attend continuing education (CE) lectures and workshops to maintain licensure, certification, or registration.

3. _____ An additional 20 new questions are added to each VTNE, but these additional questions do not count toward the final score of the candidate.

4. _____ Veterinary technicians are prohibited from entering drug prescriptions onto the patient's record.

5. _____ According to the American Association of Veterinary State Boards (AAVSB) Veterinary Technology State Practice Act Model, a veterinary technician may provide a patient's chances of recovery to a client.

6. _____ Routine dental procedures are often performed by veterinary technicians.

7. _____ The father of veterinary technology in the United States is Walter Emmett Collins.

8. _____ Most U.S. educated veterinarians have completed at least 8 years of post–high school study.

9. _____ In order to call himself or herself a specialist, a veterinarian must be board certified by a specialty organization.

10. _____ Because animals are often messy, uniforms are uncommon in small animal veterinary practices.

11. _____ The veterinary technician's professional apparel must include a watch with a second hand.

12. _____ The medical record is a legal document owned by the client but housed at the veterinary practice or supervising institution.

13. _____ Your e-mail address does not reflect on your level of professionalism.

14. _____ All states regulate the practice of veterinary medicine, but not all states regulate veterinary technology.

15. _____ The unlicensed practice of veterinary medicine is a criminal offense.

16. _____ Violations of laws or regulations may be punishable by fines or imprisonment.

17. _____ Someone convicted of crimes of moral turpitude may be denied a license to practice veterinary technology.

18. _____ Most jurisdictions require professional licensees, including veterinary technicians, to complete continuing education to renew their licenses.

19. _____ In virtually every state, a licensee may be prosecuted and disciplined for misconduct, even if the licensee's misconduct did not cause any harm to an animal.

20. _____ A veterinary technician may legally be the signatory on a document requiring the veterinarian's signature.

21. _____ A licensee may be prosecuted and disciplined for misrepresentation, which may include telling a client that a certain treatment will cure a patient.

22. _____ A licensee may be prosecuted and disciplined for animal abuse, animal neglect, or animal cruelty.

23. _____ An unlicensed veterinarian may function as a veterinary technician.

24. _____ Any licensed person who assists an unlicensed person in performing tasks that the statute includes as the practice of the profession may be aiding unlicensed practice.

25. _____ Many states have continuing education requirements for veterinary technicians.

26. _____ If a licensee is found guilty of malpractice, the board can direct a monetary award be paid to the animal's owner.

27. _____ The patient does not have to suffer any injury for the professional to be disciplined for malpractice.

28. _____ Veterinarians can be found negligent or guilty of malpractice because of the actions of a staff member.

29. _____ Whenever a veterinary technician is disciplined by a licensing board for exceeding the technician's authorized scope of practice, the veterinarian responsible for supervising the technician may also be disciplined.

30. _____ When you are summoned to a disciplinary hearing by the board, an attorney must be appointed by the board to represent you.

31. _____ The Occupational Safety and Health Act confirms that all workers have a fundamental right to a safe workplace.

32. _____ Veterinarians are prohibited from using controlled substances in the practice of veterinary medicine.

33. _____ Private veterinary hospitals are inspected by the USDA under the Animal Welfare Act.

EXERCISE 1.6 MULTIPLE CHOICE: COMPREHENSIVE

Instructions: Circle the one correct answer to each of the following questions.

1. Which organization or agency accredits veterinary technology programs in the United States?
   a. State boards
   b. NAVTA
   c. AVMA
   d. AAHA

2. Which of the following is a recognized area of specialty for a veterinary technician?
   a. Veterinary otolaryngologist
   b. Veterinary psychologist
   c. Veterinary pulmonologist
   d. Veterinary behavior technician

3. Which organization or agency has established veterinary technician specialties?
   a. State boards
   b. NAVTA
   c. AVMA
   d. AAHA

4. What was the average salary for veterinary technicians nationwide in 2015?
   a. $18,500
   b. $22,500
   c. $33,280
   d. $40,500

5. Approximately how many recommended and essential tasks are listed in the CVTEA handbook?
   a. 250
   b. 350
   c. 450
   d. 550

6. One of the most important duties for the veterinary technician in surgery is
   a. scrubbing the patient.
   b. washing the instruments.
   c. administering anesthesia.
   d. placing the catheter.

7. What is the format of the VTNE?
   a. Essay questions
   b. Multiple choice questions
   c. Short answer questions
   d. Short answer and multiple choice questions

8. Where are the VTNEs administered?
   a. Veterinary technology schools
   b. Veterinary schools
   c. Board of Veterinary Medicine auditoriums
   d. Prometric Testing Centers

9. To whom does a veterinary technology student apply to take the VTNE?
   a. AAVSB
   b. AVMA
   c. State Board of Veterinary Medicine
   d. PES

10. Which of the following merits the highest priority in patient intervention?
    a. Chronic pain
    b. Acute pain
    c. Inadequate oxygenation
    d. Diarrhea

11. Which U.S. veterinary school awards the VMD degree rather than the DVM?
    a. University of Virginia
    b. University of Georgia
    c. Tufts University
    d. University of Pennsylvania

12. The designation of VTS (veterinary specialist) is awarded by which of the following types of organizations?
    a. An academy
    b. A college
    c. A board
    d. A society

13. Animals used in research facilities and teaching institutions are registered by which government agency?
    a. AVMA
    b. AWA (USDA)
    c. HSUS
    d. Board of Veterinary Medicine

14. Graduates of AVMA and CVMA accredited programs must complete how much additional training in a registered facility before they are eligible for the Level 1 ALAT examination?
    a. 2 years
    b. 1 year
    c. 6 months
    d. 90 days

15. Which of these organizations wrote the veterinary technician code of ethics, the veterinary technician oath, and the veterinary technician portion of the Model Practice Act?
    a. AVMA
    b. CVTEA
    c. NAVTA
    d. AALAS

16. When is National Veterinary Technician week?
    a. The first week in November
    b. The third week in October
    c. The second week in May
    d. The second week in February

17. Who has the ultimate decision-making authority over the care provided to an owned animal?
    a. The attending veterinarian
    b. The state
    c. The owner
    d. The veterinary technician

18. What is the overriding purpose of the board of veterinary medicine?
    a. To protect the public
    b. To protect the animals
    c. To protect the veterinary profession
    d. To protect the veterinary and veterinary technology professions

19. Malpractice is also known as _____.
    a. Unprofessional conduct
    b. Negligence
    c. Misrepresentation
    d. An illegal act

20. Conduct that increases the risk that negligence will occur, even if negligence has not yet actually occurred, is known as _____.
    a. Malpractice
    b. Unprofessional conduct
    c. Incompetence
    d. Practicing beyond the scope of veterinary medicine

21. What is considered the most severe penalty a board may impose?
    a. Revocation of a license
    b. Monetary fine
    c. Imprisonment
    d. Closing of the hospital

22. What is the term for the public censure of a licensee without suspension or probation?
    a. Ridicule
    b. Dunking
    c. Prohibition
    d. Reprimand

23. Which act establishes that licensees have an IACUC (Institute of Animal Care and Use Committed)?
    a. Animal Welfare Act
    b. Occupational Safety Act
    c. Controlled Substance Act
    d. Medical Waste Tracking Act

24. The Horse Protection Act protects horses against which procedure?
    a. Slaughter
    b. Soring
    c. Castration without anesthesia
    d. Nerving

25. Which government agency enforces the Endangered Species Act?
    a. USDA
    b. DEA
    c. Commerce department
    d. FWS

EXERCISE 1.7 FILL IN THE CHART: IDENTIFY LEVELS OF SUPERVISION

Use check marks to indicate which type of supervision is required for the licensed, registered, or certified veterinary technician in order to perform the following tasks.

Task	Immediate Supervision	Direct Supervision	Indirect Supervision
Euthanasia			
Intravenous catheterizations			
Dental procedures			
Inducing anesthesia			
Blood collection			
Radiography			
Applying a splint			
Handling biohazardous waste			
Dental extraction not requiring a section of the tooth			
Administering immunologic agents by parenteral routes			

EXERCISE 1.8 CASE STUDY: PROFESSIONAL ETHICS

1. You moved to a small town in a state that requires veterinary technicians to be licensed by the board. You secure a job in a two-veterinarian clinic; you are the only LVT in the practice and obtain a license. You spend the first week shadowing the veterinarians in the examination rooms with clients and assisting with canine and feline spays. The practices appear to provide quality medicine and surgery. The following week, you are left alone in the treatment area to collect samples, perform lab tests, and administer medications. You notice that an assistant is taking dogs and cats in and out of a room in the rear of the clinic, and when you walk in, you find someone you have not met performing castrations. When you ask the assistant about the situation, you are told that although he is not a veterinarian, he has worked at the practice for more than 25 years and has always performed neuters in the practice.

   a. How should you respond to this situation?

   _____

   _____

   _____

   b. Should you say anything to the veterinarians? You are still in your probationary period.

   _____

   _____

   _____

   c. What are your legal and/or ethical responsibilities in this situation?

   _____

   _____

   _____

   _____

   _____

   _____

2 Veterinary Practice Management

LEARNING OBJECTIVES

When you have completed this chapter, you will be able to:
1. Pronounce, spell, and define each of the key terms in this chapter.
2. List the terms used to describe various types of veterinary facilities.
3. List the roles and responsibilities of each member of the veterinary health care team.
4. Describe the basic flow of clients, patients, and employees through a typical veterinary hospital.
5. Outline the key elements of effectively working with clients, including the importance of communication skills, myths about communication skills, and how to diffuse the anger of difficult clients.
6. Describe the major job management functions needed to run a veterinary hospital effectively.
7. Describe the primary components of excellent practice management.
8. List examples of stressors in the veterinary workplace, and describe ways to ameliorate the effects of those stressors on personnel.
9. Describe the major areas in which veterinary practices employ internal and external marketing techniques.
10. List some of the major tasks associated with good financial management.
11. List reasons why management and financial analysis are important to the business of veterinary medicine.
12. Discuss the importance of efficient operations for practice revenue.
13. Discuss key areas in which computerization adds to the efficiency and productivity of a veterinary practice.

EXERCISE 2.1 DEFINITIONS

Instructions: Define each term in your own words.

1. Clinic: _____

   _____

2. Outpatient: _____

   _____

3. Strategic planning: _____

   _____

4. Walk-in system: _____

   _____

5. Appointment system: _____

   _____

10

6. Consultation: _____

_____

7. Referral facility: _____

_____

8. AAHA: _____

_____

9. CVPM: _____

_____

EXERCISE 2.2 MATCHING #1: KEY TERMS AND DEFINITIONS RELATED TO FINANCES

Instructions: Match each term in column A with its corresponding definition in column B by writing the appropriate letter in the space provided.

Column A

1. _____ Cash flow
2. _____ Accounts receivable
3. _____ Petty cash
4. _____ Net income
5. _____ Profits
6. _____ Gross revenue

Column B

A. Money owed to the practice by the client for the sale of goods and services.

B. The total money taken in by a practice before subtracting expenses incurred.

C. The amount of money left over after all business expenses are subtracted from the gross revenue.

D. The measurement of the amount of money coming into and going out of a practice.

E. The total amount of money brought in by a practice minus all expenses incurred and taxes paid.

F. A small amount of discretionary funds that are used to make small purchases for which it is not practical to write a check or use a credit card.

EXERCISE 2.3 MATCHING #2: KEY TERMS AND DEFINITIONS RELATED TO VETERINARY FACILITIES

Instructions: Match each term in column A with its corresponding definition in column B by writing the appropriate letter in the space provided.

Column A

1. _____ On-call emergency service
2. _____ Veterinary teaching hospital
3. _____ Haul-in facility
4. _____ Specialty facility
5. _____ Hospital
6. _____ Mobile facility
7. _____ Referral facility
8. _____ Emergency facility
9. _____ Office
10. _____ Clinic

Column B

A. A facility in which the practice conducted may include inpatient as well as outpatient diagnosis and treatment.

B. A practice that conducts its work from a vehicle that can make farm or house calls.

C. A facility that consists of a large staff of DVMs who provide clinical and hospital services, but who also perform significant research, along with educating professional veterinary students.

D. A facility that is set up to allow large animals to be brought to the practice for examination or treatment.

E. A facility in which the practice conducted typically includes inpatient as well as outpatient diagnosis and treatment.

F. A facility in which veterinarians with a special interest in a specific species or area of veterinary medicine provide services.

G. A practice that is limited in the service it provides, as it does not have the facilities to perform inpatient diagnostics or treatment.

H. A facility in which the primary function is to treat and monitor critically ill or injured animals.

I. An option provided by some veterinary facilities that will treat emergencies but do not necessarily have veterinarians and staff on the premises during all operating hours.

J. A facility where services are provided by board certified veterinary specialists.

EXERCISE 2.4 MATCHING #3: EMPLOYEE POSITIONS

Instructions: Match each job duty in column A with the name of the veterinary personnel who would perform each duty (in a well-run practice) in column B by writing the appropriate letter in the space provided. Each answer can be used more than once.

Column A

1. _____ Basic animal husbandry
2. _____ Performing surgery
3. _____ Updating client and patient information
4. _____ Animal restraint
5. _____ Making appointments
6. _____ Patient assessment
7. _____ Client education
8. _____ Filling prescriptions

Column B

A. Veterinarian

B. Veterinary technician/technologist

C. Veterinary assistant

D. Receptionist

E. Kennel attendant

EXERCISE 2.5 MATCHING #4: MARKETING

Instructions: Indicate whether each of the following activities would be considered internal marketing or external marketing by writing an "I" for internal or an "E" for external in the space provided.

1. _____ Sending out vaccine reminders

2. _____ Sponsoring a little league team

3. _____ Personal appearance of staff

4. _____ Sincere care for and concern about each client

5. _____ Creating a Facebook page for the practice

6. _____ Sending out newsletters

7. _____ Placing an advertisement in the Yellow Pages

8. _____ One-stop shopping

9. _____ A clean and attractive facility

10. _____ A sign outside the practice

EXERCISE 2.6 TRUE OR FALSE: COMPREHENSIVE

Instructions: Read the following statements and write "T" for true or "F" for false in the blanks provided. If a statement is false, correct the statement to make it true.

1. _____ For a veterinary practice to be successful, most of the staff will play some type of role related to management.

2. _____ The types of staff positions that are needed will vary greatly, depending on the size and type of practice.

3. _____ When it comes to naming veterinary facilities, the terms *hospital, clinic,* and *office* can be used interchangeably.

4. _____ When it comes to delegating tasks, the best-run clinics assign tasks to the lowest paid person who can legally and competently complete the task.

5. _____ In most well-run veterinary practices, job duties are performed by any staff member who is available to accomplish the task.

6. _____ Pet owners who have owned pets previously usually have a good understanding of the care their pet needs.

7. _____ A separate entrance and exit to the veterinary practice should be provided to make it easier for clients to enter and exit the practice.

8. _____ To save time during an appointment, it is OK to have a client restrain his or her own pet.

9. _____ If laboratory samples (e.g., blood, urine) need to be collected during an appointment, the patient should be taken to the treatment area.

10. _____ As long as clients wear the proper personal protective equipment, they can accompany their pet into the radiology suite.

11. _____ When discharging an animal and reviewing home care instructions with the client, it is best to have the client pay their bill before their pet is brought out to them.

12. _____ Anyone entering the operating room during surgery should be wearing the appropriate clothes, shoes, cap, and mask.

13. _____ In a mixed-animal practice, the same examination rooms are used for large animal and small animal patients.

14. _____ Many larger equine practices have a single room used for anesthetic induction and anesthetic recovery.

15. _____ Job descriptions should be used for hiring new employees and for replacing existing employees.

16. _____ If an applicant submits a résumé and cover letter to a practice, there is no need to have them also complete a job application.

17. _____ When a practice hires a new staff member who has many years of experience from previous work at a different clinic, training is not necessary.

18. _____ Stress can be caused by both positive and negative life events.

19. _____ The terms *marketing* and *advertising* mean the same thing.

20. _____ The main goal of external marketing is to attract new clients to the practice.

21. _____ If a client does not respond to the first reminder they are sent, the practice should follow up by sending a second reminder and even a third reminder, if needed.

22. _____ Veterinary practices are relying less on the use of Yellow Book advertisements as a marketing tool.

23. _____ Newspaper advertisements are a good marketing tool for a practice that is located in a larger metropolitan area.

24. _____ The money that a veterinary practice owes for the purchase of a new piece of equipment would be considered an asset of the practice.

25. _____ To ensure that clients pay their bills in full at the time of service, clinics should not offer payment options to clients.

26. _____ If a pet is brought to the clinic with life-threatening injuries, the pet should be stabilized before a treatment plan/estimate is prepared.

27. _____ Pet insurance works in a similar manner to human health insurance.

28. _____ Ideally, physically counting the inventory in a veterinary practice should be done once a year.

29. _____ Some veterinary practices have completely eliminated paper medical records and replaced them with electronic medical records.

EXERCISE 2.7 MULTIPLE CHOICE: COMPREHENSIVE

Instructions: Circle the one correct answer to each of the following questions.

1. Increased competition, new technology, increasing numbers of malpractice threats, and shifting client expectations have
   a. Caused many veterinary practices to go out of business
   b. Made effective management of a veterinary practice more complex
   c. Caused a significant drop in client compliance
   d. Caused many veterinary practices to hire more staff

2. In a typical veterinary practice, the person who acts as the chief executive officer and delegates areas of responsibility is usually the
   a. Financial manager
   b. Veterinarian-owner
   c. Hospital administrator
   d. Practice manager

3. The individual typically responsible for all activities of the practice and running the hospital in conjunction with the practice's owner(s) is referred to as the
   a. Office manager
   b. Practice manager
   c. Hospital administrator
   d. Associate veterinarian

4. The best way to ensure that all of the major pieces of equipment in a veterinary practice are cleaned and maintained on a regular basis is to
   a. Assign each member of the team a specific piece of equipment to clean and maintain
   b. Make sure that every member of the team takes part in equipment cleaning and maintenance during downtime
   c. Hire an outside vendor to clean and maintain the equipment, as most of it is very complex and expensive
   d. Assign one person in the practice to clean and maintain all of the equipment on a regular basis

5. To minimize the amount of time clients have to wait in the reception area, there should be _____ examination rooms available for each veterinarian working on a particular day.
   a. One
   b. Two
   c. Three
   d. Four

6. Placement of the laboratory and pharmacy in a central location is very important because
   a. They can be used in place of an examination room during busy periods
   b. They are often used for examining and treating both outpatients and hospitalized patients
   c. They are both important profit centers for the practice
   d. This is where the material safety data sheets should be located

7. Practices need to get the maximum use out of their storage area because
   a. This space is usually cluttered and disorganized
   b. The practice must have enough inventory on hand to meet their clients' needs
   c. This space typically generates very little income
   d. It will reduce the chance that inventory becomes outdated

8. It is more common to perform a necropsy when a large animal dies than when a small animal dies because
   a. There is a need to determine if the rest of the herd is threatened
   b. Large animals are a lot more expensive to replace than small animals
   c. When a large animal dies, the owners are more likely to file a lawsuit against the practice
   d. Most small animal owners cannot afford to pay for a necropsy if their pet dies

9. A client's judgment regarding the quality of medicine provided at a veterinary practice is generally based on
   a. The cost of the care provided
   b. The amount of time the doctor spends with them
   c. The health status of their pet
   d. The level of service the client receives

10. One of the most common selection criteria used by clients when choosing a veterinary practice is
    a. The fees charged
    b. The location
    c. The number of staff
    d. The hours of operation

11. Complaints against veterinary practices are usually caused by
    a. Long wait times in the examination room and/or reception area
    b. The staff or DVM making a medical mistake
    c. The fees charged
    d. Ineffective communication

12. Which one of the following practices should be the most successful when it comes to annual strategic planning for the practice?
    a. The practice in which all staff are involved in the planning
    b. The practice in which the owner does all the planning
    c. The practice in which the management team does all the planning
    d. The practice in which the manager and doctors do all the planning

13. A document that is a visual representation of how authority and responsibility flow between the various areas of the practice or practice staff is called a(n)
    a. Job description
    b. Business plan
    c. Organizational chart
    d. Employee manual

14. It is best to base the employee's pay on
    a. Performance
    b. Seniority
    c. Experience
    d. Education

15. One of the most important reasons for holding regular employee evaluations is to
    a. Reprimand the employee for not following practice protocols
    b. Judge whether or not the employee's goals were met
    c. Determine if the employee deserves a raise
    d. Improve the employee's performance

16. Which one of the following statements is the most accurate when it comes to describing marketing for a veterinary practice?
    a. Any effort the practice makes to increase sales and generate a profit
    b. Any effort the practice makes to retain or obtain clients and make the practice more visible in the community
    c. Advertising the services the practice offers using tools such as Yellow Book ads and a website
    d. Any effort the practice makes to offer new and different products and services to existing and new clients

17. When it comes to the sales of products such as pet food, the veterinary practice is at an advantage over feed stores and grocery stores because
    a. The veterinary clinic usually offers a wider selection than other stores
    b. Practice employees can educate clients about the food they purchase
    c. The pet food sold at a veterinary practice is usually higher quality
    d. The veterinary practice has a lower overhead

18. A veterinary practice's website should
    a. generate a return on investment
    b. be developed by an outside professional
    c. be updated on a regular basis
    d. include a list of commonly phone-shopped fees

19. One of the financial tasks that many practices will not do on their own is
    a. Establish KPIs
    b. Determine profitability
    c. Calculate the practice's net worth
    d. Prepare a yearly tax return

20. A financial report that lists a practice's assets and liabilities is called a(n)
    a. Balance sheet
    b. Net worth statement
    c. Profit and loss statement
    d. Income statement

21. A financial report used to evaluate the financial performance of a practice for a specified period of time is called a(n)
    a. Profitability statement
    b. Cash flow statement
    c. Net revenue statement
    d. Income statement

22. When determining the financial success of a veterinary practice, the _____ is the most important indicator.
    a. Average transaction charge
    b. Gross revenue
    c. Profitability
    d. Net revenue

23. One of the main reasons inventory management is so important in a veterinary practice is that
    a. Inventory is a significant expense for a practice
    b. Inventory accounts for most of the revenue generated by a practice
    c. Extra inventory must be kept on hand to ensure the practice never runs out of anything
    d. Most items kept in inventory have a slim profit margin

EXERCISE 2.8 CASE STUDY #1: VETERINARY PRACTICE MANAGEMENT

1. You are the head credentialed veterinary technician in a small animal private practice and the supervisor in charge of supervising all veterinary assistants. This role includes hiring, training, and disciplining the veterinary assistants that you supervise. The practice has only been open for one year, and business has grown steadily to the point where some members of the staff are becoming overwhelmed. Because of this, you speak to the hospital administrator about adding an additional veterinary assistant position. The hospital administrator is supportive of this idea and charges you with the task of creating a job description for the new veterinary assistant position. Create a short job description for a new veterinary assistant employee, making sure that you include all six components of a well-written job description.

_____

_____

_____

_____

_____

_____

_____

_____

_____

_____

_____

_____

_____

_____

17

2. Now that you have a job description for the position, describe how you will attract applicants.

_____

_____

_____

_____

_____

_____

3. You have invited several applicants for a face-to-face interview. What three things should you obtain from the applicants to give you more detailed information about the applicant's skills and experience?

Item #1 _____

Item #2 _____

Item #3 _____

4. As you are preparing to interview the applicants, you make sure to review the types of questions that are illegal to ask during a job interview. Give two examples of questions that cannot be asked of an applicant during a job interview.

_____

_____

_____

_____

_____

5. After going through the application and interview process, a decision was made to hire Lilly Rainsworth as the new veterinary assistant. Lilly starts out very well at the new clinic and seems to be really catching on, but after she has been there for about six months, you notice her attitude start to change from good to bad, and she is starting to take too many days off work. She also seems to "fly off the handle" any time something does not go exactly as planned. What do you think could be the problem with Lilly, and how might you go about dealing with this problem?

_____

_____

_____

_____

_____

_____

_____

EXERCISE 2.9 CASE STUDY #2: DIFFUSING ANGER

Cutie, a 12-year-old, female, spayed poodle mix was presented for a dental cleaning. A minimum patient database was acquired, and Cutie was prepared for the dental cleaning in a routine manner. The dental cleaning was performed, and during the course of the procedure, 15 teeth had to be extracted because of advanced periodontal disease. The client was not informed prior to the procedure because the possibility of extractions was discussed at the preop interview.

When the owner was notified of the number of teeth that were extracted, he became agitated and very angry, and said, "Great! Now she will never be able to eat normally! It is all your fault!"

1. What could you do to diffuse this client's anger in this situation?

_____

_____

_____

_____

_____

_____

3 Veterinary Medical Records

LEARNING OBJECTIVES

When you have completed this chapter, you will be able to:
1. Pronounce, define, and spell all the Key Terms in this chapter.
2. List and describe the primary and secondary purposes of the medical record.
3. Explain the legal issues related to ownership of medical records, release of medical information, and maintenance of medical records.
4. Describe methods for formatting medical records and explain their respective advantages and disadvantages.
5. List and describe each component of the problem-oriented veterinary medical record (POVMR).
6. Explain each portion of the technician SOAP note, including the types of information included in each portion, and describe how each portion correlates to the steps in the veterinary technician practice model (presented in Chapter 1).
7. Describe the importance of cage cards, discharge instructions, and summary and medication administration/order record (MAOR) forms and why they are valuable in organizing the care of hospitalized veterinary patients.
8. Compare and contrast the types of filing systems commonly used for paper medical records.
9. Explain the advantages and disadvantages of electronic medical record keeping.
10. List and describe the types of paper-based forms and logs commonly used in veterinary practice.
11. Describe methods for collecting and storing medical information in ambulatory veterinary medical practices.

EXERCISE 3.1 FILL-IN-THE-BLANK: KEY TERMS AND DEFINITIONS

Instructions: Fill in each of the spaces provided with the missing key term or definition that completes the sentence. Acronyms may be used when appropriate.

1. The physical folder for each veterinary patient and the total body of information that comprises each animal's health history is called the _____ _____.

2. Interaction between veterinarians and their clients and patients is conducted under the _____ _____ _____ _____, and medical records must be maintained for all patients with whom this relationship exists.

3. Through the use of the _____ veterinary medical record, an organized approach to clinical veterinary care is achieved, as information is grouped by problem, and each problem is assigned a number and addressed individually.

4. The _____ _____ veterinary medical record is a medical record format in which patient information is grouped by subject matter, clinical observations are entered as they become evident, and progress note paragraphs are written in chronologic order.

5. The _____ refers to the collective information that identifies an individual patient, such as the species, breed, gender, reproductive status, age, color, and distinctive markings.

6. Recorded information, such as a patient's date of birth, preventive medicine program, behavior, previous conditions, and known allergies, is included as part of the _____ _____ in a comprehensive medical record.

7. A structured system of documenting patient evaluation and assessment in the progress notes is called the _____ format.

8. Patient information, such as presenting complaint, current medications, location and character of problems, treatment efforts, and recent changes in the environment, may be included as part of the _____ _____ in a comprehensive medical record.

9. Major medical disorders experienced by a patient during its lifetime are included in the _____ _____ list, which serves as an index to the patient's medical history.

10. Veterinary practices will often use the _____ _____ list to assist the veterinary health care team when working through current patient problems.

11. The ongoing daily management of hospitalized patients is documented in _____ _____ so that therapeutic treatment and plans may be evaluated and adjusted accordingly.

12. Hypothermia, altered mentation, inappropriate elimination, and risk of infection are examples of _____ _____, according to the veterinary technician practice model.

13. To ensure that a hospitalized patient is given the treatments, diagnostic tests, and diet requested by the veterinarian, the _____ or ward treatment sheet is used.

14. A _____ is a collection of all available information that would contribute to the diagnostic process of a patient when originally seen for a particular problem.

EXERCISE 3.2 MATCHING #1: TECHNICIAN SOAP NOTES

Instructions: Match each set of patient information with the appropriate component of technician SOAP progress notes by writing the appropriate letter in the space provided. Note that each answer can be used more than once.

Column A

1. _____ Temperature, weight, capillary refill time

2. _____ Awake, standing, wagging tail

3. _____ Limited daily exercise, cold compresses to injury

4. _____ Heart rate, respiratory rate, skin retraction time

5. _____ Cardiac insufficiency, hypotension, decreased perfusion

6. _____ Antibiotics prescribed, hypoallergenic diet, follow-up appointment

7. _____ Anxiety, acute pain, reduced mobility

8. _____ Lethargic, not eating well, lying in right lateral recumbency

Column B

A. Subjective

B. Objective

C. Assessment

D. Plan

EXERCISE 3.3 MATCHING #2: TECHNICIAN EVALUATIONS

Instructions: Match the clinical observations/assessments of a canine patient in column A with the appropriate Physiologic Need based on the Hierarchy of Patient's Physiologic Needs in column B.

Column A

1. _____ Bleeding gingiva, halitosis, difficulty chewing

2. _____ Body temperature of 94° F, acute abdominal pain, chemistry panel K+ = 1.2 mmol/L

3. _____ Anxious, fearful, displays submissive urination

4. _____ Deep sores caused by licking and scratching at ears; owner won't use an Elizabethan collar as directed

5. _____ Restless at night, gets up slowly, pants heavily when exercised

6. _____ Dyspnea, blue mucous membranes, oxygen level 89% on pulse oximetry

7. _____ Delayed recovery of skin tenting, weak peripheral pulse, tacky mucous membranes

8. _____ Moaning frequently, reluctant to move, tail tucked between legs

9. _____ Urinating in the house, urinating more frequently, unable to hold urine overnight

Column B

A. Priority 1—Oxygenation

B. Priority 2—Critical Safety and/or Severe Pain

C. Priority 3—Hydration

D. Priority 4—Elimination

E. Priority 5—Nutrition

F. Priority 6—Noncritical Safety

G. Priority 7—Chronic Pain or Mild-Moderate Acute Pain

H. Priority 8—Activity

I. Priority 9—Utility

EXERCISE 3.4 TRUE OR FALSE: COMPREHENSIVE

Instructions: Read the following statements and write "T" for true or "F" for false in the blanks provided. If a statement is false, correct the statement to make it true.

1. _____ The medical record can be used as a legal document in a court of law and can be of critical importance in defending against malpractice suits.

2. _____ Completed consent and authorization forms provide veterinary practices with legal evidence of informed consent and can be signed by a pet owner of any age.

3. _____ Entries in written records may be corrected using correction fluid, provided the entry is signed and dated by the person who made the error, with a brief explanation of the correction.

4. _____ Only approved, standard abbreviations should be used in medical record keeping.

5. _____ Veterinary medical records are the property of the pet owner because the client purchased the veterinary services that generated the medical information.

6. _____ The owner of an animal should not be required to sign an authorization form to obtain a copy of his or her pet's record for himself or herself.

7. _____ If a veterinarian diagnoses a reportable disease, permission from the client to release the patient's record must be obtained prior to alerting local, state, and federal agencies.

8. _____ When using source-oriented veterinary medical records, clinical observations are entered as they become evident so that the most recent information is located last.

9. _____ The American Animal Hospital Association (AAHA) endorses the use of problem-oriented medical record keeping for practices seeking AAHA certification.

10. _____ When recording physical examination results, abbreviations such as "BAR" and "WNL" should not be used because they may be interpreted differently by other veterinary health care providers.

11. _____ The POVMR working problem list helps veterinarians and veterinary technicians think critically, identify and prioritize problems, and formulate an understanding of the patient's reactions to an illness.

12. _____ Medication administration/order records should include the patient's full name, patient I.D. number and/or signalment, and any known allergies that the patient may have.

13. _____ When documenting treatments on an MAOR, an "X" should be placed in the appropriate column at the time that the medication is administered to the patient.

14. _____ Medications given during surgical or anesthetic procedures should be entered on the MAOR along with all other medications that the patient receives.

15. _____ When using the alphabetic system of medical record filing, a major disadvantage is that a client cross-reference list must be generated and maintained.

16. _____ The American Animal Hospital Association requires that paper records for each patient should be stored in standard 8- × 10-inch folders.

17. _____ The primary medical record collection should include active records covering a 3-year period.

18. _____ A recommended practice for purging files is to remove and shred all records that have been inactive for 4 years or more.

19. _____ According to the Federal Comprehensive Drug Abuse and Control Act, an inventory of all controlled substances must be made on an annual basis.

20. _____ Controlled drugs that are considered the most addictive are in the Schedule V category.

21. _____ A log is a hard-copy document noting specific procedures.

22. _____ According to DEA regulations, Schedule II controlled drugs must be maintained in a separate inventory record.

23. _____ Practices must keep 12 different types of logs.

24. _____ Electronic record entries made within the first 24 to 48 hours of patient care are regarded as the primary document.

25. _____ An accepted medical record-keeping practice for ambulatory practitioners is to make handwritten notes on carbonized invoice sheets that are loaded into a sturdy metal dispenser.

EXERCISE 3.5 SHORT ANSWER: PROBLEM-ORIENTED VETERINARY MEDICAL RECORDS (POVMR)

Instructions: Provide a short answer to each of the following questions in the space provided.

1. In what way does the POVMR provide a more organized approach to clinical veterinary care than a SOVMR?

   _____

   _____

   _____

2. Although the POVMR includes SOAP notes that may be written by both veterinarians and veterinary technicians, the focus of their assessments is different. How does the focus of these assessments differ?

   _____

   _____

   _____

3. What are the four general components most commonly included in the POVMR?

   i. _____

   ii. _____

   iii. _____

   iv. _____

4. The working problem list is an important component of the POVMR that helps the veterinary health-care team work through current problems. Explain the difference between the master problem list and the working problem list.

   _____

   _____

   _____

5. Why is the working problem list helpful to the veterinarian and veterinary technician?

   _____

   _____

   _____

6. The POVMR may include a Medication Administration/Order record (MAOR) to assist the veterinary health-care team carry out treatment orders of hospitalized patients efficiently. Describe the general format used and summarize the types of information that should be included on MAORs.

   _____

   _____

   _____

_____

_____

_____

_____

_____

_____

_____

7. The plan for patient care is an accumulation of interventions developed by the veterinary technician for each evaluation listed in the assessment portion of the SOAP.

   a. What is the ultimate goal of developing a patient care plan?

   _____

   b. Give several examples of the general types of interventions that would be considered part of the care plan.

   _____

8. POVMR discharge instructions provide pet owners with the information and resources to continue any prescribed homecare and monitoring of their pet. Summarize the information and procedures that should be included when discharging a hospitalized patient, so that a desirable outcome for both the patient and owner may be achieved.

_____

_____

_____

_____

_____

_____

_____

_____

_____

4 Occupational Health and Safety in Veterinary Hospitals

LEARNING OBJECTIVES

When you have completed this chapter, you will be able to:
1. Pronounce, define, and spell all the Key Terms in this chapter.
2. Do the following regarding safety in the veterinary hospital:
   - Explain the acronym OSHA, and describe the role it plays in the development of safety programs in veterinary practices.
   - List the safety rights and responsibilities of *employees* in the workplace.
   - List the safety rights and responsibilities of workplace *leaders*.
3. List common workplace hazards in a veterinary facility, describe precautions that can be taken to reduce the risk of these hazards, and do the following:
   - Explain proper methods for lifting objects and animals.
   - List hazards associated with the use of ethylene oxide, formalin, glutaraldehyde, anesthetic gases, and compressed gases.
   - Describe the requirements of the OSHA "right to know" law.
   - Explain the acronym SDS and describe the components of an SDS.
4. Do the following regarding medical and animal-related hazards:
   - List hazards related to the capture and restraint of small and large animals.
   - Explain risks associated with excessive noise and methods taken to minimize these risks.
   - Describe hazards related to bathing and dipping animals and explain methods to minimize these risks.
   - Define the term *zoonotic disease,* and list zoonotic and nonzoonotic diseases commonly encountered in veterinary practices.
5. Explain the importance of wearing goggles, gloves, and a surgical mask when performing dental procedures on animals.
6. List methods to minimize the risks associated with exposure to radiation, anesthetic gases, and medical waste.
7. List the equipment and supplies needed to protect veterinary personnel when handling hazardous pharmaceuticals such as chemotherapeutic drugs, and describe methods for safely handling contaminated bedding and waste from oncology patients.

EXERCISE 4.1 MATCHING #1: KEY TERMS—INFECTIOUS AGENTS

Instructions: Match each term in column A with its corresponding definition in column B by writing the appropriate letter in the space provided.

Column A

1. _____ *Giardia*
2. _____ Lyme disease
3. _____ Panleukopenia
4. _____ Parvoviral enteritis
5. _____ Rabies
6. _____ Ringworm
7. _____ Sarcoptic mange
8. _____ Toxoplasmosis

Column B

A. A zoonotic viral disease that can affect any warm-blooded animal; spread by contact with saliva.

B. A condition of dogs caused by a highly infectious agent.

C. A tick-transmitted condition caused by *Borrelia burgdorferi*.

D. This zoonosis can cause hydrocephalus and mental retardation by affecting the human fetus.

E. A protozoan; can be contracted by drinking contaminated water.

F. A skin condition caused by a mite of zoonotic concern.

G. A highly contagious viral disease that infects cats but not dogs.

H. A zoonotic skin condition caused by the agent *Microsporum* sp.

EXERCISE 4.2 MATCHING #2: KEY TERMS—ACRONYMS

Instructions: Match each acronym in column A with its corresponding description in column B by writing the appropriate letter in the space provided.

Column A

1. _____ CDs
2. _____ SDS
3. _____ OSHA
4. _____ PPE
5. _____ WAGS

Column B

A. Occupational Safety and Health Administration—A federal agency that ensures safety for American workers.

B. Waste anesthetic gases—Risks associated with long-term exposure to these substances can be reduced by scavenging systems.

C. Safety data sheet—Sections covering the health risks, protective equipment, and disposal requirements for products.

D. Cytotoxic drugs—Pharmaceutical agents used to treat cancer.

E. Personal protective equipment—Appropriate items that should be worn when working with hazardous materials.

EXERCISE 4.3 MATCHING #3: KEY TERMS—CONDITIONS

Instructions: Match each condition in column A with the correct associated statement in column B by writing the appropriate letter in the space provided.

Column A

1. _____ Carpal tunnel syndrome
2. _____ Cutaneous larval migrans
3. _____ Visceral larval migrans
4. _____ Diarrhea and cramping
5. _____ Toxoplasmosis

Column B

A. A zoonotic infection caused by the roundworm larvae resulting in a cyst-like growth; can result in blindness if the eye is involved.

B. A zoonotic infection caused by the hookworm parasite, characterized by red itchy lines on the skin that lengthen as the parasite moves from one part of the body to another subcutaneously.

C. A protozoal infestation that can be transmitted by eating raw or undercooked meat.

D. An ergonomic injury.

E. Characteristic of a zoonotic infection caused by the subclass of protozoal agents known as coccidia.

EXERCISE 4.4 MATCHING #4: CLASSIFICATION OF MEDICAL WASTE

Instructions: Match each item in column A with the appropriate classification in column B by writing an "A" (for medical waste) or a "B" (for normal trash) in the space provided.

Column A

1. _____ A needle used to draw blood for a heartworm test.
2. _____ Waste from a patient infected with canine distemper virus.
3. _____ Bloody gauze sponges used on a patient infected with brucellosis.
4. _____ A bacterial culture plate used to culture *Pseudomonas* spp.
5. _____ An IV catheter used to deliver a chemotherapy drug.
6. _____ Tissues from a rabies suspect before receipt of test results.
7. _____ Urine and feces from a patient that received a chemotherapy agent earlier in the day.
8. _____ The uterus and ovaries of a patient that was spayed that day.
9. _____ A scalpel blade used to remove a fatty tumor from a dog.
10. _____ A blood tube used to draw blood for a thyroid hormone assay in a cat.

Column B

A. Medical waste

B. Normal trash

EXERCISE 4.5 FILL-IN-THE-BLANK: COMPREHENSIVE

Instructions: Fill in each of the spaces provided with the missing word or words from the following list to complete the sentence.

Use the following key terms to fill in the blanks:

A. Ergonomic injury

B. Hazardous chemical

C. Ground-fault circuit interrupter

D. Hazardous materials plan

E. Hospital Safety Manual

F. "Right to know" law

1. Instructions on how the practice will maintain hazardous material documents and proper protective policies within the clinic should be detailed in the _____.

2. Enforced by OSHA, the _____ requires that the employee wear all appropriate PPE when handling hazardous chemicals.

3. Technicians should vary their arm and hand positions and posture often to avoid repetitive actions that can lead to a(n) _____.

4. Safety-related policies adopted by a clinic should be found in the clinic's _____.

5. Drugs and medications are considered a type of _____.

6. When working around a wet area, any electrical appliances should be plugged into a _____.

EXERCISE 4.6 TRUE OR FALSE: COMPREHENSIVE

Instructions: Read the following statements and write "T" for true or "F" for false in the blanks provided. If a statement is false, correct the statement to make it true.

1. _____ An employee is required to admit an OSHA inspector regardless of whether the practice owner is present or not.

2. _____ It is appropriate to plug an autoclave into a surge suppressor to protect it from electrical fluctuations.

3. _____ When disposing of a fluorescent light bulb that is too long to fit in the trash, it is acceptable to wrap it in a protective wrap such as brown paper and break it, as long as the pieces are kept in a confined area.

4. _____ Flammable material should be stored a minimum of 3 feet from a water heater.

5. _____ Never attempt to fight a fire, regardless of its size, if you are unsure how to properly use the fire extinguisher.

6. _____ If you are confronted by an armed person attempting to steal controlled drugs, you should never open the controlled substance cabinet; you should instead try to escape and call the police.

7. _____ Whereas a clinic is required to provide safety equipment, it is the employee's decision as to whether or not to wear it.

8. _____ Water should be added to the concentrate when making a cleaning solution.

9. _____ Unless the SDS indicates otherwise, use a detergent when cleaning up a spill.

10. _____ Ethylene oxide, although a potential carcinogen, is an excellent cold sterilization solution.

11. _____ For optimal safety, an animal restrainer should focus her or his attention on the procedure being performed.

12. _____ Glutaraldehyde is a cold-sterilization solution used to sterilize instruments without the use of steam.

13. _____ The most common type of injury in the veterinary setting is animal-related.

14. _____ Noise from barking is irritating and frustrating but will not damage your hearing.

15. _____ The spray attachment on the tub should be used as an emergency eye flush because it offers more control.

16. _____ Ringworm is caused by a zoonotic parasite.

17. _____ Roundworm eggs in the soil can remain viable for long periods of time.

18. _____ Pregnant women should be advised to avoid contact with cats to prevent contracting toxoplasmosis.

19. _____ Panleukopenia has zoonotic potential.

20. _____ It is possible to carry pathogens home to personal pets.

21. _____ Long-term exposure to low doses of radiation is considered relatively safe.

22. _____ Sunlight can cause false dosimetry badge readings.

23. _____ Portable x-ray units are considered less dangerous because of their limited power.

24. _____ It is permissible to dispose of used x-ray developing chemicals down the drain.

25. _____ You should wear your dosimetry badge at all times during your shift.

26. _____ The best method to reduce the amount of WAG exposure is to use a proper scavenging system.

27. _____ An absorption waste anesthetic gas scavenging canister should be checked for saturation by weighing it.

28. _____ Compressed gas cylinders can be stored anywhere in the clinic as long as they are empty.

29. _____ Used soda lime crystals should be disposed of as medical waste.

30. _____ Needles should be removed from syringes before depositing them in the sharps container to prevent overfilling.

31. _____ A biologic safety cabinet should be used when preparing chemotherapy drugs.

EXERCISE 4.7 MULTIPLE CHOICE: COMPREHENSIVE

Instructions: Circle the one correct answer to each of the following questions.

1. OSHA's "right to know" law requires all of the following EXCEPT
   a. Employees to be informed of all chemicals they may be exposed to
   b. Employer to eliminate all hazards in the workplace
   c. Employees to wear all PPE prescribed by the manufacturer
   d. Employer to provide PPE at no cost to all employees

2. If your clinic has more than 10 employees, you are entitled to all of the following except to
   a. See data that applies to your safety
   b. Be informed about the types of accidents that occurred in the clinic
   c. Be given information regarding other staff members
   d. View a summary of work injuries/illnesses

3. Which of the following is considered an acceptable method of providing clinic-specific training to employees?
   a. Staff meetings
   b. Continuing education courses
   c. On-the-job training
   d. All of the above

4. Flammable materials should always be stored at least _____ feet away from a furnace or other ignition source.
   a. 3
   b. 5
   c. 6
   d. 8

5. The _____ includes instructions for organizing and maintaining a clinic's "right to know" documents.
   a. OSHA poster
   b. Hazardous material plan
   c. Safety data sheet
   d. Centers for disease control and prevention website

6. The chemical formalin is primarily used for
   a. Tissue preservation
   b. Disinfection
   c. Antisepsis
   d. Gas sterilization

7. The most common type of injury in a veterinary clinic is
   a. Strained/sprained back from improper lifting
   b. Carpal tunnel syndrome
   c. Slip and fall
   d. Animal-related

8. The best way to protect yourself from animal-related injuries is to
   a. Show you are not afraid
   b. Get training and practice
   c. Use force
   d. Try to outwit the animal

9. A zoonotic disease that is associated with joint pain and fever is
   a. Rabies
   b. *Toxoplasmosis*
   c. Lyme disease
   d. *Giardiasis*

10. _____ larva can migrate to virtually any organ and develop into visceral larval migrans.
    a. Roundworm
    b. Hookworm
    c. Protozoa
    d. Sarcoptic mange

11. *Toxoplasma* eggs sporulate and become infectious _____ after they are passed.
    a. Immediately
    b. 2 to 4 hours
    c. 2 to 4 days
    d. 2 to 4 weeks

12. This parasite can cause cutaneous larval migrans in humans:
    a. Roundworm
    b. Hookworm
    c. Protozoa
    d. Sarcoptic mange

13. A zoonotic pathogen that can be acquired by drinking contaminated water is
    a. Ringworm
    b. Roundworm
    c. *Giardia*
    d. *Toxoplasma*

14. A pathogen found in the mouth of animals that can lead to cardiac and pulmonary problems in both humans and animals is
    a. *Pasteurella multocida*
    b. *Escherichia coli*
    c. *Toxoplasma gondii*
    d. *Borrelia burgdorferi*

15. When taking a diagnostic radiograph, the x-ray beam should be collimated to
    a. The size of the whole area of interest
    b. The size of the cassette
    c. Larger than the size of the cassette
    d. Smaller than the size of the cassette

16. When taking diagnostic radiographs, the dosimetry badge should be worn
    a. On your collar under the apron
    b. On your collar outside the apron
    c. On the waist tie outside the apron
    d. On your belt under the apron

17. According to OSHA, the level of waste halogenated anesthetic agents in the clinical air should not exceed
    a. 2 parts per million
    b. 2 pounds per square inch
    c. 2 cm of water
    d. 2%

18. The source of the majority of anesthetic gas in the room during a procedure is
    a. Animal exhalation
    b. Leaks in the endotracheal tube
    c. Leaks in the machine
    d. Improper ventilation in the room

19. Which type of scavenging system requires weighing and replacement of components?
    a. Passive exhaust
    b. Active removal
    c. Absorption
    d. Accumulation

20. To prevent unnecessary exposure to WAGs when recovering a patient, you should do all of the following except
    a. Keep the number of recovering animals in one room to a minimum
    b. Keep your face away from the animal's face
    c. "Flush" the system before extubation
    d. Extubate the animal as quickly as possible

21. Which of the following materials is considered hazardous?
    a. IV catheter removed after a spay procedure
    b. Bandaging from a declaw procedure
    c. Scalpel blade used for a celiotomy
    d. Blood tubes from a dog infected with parvovirus

EXERCISE 4.8 CASE STUDY #1: FIRE AND EVACUATION

It is a busy Monday morning at the hospital where you work. The phones are ringing off the hook, the doctors are in rounds, appointments are about ready to start, and the other technicians are busy treating patients. Suddenly you smell smoke and notice it is coming from the laundry area. Apparently lint has clogged the outlet hose of the clothes dryer and caught on fire from the heat generated by the dryer. Smoke is billowing out into the room, and you can see flames through the glass door of the dryer. The fire does not appear to have spread or to involve the building, and at this point you do have a means of escape.

1. List the steps you should take to ensure everyone's safety. Keep the following in mind:
    - Your clinic does not have an automated fire alarm system.
    - You know where the fire extinguishers are located and have been trained on their use.

_____

_____

_____

_____

_____

_____

_____

_____

_____

_____

_____

_____

_____

_____

EXERCISE 4.9 CASE STUDY #2: RIGHTS AND RESPONSIBILITIES UNDER OSHA

Monday afternoon is just as busy as the morning *was (see case study #1). You* have been asked to perform a variety of diagnostic tests, treat the hospitalized patients, and prepare several patients for release. In the process of taking thoracic radiographs on a patient, you notice that the lead glove on your left hand has a hole in it. The patient you are imaging is a wiggly little terrier that is very hard to hold. You decide to take off the lead gloves so you can hold it more easily. In the process of taking the radiographs, the patient bites you on the right forefinger, producing a painful, bleeding wound.

1. Considering your rights and responsibilities under the Occupational Safety and Health Act, what are you obligated to do as an employee of the practice under these circumstances?

_____

_____

_____

2. What is your employer required to do under the Occupational Safety and Health Act?

_____

_____

_____

5 | Animal Behavior

LEARNING OBJECTIVES

When you have completed this chapter, you will be able to:

1. Pronounce, spell, and define all key terms in the chapter.
2. Explain why behavior problems can be life-threatening to pets.
3. Summarize the veterinary technician's role in supporting behavioral health.
4. List steps taken when gathering information for a behavioral history.
5. Do the following regarding learning and animal behavior modification:
   - Explain how animals learn and whether or not their behavior, like that of humans, is based on a moral code of conduct.
   - Differentiate between positive reinforcement, positive punishment, negative reinforcement, and negative punishment.
   - Explain the relationship between operant behaviors and continuous and intermittent reinforcement.
   - Describe why extinction of a behavior is difficult to achieve.
   - Distinguish between the following: desensitization, counter conditioning, counter commanding, and flooding.
6. Do the following regarding preventing behavior problems:
   - Describe each step in the Five-Step Positive Proaction Plan. List the criteria required for effective discipline.
   - Explain the importance of habituating young animals to handling.
   - Explain some of the challenges in habituating older animals to handling.
   - Describe ways in which a veterinary technician can assist a client in selecting a pet.
   - Describe the role medication plays in treating behavior problems.
7. Do the following regarding canine and feline development and behavior:
   - Describe the four stages of canine and feline development.
   - List important canine and feline behaviors that owners should be able to interpret correctly.
   - Explain how a veterinary technician's understanding of animal behavior can create a safer environment for workers, pet owners, and pets.
   - Describe methods for introducing a new dog or cat to existing pets.
   - List common behavior problems in dogs and cats and describe methods for addressing them.
   - Describe common circumstances in the dog and cat in which aggression can be problematic for the pet owner.
8. Do the following regarding equine behavior:
   - Explain how being a prey species influences the behavior of horses and their desire to be in a herd.
   - Describe how hierarchy affects the behavior of individual animals within a herd of horses.
   - Describe normal sexual behavior in mares and stallions.
   - Describe the behavior of mares with foals and explain why foal rejection is a behavior emergency.
   - List three common stable vices in horses.
9. Do the following regarding cattle and small ruminant behavior:
   - Describe how hierarchy affects the behavior of individual animals within a herd of cattle, sheep, or goats.
   - Describe how aggression commonly manifests in cattle, sheep, and goats.
   - Describe normal sexual and maternal behaviors in farm animals.
   - Describe common behavior problems in domestic livestock.

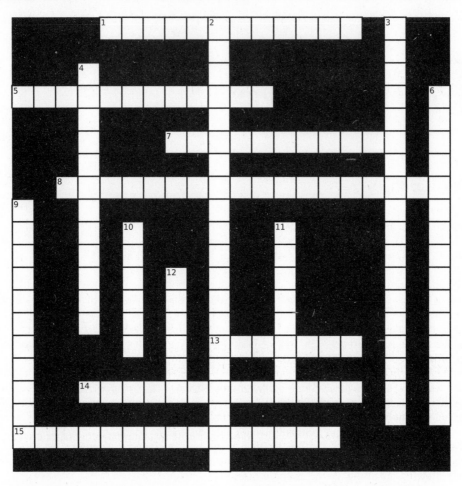

Across

1   A superior position in a rank order or social hierarchy. (2 words)
5   Grooming performed by one animal upon another of the same species.
7   Having given birth only one time or being pregnant for the first time.
8   Occurs when an animal is highly motivated to perform a particular behavior but is for some reason prevented from doing so. (2 words)
13 This emotional response leads to a physiologic response similar to that of fear.
14 Providing a puppy with pleasant experiences with people, situations, and other animals.
15 A wolf pack will form this, but free-ranging dogs generally do not. (2 words)

Down

2   Cheek and tail rubbing in cats are two examples of these. (2 words)
3   A dog that is acting as if it is sorry for its actions is exhibiting this. (2 words)
4   Two dogs, two sheep, and two horses are three examples of these.
6   A lower position in a rank order or social hierarchy. (2 words)
9   Having given birth more than one time.
10 May lead to weight loss, changes in the white blood cell counts, and decreased immunity to disease.
11 Occurs when an individual is motivated to perform two opposing behaviors.
12 A fear of thunder is an example of this.

EXERCISE 5.2 MATCHING #1: TERMS AND DEFINITIONS

Instructions: Match each term in column A with its corresponding definition in column B by writing the appropriate letter in the space provided.

Column A

1. _____ Affiliative behaviors

2. _____ Conflict

3. _____ Frustration

4. _____ Stress

5. _____ Social hierarchy

Column B

A. Seen in herd animals.

B. The result of chronic fear or anxiety from which there is no escape.

C. Experienced by the animal by the sudden withdrawal of reinforcement of a previous long-term behavior that received reward.

D. Behaviors performed by two animals that include cheek and tail rubbing.

E. When an individual is motivated to perform two opposing behaviors.

EXERCISE 5.3 MATCHING #2: TYPES OF AGGRESSION

Instructions: Match each term in column A with its corresponding statement in column B by writing the appropriate letter in the space provided.

Column A

1. _____ Idiopathic aggression

2. _____ Food-related aggression

3. _____ Irritable aggression

4. _____ Maternal aggression

5. _____ Predatory aggression

6. _____ Inter-dog aggression

7. _____ Territorial aggression

Column B

A. More common in older dogs.

B. Unpredictable and severe, occurring in the absence of stimuli.

C. Only seen in unspayed females.

D. Consistent with hunting behavior.

E. Occurs only in the presence of a high-value food item.

F. May result from changing the dog hierarchy within a household.

G. Demonstrated only in a particular area when approached by a perceived threat.

Instructions: Answer the questions about each photo.

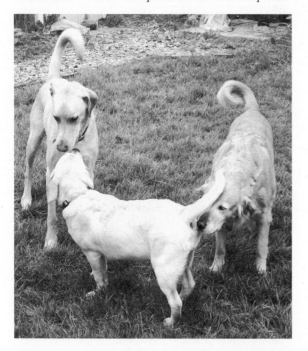

1. a. Which of the dogs in this photo is exhibiting a dominant role? What is typical behavior of a dog assuming a dominant role?

_____

_____

_____

_____

   b. Which of the dogs in this photo is exhibiting a submissive role? What behavior is typical of a dog assuming a submissive role?

_____

_____

_____

_____

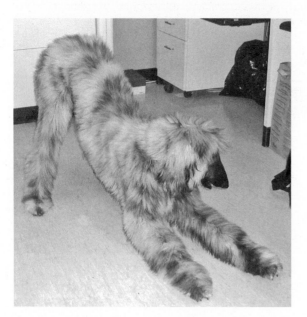

2. What behavior is this dog exhibiting? How do you know?

_____

_____

_____

_____

_____

Chapter **5 Animal Behavior**

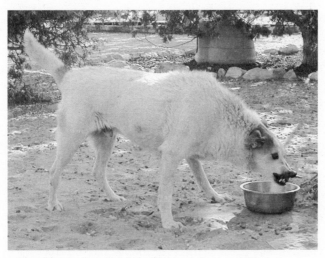

3. What behavior is this dog exhibiting? How do you know?

_____

_____

_____

_____

_____

_____

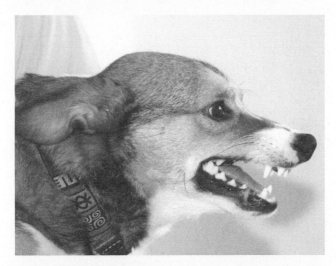

4. Is this dog exhibiting fear-related aggression or dominance aggression? How do you know?

_____

_____

_____

_____

_____

_____

5. Is this cat relaxed or aggressive? How do you know?

_____

_____

_____

_____

_____

_____

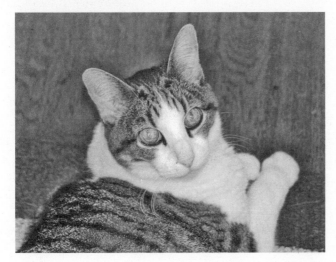

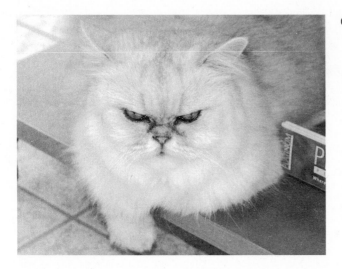

6. a. Is this cat relaxed or aggressive? How do you know?

_____

_____

_____

_____

b. How does this behavior differ from fearful behavior?

_____

_____

_____

_____

EXERCISE 5.5 TRUE OR FALSE: COMPREHENSIVE

Instructions: Read the following statements and write "T" for true or "F" for false in the blanks provided. If a statement is false, correct the statement to make it true.

1. _____ Questions about pet behavior should be included on any client history form.

2. _____ Client education about pet behavior problems is vital to preventing problems.

3. _____ A veterinary technician specialty in behavior does not currently exist.

4. _____ Dogs have a strong sense of "right" and "wrong," which affects their behavior.

5. _____ Punishment and negative reinforcement are the same thing.

6. _____ Flooding is a technique used to treat fearful behavior.

7. _____ If food rewards are used to train a dog, they must be used forever.

8. _____ Chewing is a behavior that is self-reinforcing.

9. _____ Providing adequate exercise is important in preventing unwanted dog behaviors.

10. _____ A dog that has defecated in the house and looks guilty when you come home knows it did wrong.

11. _____ Used alone, medications rarely solve behavior problems.

12. _____ During the socialization period, puppies develop a substrate preference for elimination.

13. _____ Selegiline should not be given with fluoxetine.

14. _____ Dogs become sexually and socially mature by 6 months of age.

15. _____ When puppies are presented to the clinic, you should take time to praise and provide food rewards for good behavior.

16. _____ Choke collars are very useful for training a large dog to walk on a leash.

17. _____ The best initial response to a dog exhibiting fear is to prevent its exposure to any of the things that cause the fear.

18. _____ A dog with a thunderstorm phobia may become very destructive or injure itself.

19. _____ All dog aggression is considered abnormal.

20. _____ Neutering will produce a dramatic decrease in all types of canine aggression.

21. _____ Any breed of dog may develop aggression.

22. _____ A female dog may also lift her leg to urinate.

23. _____ Aggression is very common when a new cat is added to a household with a resident cat.

24. _____ A cat carrier should not be taken out of the closet until the very minute it will be needed to take the cat to the veterinary clinic.

25. _____ Food rewards can be used to make cats more comfortable in the veterinary clinic.

26. _____ Declawing cats is cruel and painful and should never be performed.

27. _____ Even when no fighting occurs, when one cat in a household spends the majority of its time hiding from the other cat, it is a sign that the cats are not getting along.

28. _____ While sitting on their owner's lap and being petted, cats will sometimes bite.

29. _____ Redirected aggression is a rare and unimportant problem in cats.

30. _____ A cat that dislikes its litter will neither defecate nor urinate in the box.

31. _____ Older cats that vocalize in a random and purposeless way may be exhibiting signs of feline cognitive dysfunction.

32. _____ The main advantage of a hierarchy in social animals is that it allows them to gang up on predators.

33. _____ A frightened horse may injure its handler.

34. _____ Visual cues are the primary means by which mare and foal recognize each other.

35. _____ Cribbing is not seen in free-ranging horses.

36. _____ When fighting, horses may kick out with both front legs.

37. _____ Most equine aggression toward humans is a learned response related to fear.

38. _____ When approaching sheep in a pen, the most dominant animal will be at the front of the flock.

39. _____ Dairy bulls are notoriously aggressive toward humans.

Instructions: Circle the one correct answer to each of the following questions.

1. Which term refers to the process by which an association between two events is broken?
   a. Punishment
   b. Negative reinforcement
   c. Extinction
   d. Intermittent reinforcement

2. What is the term for changing an animal's emotional response to a stimulus?
   a. Counter conditioning
   b. Systematic desensitization
   c. Negative reinforcement
   d. Classical conditioning

3. What is the process by which you substitute an alternative behavior that is incompatible with the problem behavior?
   a. Counter conditioning
   b. Systematic desensitization
   c. Classical conditioning
   d. Positive reinforcement

4. Learned helplessness may result from which training technique?
   a. Systematic desensitization
   b. Negative reinforcement
   c. Counter conditioning
   d. Flooding

5. Exposing an animal frequently to nonthreatening stimuli, such as strangers, nail trimming, grooming, and handling, is an example of which process?
   a. Counter conditioning
   b. Operant conditioning
   c. Habituation
   d. Systematic desensitization

6. Giving a dog a food reward after each nail is trimmed is an example of which process?
   a. Operant conditioning
   b. Classical conditioning
   c. Flooding
   d. Systematic desensitization

7. Which of the following is classified as a tricyclic antidepressant (TCA)?
   a. Clomicalm
   b. Valium
   c. Reconcile
   d. Anipryl

8. How long does the neonatal period last in puppies?
   a. 8 weeks
   b. 6 weeks
   c. 4 weeks
   d. 2 weeks

9. At what age does the socialization period start in puppies?
   a. 8 weeks
   b. 6 weeks
   c. 4 weeks
   d. 2 weeks

10. A dog in your clinic that is lip licking, yawning, and looking away from you is exhibiting behavior indicating that it is
    a. Sleepy
    b. Anxious
    c. Aggressive
    d. Hungry

11. Most problem behaviors seen in the clinic are caused by which of the following?
    a. Disease
    b. Lack of training
    c. Fear
    d. Learned aggression

12. When a healthy dog refuses a highly palatable food treat, it is usually because the dog is
    a. Not hungry
    b. Fearful
    c. Aggressive
    d. Carsick

13. When playing with a dog, the second its teeth contact your skin, the owner should
    a. Walk away from the dog
    b. Pin it to the ground and growl
    c. Smack it on the face
    d. Throw a toy in another direction

14. Which best describes the Gentle Leader?
    a. Choke collar
    b. Body harness
    c. Stiff leash
    d. Head halter

15. Fears are best treated by using which of the following?
    a. Cognitive dysfunction
    b. Classical conditioning
    c. Systematic desensitization
    d. Flooding

16. Which drug is FDA approved for the treatment of separation anxiety in dogs?
    a. Reconcile
    b. Valium
    c. Anipryl
    d. Ovaban

17. Which drug is FDA approved for the treatment of canine cognitive dysfunction?
    a. Reconcile
    b. Valium
    c. Anipryl
    d. Ovaban

18. At what age does the sensitive period for socialization in the kitten occur?
    a. Weeks 2 to 7
    b. Weeks 4 to 16
    c. Weeks 8 to 10
    d. Weeks 12 to 18

19. A cat with its body arched, tail erect, and ears flattened to its head is exhibiting which behavior?
    a. Predatory aggression
    b. Greeting
    c. Dominant aggression
    d. Fear aggression

20. Two cats staring at one another from 3 feet apart are exhibiting which behavior?
    a. Aggression
    b. Fear
    c. Greeting
    d. Acceptance

21. When two cats are interacting and one hisses, the hissing cat is exhibiting which behavior toward the other cat?
    a. Submission
    b. Aggression
    c. Fear
    d. Acceptance

22. What is the position of the ears in an aggressive horse?
    a. Erect and forward
    b. Pinned back facing outward
    c. Swiveling front and back
    d. Rotated backward

23. Which of the following is a greeting call used by the horse?
    a. Snort
    b. Squeal
    c. Nicker
    d. Whinny

24. The vomeronasal organ is involved in which behavior in the horse?
    a. Aggression
    b. Olfaction
    c. Vision
    d. Touch

25. The horse hierarchy in a pasture is mostly determined by which factor?
    a. Individual temperament
    b. Size
    c. Age
    d. Sex

26. What is it called when mares do not show behavioral signs of estrus?
    a. False heat
    b. Anestrus
    c. Silent heat
    d. Pseudocyesis

27. Self-mutilation is a behavior problem that occurs most commonly in
    a. Geldings
    b. Mares
    c. Foals
    d. Stallions

28. Today's management practices usually result in the foal being weaned at what age?
    a. 8 to 9 months
    b. 4 to 6 months
    c. 6 to 8 weeks
    d. 4 to 6 weeks

Mrs. Benjamin Franklin and her three children, ages 14, 8, and 6 years, have brought their 16-week-old male Springer Spaniel puppy to your veterinary clinic for its final booster vaccination. You ask how housebreaking is progressing, and she starts to cry. She is thinking of getting rid of the pup because it continues to poop and pee in the house. They brought the pup home 6 weeks ago from the breeder. They feed it free-choice, and it has constant access to water. They let it out in the yard four times a day, including just before bedtime. When Ben finds an accident in the house, he rubs the pup's face in it and screams "Bad dog!" The pup is closed up in the kitchen overnight and has also begun chewing the legs on the kitchen chairs.

1. What is she doing wrong? What advice do you have for her on fixing this situation?

_____

_____

_____

_____

_____

_____

_____

_____

_____

_____

_____

_____

_____

EXERCISE 5.8 CASE STUDY #2: INAPPROPRIATE URINATION IN A MULTICAT HOUSEHOLD

Mrs. Davis has a 3-year-old neutered male cat named Moony. Recently, she got married, and her new husband moved in with his 4-year-old spayed female cat, Sunny. Initially she locked Moony in a bedroom and gave Sunny run of the house. Two weeks ago she let Moony into the rest of the house. The two cats initially ignored one another. Sunny hid most of the time once Moony started roaming the house, although no hissing or fighting was seen. Recently, Mrs. Davis started finding small amounts of urine running down the umbrella stand, coat rack, drapes, and walls. The single litter box in the bathroom is still being used. She has no idea which cat is no longer using the litter box. She is very unhappy and wants your advice.

1. What should you tell her to do?

_____

_____

_____

_____

_____

_____

_____

_____

_____

_____

_____

_____

_____

EXERCISE 5.9 CASE STUDY #3: CHOOSING A NEW PET

Mr. Thomson and his family have come to the clinic with their dog, Victoria, for a routine visit. During the course of the visit, he informs you that they would like to get a companion for Victoria but are unsure where to begin. One way you could help them make this decision would be to guide them as to what species, breed, and gender might be appropriate for their family.

1. What are some other ways you could assist them so that they can find a healthy pet with behavioral characteristics that are a good fit for their family?

_____

_____

_____

_____

_____

43

6 Restraint and Handling of Animals

LEARNING OBJECTIVES

When you have completed this chapter, you will be able to:

1. Pronounce, spell, and define all the Key Terms in this chapter.
2. List three indications for animal restraint, and describe methods for approaching dogs and cats before attempting restraint.
3. Do the following regarding canine and feline capture and restraint:
   - List the actions taken to diminish stress in dogs and cats during physical examinations and hospitalization.
   - List some of the equipment and the methods used in capturing and restraining both cooperative and uncooperative dogs and cats.
   - List the advantages and disadvantages of chemical restraint in dogs and cats.
   - Describe various positions for restraining cats and dogs, specifically for nail trimming and venipuncture of the cephalic vein.
4. Do the following regarding equine capture and restraint:
   - Explain the principles that affect equine perception and behavior.
   - Describe the physical abilities of horses and how these affect the ways in which horses are handled.
   - Describe methods for approaching and capturing adult and juvenile equine patients, including using restraint equipment, diversions, and pharmaceutical products, and identify special restraint techniques for horses and the circumstances in which they are used.
5. Do the following regarding capture and restraint of cattle:
   - Describe the principles that affect cattle behavior, and list principles used to move cattle and individuals in an effective and low-stress manner.
   - Explain the differences in housing between dairy and beef cattle, and describe how these differences affect methods to handle and restrain them.
   - List the types of bulls known to be particularly dangerous to handle.
   - List the equipment used to restrain cattle in general and to restrain specific parts of their body. Also, describe the circumstances of their use.
6. Describe methods for observing and approaching swine of each gender and age group, and discuss methods used to capture and restrain adult and young pigs.
7. Do the following regarding small ruminant capture and restraint:
   - Describe the behavioral tendencies of small ruminants, and explain how these influence the approach and capture of herds.
   - List the factors that affect levels of aggression in camelids and describe how aggression presents in these species.
   - Describe the approach, capture, and restraint of individual sheep, goats, and camelids.
   - List additional restraint techniques used in camelids but not in sheep or goats.
8. Describe restraint and handling techniques used with birds, small mammals, and reptiles.

EXERCISE 6.1 TERMS AND DEFINITIONS: ANIMAL RESTRAINT

Instructions: Define each term in your own words.

(Note: Terms #1 through #3 are behaviors seen during approach or capture.)

1. Displacement behavior

   _____

   _____

2. Fight-or-flight response

   _____

   _____

   _____

3. Fear biting

   _____

   _____

4. Double-barrel kick

   _____

   _____

5. Cow kick

   _____

   _____

6. Diversionary restraint

   _____

   _____

7. Humane twitch

_____

_____

8. Cross-tie

_____

_____

9. Hobbles

_____

_____

10. Tail tie

_____

_____

11. Stocks

_____

_____

12. Twitch

_____

_____

13. Cradle

_____

_____

EXERCISE 6.2 MATCHING #1: KEY TERMS AND DEFINITIONS

Instructions: Match each term in column A with its appropriate definition in column B by writing the appropriate letter in the space provided.

Column A

1. _____ Aggression
2. _____ Binocular vision
3. _____ Blind spots
4. _____ Displacement behaviors
5. _____ Diversionary restraint
6. _____ Fear biting
7. _____ Fight-or-flight response
8. _____ Flight zone
9. _____ Point of balance
10. _____ Tortoise
11. _____ Turtle

Column B

A. Vision in which both eyes are used synchronously to produce a single image.

B. A land turtle.

C. Yawning, scratching, and licking of the lips in a fearful dog represents this.

D. A behavior with intent to harm.

E. Unlike cattle raised for production, pet cattle do not have one of these.

F. Tapping lightly on the horse's head or use of a twitch in a horse represents this.

G. Chasing a dog into a corner may result in this.

H. A marine reptile with a toothless, horny beak and a shell of bony dermal plates.

I. A state of alert when a threat is perceived.

J. The areas directly behind a horse, directly in front of its nose, and between its eyes.

K. A specific location on an animal's anatomy from where an animal-care professional's step in either direction would cause the animal to move in the opposite direction.

EXERCISE 6.3 MATCHING #2: RESTRAINT TECHNIQUES FOR EXOTIC SPECIES

Instructions: Match each species in column A with the technique used to restrain it in column B by writing the appropriate letter in the space provided.

Column A

1. _____ Raptors
2. _____ Hedgehogs
3. _____ Hamsters
4. _____ Lizards
5. _____ Small- to medium-size psittacine birds
6. _____ Mice
7. _____ Sugar gliders
8. _____ Snakes
9. _____ Rabbits and chinchillas
10. _____ Gerbils
11. _____ Large psittacine birds
12. _____ Turtles
13. _____ Ferrets

Column B

A. Cover the head with a leather hood and restrain the body with leather gloves and a towel.

B. Control the head with the thumb and index finger, being careful not to damage the large eyes.

C. Scruff the neck and dorsum and restrain the tail with the pinky finger.

D. Restrain the head and the torso with one hand, and use the other hand to restrain the tibiotarsus of both legs.

E. Grasp the plastron and carapace with a "sandwich"-type grip with one hand, and grasp the head behind the mandibles with the other hand.

F. Scruff the neck, being careful not to make the skin too taught around the face.

G. Carry like a football with the head in the crook of the arm and one arm supporting the chest and hindlimbs.

H. Control the head with one hand, support the trunk with the other hand and forearm, and hold the tail between the arm and body.

I. Gently scruff the neck, hold the body in a vertical position, and stabilize the hindlimbs with the other hand.

J. Restrain with leather gloves to avoid injury from the quills.

K. Control the head with the thumb and middle finger, with an index finger on top of the head. Control the rest of the body with the other hand.

L. Wrap the torso in a towel so the handler can concentrate on the head, beak, and feet.

M. Control like a hamster, being very careful not to grab the tail.

Instructions: Answer the questions about each photo.

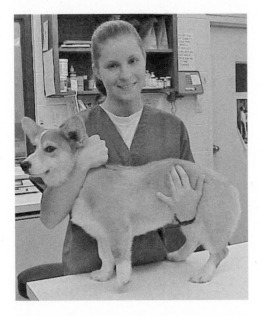

1. Examine this technician's restraint technique of a dog. Why does she have her arms in these specific locations? What advantages do these positions afford?

   _____

   _____

   _____

   _____

   _____

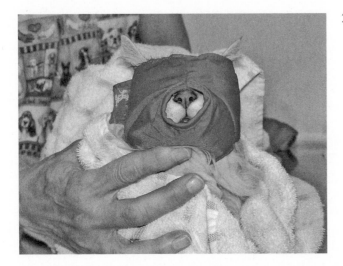

2. When applying a cat muzzle such as this one, what principles must be followed to ensure your safety and the animal's safety?

   _____

   _____

   _____

   _____

   _____

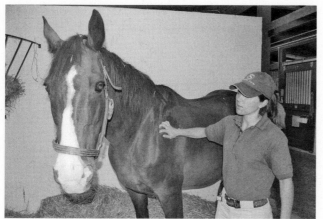

3. What principles are this technician following when approaching this horse to minimize the risk of injury?

_____

_____

_____

_____

_____

_____

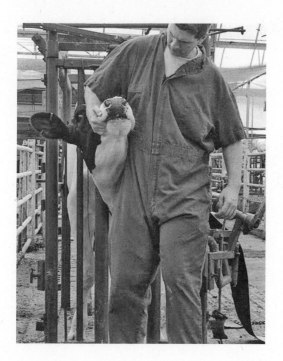

4. Describe the technique being used by this technician to open a cow's mouth for administration of oral fluids or boluses.

_____

_____

_____

_____

_____

_____

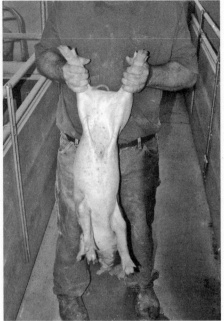

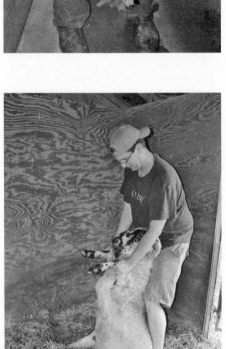

5. This technique (holding the pig by its rear legs) is used to restrain larger nursery pigs or small pigs. What alternative techniques can be used for small pigs?

_____

_____

_____

_____

_____

_____

6. This sheep is being restrained by "flipping." Explain how this is done.

_____

_____

_____

_____

_____

_____

EXERCISE 6.5 TRUE OR FALSE: COMPREHENSIVE

Instructions: Read the following statements and write "T" for true or "F" for false in the blanks provided. If a statement is false, correct the statement to make it true.

1. _____ Practice owners are responsible for any injuries incurred by veterinary personnel and clients during the performance of veterinary procedures.

2. _____ Corrective training methods that can improve a pet with dominance aggression can also improve a pet with fear-related aggression.

3. _____ Cats should be acclimated to the carrier prior to being loaded up for a visit to the veterinary clinic.

4. _____ You should ask every owner if his or her pet is "nice" before grabbing it.

5. _____ An animal that freezes when you go to pick it up is no longer stressed.

6. _____ Cats tend to be more stressed on the examination table than in the carrier.

7. _____ Most dogs respond favorably to vocal reassurance.

8. _____ A towel is a useful restraint device for working with cats.

9. _____ Kittens are generally harmless and are easily restrained in a veterinary clinic.

10. _____ Lift tables are very useful for examining large dogs.

11. _____ Because dogs are comfortable with their owners, the owner should be encouraged to hold his or her dog for examination.

12. _____ Many dogs behave better with minimal restraint.

13. _____ When positioning a dog for cephalic venipuncture, it should be in lateral recumbency or sitting.

14. _____ The best position to put a dog in when trimming its nails is lateral recumbency.

15. _____ Race horses may become protective of their stalls and act aggressively when a stranger enters.

16. _____ Horses can kick with both front and hind legs.

17. _____ It is best to enter a stall quickly and grab a horse's halter before it has a chance to react.

18. _____ The best way to catch a foal is to stand between the mare and the foal.

19. _____ It is recommended that the lead rope be wrapped around the arm to help control the horse.

20. _____ It is counterproductive to attempt any procedures when the twitch is initially applied.

21. _____ The best way to restrain a foal is to place an arm around its chest and hind end and lift it off the ground.

22. _____ Dairy cattle tend to have shorter flight zones than beef cattle.

23. _____ The best way to move cattle is to herd them from behind.

24. _____ Cows do not have upper incisors.

Chapter **6** **Restraint and Handling of Animals**

25. _____ When moving pigs in a pen, they can become agitated and may become hyperthermic.

26. _____ After the animal has been moved into a smaller pen, the first step of restraint for all small ruminant species is to control the head.

27. _____ One problem when restraining birds is if they get loose, they may fly into windows and injure themselves.

28. _____ Birds do not have a diaphragm.

29. _____ Rabbits cannot breathe through their mouths like dogs.

30. _____ Hedgehogs can shoot their quills into enemies like a porcupine.

31. _____ Hedgehogs generate frothy sputum, which they lick onto their spines.

32. _____ Restricting the movement of an iguana's thorax will cause it to suffocate.

33. _____ Some turtle species are poisonous.

34. _____ The towel is the preferred method for restraining medium to large lizards.

EXERCISE 6.6 MULTIPLE CHOICE: COMPREHENSIVE

Instructions: Circle the one correct answer to each of the following questions.

1. Most of the aggressive behaviors seen in dogs and cats in the clinic are a result of which of the following?
   a. Dominance
   b. Fear
   c. Poor training
   d. Disease

2. When a fearful pet displays warnings as you approach its cage, the situation can be improved by doing which of the following?
   a. Backing up
   b. Feeding it
   c. Putting a snare around its neck
   d. Grabbing it with gloves

3. What can be sprayed onto towels, muzzles, and other equipment to make a dog feel more comfortable in the veterinary clinic?
   a. Citronella
   b. Doggieway
   c. Beef broth
   d. Dog Appeasing Pheromone

4. A clear, hollow plastic ball that fits over a dog's head is known as the
   a. Air Muzzle
   b. Space Helmet
   c. Birdcage
   d. Fish bowl

5. When holding off a cephalic vein for venipuncture, the holder must do which of the following?
   a. Press down into the jugular furrow
   b. Rotate the vein laterally
   c. Rotate the vein medially
   d. Hold the pet in dorsal recumbency

6. The horse's eyes are located laterally on their head. How much binocular vision do they have?
   a. 360 degrees
   b. 180 degrees
   c. 90 degrees
   d. 60 degrees

7. Most horses are traditionally and typically handled from which direction?
   a. Front
   b. Right side
   c. Left side
   d. Rear

8. What is the normal flight zone for a domestic horse in a field?
   a. 6 to 12 feet
   b. 10 to 30 feet
   c. 20 to 50 feet
   d. Domestic horses do not have a flight zone.

9. When capturing a yearling horse, the best initial move is to
   a. Rapidly grasp the halter
   b. Face it and look it in the eye
   c. Put a chain over its nose
   d. Squat down and scratch the withers

10. Which is the best place to initially touch a horse?
    a. Withers
    b. Ears
    c. Muzzle
    d. Butt

11. Physical restraint of the adult equine begins with which piece of equipment?
    a. Stocks
    b. Head chute
    c. Lariat
    d. Halter

12. What is one purpose for using a cradle on a horse?
    a. Prevent kicking
    b. Prevent cribbing
    c. Hold it still
    d. Calm it down

13. What is the point of balance of a cow?
    a. Hip
    b. Head
    c. Shoulder
    d. Flank

14. Which of the following is used to administer a bolus to a dairy cow?
    a. Teat cannula
    b. Syringe and needle
    c. Stomach tube
    d. Balling gun

15. If the jugular vein is inaccessible, what other vessel is commonly used for bovine blood collection?
    a. Coccygeal vein
    b. Cephalic vein
    c. Medial saphenous vein
    d. Facial vein

16. Lameness is a common disease of dairy cows and most commonly requires which treatment?
    a. Corrective shoes
    b. Casts
    c. Corrective trimming
    d. Surgery

17. Which of the following has the least herding instinct?
    a. Cattle
    b. Sheep
    c. Horses
    d. Pigs

18. Unlike ruminants, pigs have a genetic predisposition to which of the following?
    a. Anorexia nervosa
    b. Epilepsy
    c. Hyperthermia
    d. Laryngeal spasms

19. Which device is commonly used to restrain adult pigs for blood collection?
    a. Rope
    b. Hobbles
    c. Snare
    d. Gloves

20. Ear protection is necessary when restraining which animal?
    a. Llamas
    b. Sheep
    c. Goats
    d. Pigs

21. Restraint of potbellied pet pigs is most similar to that of
    a. Adult farm pigs
    b. Piglets
    c. Dogs
    d. Sheep

22. What is occurring when llamas and alpacas make a gurgling sound while being captured?
    a. Respiratory distress
    b. Getting ready to spit
    c. Diarrhea
    d. Colic

23. What are camelids doing when they "kush"?
    a. Spitting
    b. Rearing up
    c. Lying down
    d. Herding

24. How does a deer restraint chute differ from the one used with cattle?
    a. It rotates.
    b. It is taller.
    c. It is wider.
    d. The floor drops out.

25. What is the term for the rapid dilating and constricting of a parrot's pupils?
    a. Pinning
    b. Nystagmus
    c. Strabismus
    d. Miomydriasis

26. Being able to visualize a bird's keel while the bird is being restrained allows what to be observed?
    a. Body temperature
    b. Breathing
    c. Feces
    d. Beak

27. With which animal are leather hoods often used as part of the restraint procedure?
    a. Macaw
    b. Ferret
    c. Alpaca
    d. Falcon

28. Which animal, if improperly restrained, can break its own back while still being held?
    a. Ferret
    b. Guinea pig
    c. Hawk
    d. Rabbit

29. Which rodent is normally most aggressive to handle?
    a. Guinea pig
    b. Ferret
    c. Hamster
    d. Mouse

30. In which animal is fur slip most likely to occur?
    a. Rabbit
    b. Gerbil
    c. Sugar glider
    d. Mouse

31. Snakes often threaten by doing which of the following?
    a. Hissing
    b. Growling
    c. Curling into a ball
    d. Spitting

32. Which of the following has a plastron?
    a. Iguana
    b. Macaw
    c. Box turtle
    d. Python

EXERCISE 6.7 CASE STUDY: RECAPTURING AN ESCAPED DOG

You are walking a newly arrived German Shepherd through the clinic, and it slips out of its collar and runs out into the enclosed courtyard to cower in the bushes. Describe what you should do to recapture it.

_____

_____

_____

_____

_____

_____

_____

_____

_____

_____

_____

7 History and Physical Examination

LEARNING OBJECTIVES

When you have completed this chapter, you will be able to:

1. Pronounce, spell, and define all the Key Terms in this chapter.
2. Obtain an accurate and complete medical history in small animals by:
   - Explaining the role of the veterinary technician in obtaining the patient's medical history.
   - Listing questions commonly used to obtain a dog's or a cat's medical history.
   - Describing what a leading question is and explaining why asking the owner leading questions can lead to inaccurate historical information.
   - Describing the type of information contained in each section of the patient's medical history for dogs and cats.
   - Explaining what a patient's signalment is and how it relates to patient assessment.
   - Listing aspects of an animal's origin, background, and past medical history that may be relevant to a presenting complaint.
3. Describe the general procedures used to perform and document a physical examination in dogs and cats, including a subjective assessment of the patient in its surroundings and the measurement of temperature, pulse, and respiration.
4. Discuss methods for performing a comprehensive evaluation of each of the body systems in small animal species.
5. Obtain an accurate and complete medical history in large animals by:
   - Explaining the importance of determining owner/ agent information.
   - Describing how the signalment of a large animal relates to patient assessment.
   - Discussing the individual history and chief complaint of the large animal.
   - Discussing the medication and treatment history.
   - Describing why the process of gathering historical information on herd health differs from taking an individual's patient history.
6. List and describe unique procedures used in the physical examination of horses and ruminants.

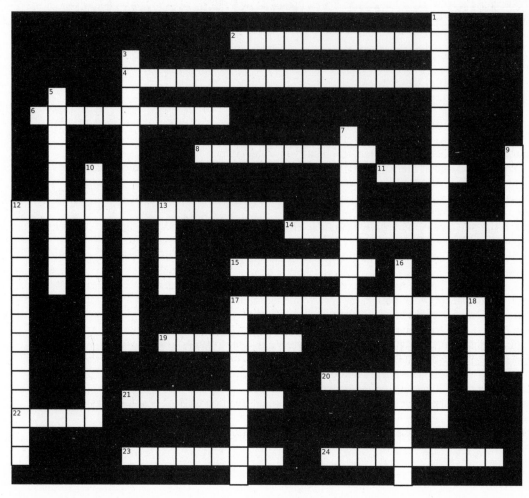

Across

2   Occurs when heat-dissipating mechanisms cannot overcome excessive ambient temperatures.
4   A method of evaluating nutritional status. (3 words)
6   Decreased circulating blood volume.
8   Enlargement of the kidneys.
11 Decreased perfusion and oxygen delivery to tissues.
12 A condition that causes a lack of lung sounds in the ventral lung fields. (2 words)
14 A physical indication of the difference between the systolic and diastolic arterial pressure. (2 words)
15 A disease condition that causes an enlarged uterus because of buildup of pus.
17 Abnormal fluid buildup within the lung tissue. (2 words)
19 Referring to the "armpit."
20 Inflammation of the large bowel.
21 Excessive grooming that damages hair and skin.
22 The nostrils.
23 Mental activity of a patient.
24 The age, sex, breed, color, and reproductive status of an animal.

Down

1   A congenital heart defect that results in "bounding" pulses. (3 words)
3   A technique used to detect abdominal gas accumulations. (2 words)
5   A result of impaired thermoregulation in any sick animal, such as a cat with chronic renal failure.
7   The presence of sugar in the urine.
9   An audible heartbeat without a pulse. (2 words)
10 A heart defect associated with narrowing of the outflow tract of the left ventricle. (2 words)
12 Abnormal movement of abdominal contents through the pelvic diaphragm. (2 words)
13 Elevated body temperature.
16 A condition that causes a lack of lung sounds in the dorsal lung fields.
17 An adjective indicating increased water consumption.
18 Referring to the ear.

Chapter **7 History and Physical Examination**

EXERCISE 7.2 MATCHING #1: MEDICAL HISTORY

Instructions: Historical information can be divided into several sections. Match each statement in column A with the corresponding section of the medical history to which it belongs in column B by writing the appropriate letter in the space provided.

Column A

1. _____ I brought Wizer in today because she started vomiting about a week ago.

2. _____ Felix has no allergies to any medications as far as I am aware.

3. _____ Pepper was feeling well until last Tuesday.

4. _____ I am giving Sparticus hairball medicine twice a week.

5. _____ Bella is 3 years old and was spayed at 6 months of age.

6. _____ I don't see any change in the amount of water Max is drinking or the amount of urine in the box.

7. _____ Rocky was vomiting about once a day for a few days but is now vomiting a couple of times a day.

8. _____ Chloe got an infection 2 years ago from a cat bite and had a cold when she was a baby.

Column B

A. Signalment

B. Background information

C. Past pertinent medical history

D. Presenting complaint

E. Last normal

F. Progression

G. Systems review

H. Medications

EXERCISE 7.3 MATCHING #2: KEY TERMS

Instructions: Match each term in column A with its corresponding definition in column B by writing the appropriate letter in the space provided.

Column A

1. _____ Ataxia

2. _____ Pruritic

3. _____ Borborygmus

4. _____ Icterus

5. _____ Stridor

6. _____ Alopecia

7. _____ Ileus

8. _____ Stertor

9. _____ Excoriation

10. _____ Halitosis

Column B

A. Inspiratory noise similar to snoring

B. Intestinal motility sound

C. Skin lesions caused by scratching

D. Harsh, high-pitched respiratory sound

E. Foul odor to the breath

F. Incoordination

G. Complete absence of intestinal motility

H. Itchy

I. Hair loss

J. Yellow mucous membranes

EXERCISE 7.4 TRUE OR FALSE: COMPREHENSIVE

Instructions: Read the following statements and write "T" for true or "F" for false in the blanks provided. If a statement is false, correct the statement to make it true.

1. _____ The medical record is a legal document.

2. _____ Congenital defects are more likely to be diagnosed in younger patients.

3. _____ There is no need to ask behavior-related questions when obtaining the history of a sick animal.

4. _____ Animals do not suffer from allergic reactions to medications.

5. _____ Pyometra occurs most commonly 2 weeks to 2 months following a heat cycle.

6. _____ Many mammary tumors in dogs are prevented by spaying before the first heat.

7. _____ Medical terminology should be avoided on the medical record.

8. _____ Hypothermia is more common in patients that are young, old, or thin.

9. _____ The heart rate in a healthy animal should be twice the pulse rate.

10. _____ An animal in hypovolemic shock will have a strong pulse pressure.

11. _____ Gingivitis is a precursor to periodontal disease.

12. _____ The nictitating membrane is also known as the third eyelid.

13. _____ Normal tracheal airflow is turbulent, and the respiratory sounds should be loud and harsh.

14. _____ Hyperemia of the gingiva is usually caused by dehydration.

15. _____ The liver cannot be palpated in a healthy animal.

16. _____ The canine uterus cannot be palpated unless it is enlarged.

17. _____ The popliteal lymph nodes are located in the caudal ventral abdomen just medial to each thigh.

18. _____ All cranial nerves can be evaluated on a neurologic examination.

19. _____ The pupillary light reflex tests cranial nerves II and III.

20. _____ Equine insurance coverage is common in the United States.

21. _____ It is acceptable to dip an animal thermometer in the horse's water bucket to provide lubrication before inserting it into the horse's rectum.

22. _____ A normal resting pulse rate in an adult horse is 17 to 27 beats per minute.

23. _____ Normal horses cannot breathe through the mouth.

24. _____ Most murmurs heard in horses are ejection murmurs and are not signs of valvular abnormalities.

25. _____ A horse's height is measured by hands, with one hand being equal to 6 inches.

26. _____ When ruminants breathe through their mouths, it is usually considered a sign of distress or heat stress.

27. _____ Pings are normal findings when auscultating a ruminant's abdomen.

EXERCISE 7.5 MULTIPLE CHOICE: COMPREHENSIVE

Instructions: Circle the one correct answer to each of the following questions.

1. Which term refers to sugar in the urine?
   a. Icterus
   b. Polyuria
   c. Glycosuria
   d. Hyperglycemia

2. What is seen in a polydipsic cat?
   a. Hypovolemia
   b. Increased drinking
   c. Ileus
   d. Increased urination

3. Which term refers to an elevated body temperature?
   a. Ileus
   b. Hypothermia
   c. Hypertension
   d. Hyperthermia

4. A cat with a body temperature of 98° F is exhibiting which of the following?
   a. Hyperthermia
   b. Hypothermia
   c. Stridor
   d. Hypovolemia

5. Which condition will cause a cat to resist having a rectal thermometer placed?
   a. Ileus
   b. Polydipsia
   c. Colitis
   d. Icterus

6. Which may be a sign of upper airway disease?
   a. Ileus
   b. Ataxia
   c. Pyometra
   d. Stertor

7. The aural temperature is taken from which site?
   a. Rectum
   b. Ear
   c. Mouth
   d. Vagina

8. From which vessel is the pulse generally taken in a dog or cat?
   a. Jugular vein
   b. Carotid artery
   c. Femoral artery
   d. Cephalic vein

9. A pulse deficit occurs in which situation?
   a. When the heart rate is less than the pulse rate
   b. When the heart rate exceeds the pulse rate
   c. Whenever the pulse slows down
   d. Whenever the pulse is weaker than normal

10. Which is caused by a cardiovascular problem?
    a. Glycosuria
    b. Stertor
    c. Colitis
    d. Shock

11. Which may cause a weak peripheral pulse?
    a. Hypovolemia
    b. Stertor
    c. Hypothermia
    d. Ileus

12. The rolling of the lower eyelid in toward the eye is known as
    a. Ectropion
    b. Entropion
    c. Hypyon
    d. Miosis

13. Which of the following will cause an eyeball to feel firm on palpation?
    a. Mucocele
    b. Ophthalmitis
    c. Glaucoma
    d. Retinitis

14. What is the medical term for pupils of different sizes?
    a. Heterotropia
    b. Cataract
    c. Mydriasis
    d. Anisocoria

15. Petechiation inside the pinna may be a sign of which disorder?
    a. Thrombocytopenia
    b. Otitis externa
    c. Hematoma
    d. Otitis media

16. Stenotic nares are commonly seen in
    a. Aortic stenosis
    b. Brachycephalic breeds
    c. Dolichocephalic breeds
    d. Arabian horses

17. Which device is used for auscultation?
    a. Otoscope
    b. Ophthalmoscope
    c. X-ray machine
    d. Stethoscope

18. Which term refers to increased fluid in the thoracic cavity?
    a. Pleural effusion
    b. Colitis
    c. Pyometra
    d. Ascites

19. Capillary refill time is used to assess which condition?
    a. Anemia
    b. Dehydration
    c. Perfusion
    d. Heart rate

20. What does a sinus arrhythmia indicate in a dog?
    a. Normal cardiac function
    b. Cardiomyopathy
    c. Congestive heart failure
    d. Shock

21. What causes the jugular veins to be distended all the way up the neck?
    a. Hypotension
    b. Increased central venous pressure
    c. Dehydration
    d. Anemia

22. Which is a sign of a bacterial skin infection?
    a. A nodule
    b. Broken hairs
    c. Pustules
    d. A mass

23. What is seen in an animal that is obtunded?
    a. Hyperactivity
    b. Head tilt and circling
    c. Weak in the rear end
    d. Not interested in surroundings

24. Nystagmus often suggests that a lesion is located where in the patient?
    a. Vestibulocochlear nerve (cranial nerve VIII)
    b. Optic nerve (cranial nerve II)
    c. Sciatic nerve
    d. Nasal passage

25. A gray coat color in a horse is associated with a higher incidence of which of the following?
    a. Obstructive urolithiasis
    b. β-mannosidase deficiency
    c. Neonatal isoerythrolysis
    d. Melanoma

26. Black walnut shavings may cause which problem in horses?
    a. Colic
    b. Laminitis
    c. Thrush
    d. Asthma

27. What is the normal rectal temperature for an adult thoroughbred horse?
    a. 98° F to 99° F
    b. 99° F to 101.5° F
    c. 100.5° F to 103° F
    d. 102° F to 104.5° F

28. From which vessel is the pulse most commonly felt in the horse?
    a. Femoral artery
    b. Carotid artery
    c. Facial artery
    d. Jugular vein

29. Which term refers to the absence of intestinal sounds and may be noted in the horse?
    a. Borborygmus
    b. Icterus
    c. Ileus
    d. Colitis

30. What is the normal eructation rate in a normal cow?
    a. 6 per hour
    b. 12 per hour
    c. 18 per hour
    d. 24 per hour

EXERCISE 7.6 FILL IN THE CHART: REGURGITATION AND VOMITING

Instructions: Asking specific questions with the goal of determining whether the dog is truly vomiting or is actually displaying regurgitation is critical to obtaining an accurate history.

Fill in the chart with the following key:

R—Rarely to never
O—Often
N—Never
S—Sometimes
A—Always

Historical Differentiation Between Regurgitation and Vomiting

	Regurgitation	Vomiting
Bile		
Digested food		
Active abdominal retch		
Hypersalivation		
Gagging		
Odynophagia		

EXERCISE 7.7 FILL IN THE CHART: REFLEX RESPONSES

Instructions: A neurologic examination of the limbs involves assessment of postural reactions, reflexes, and sensation. Fill in the chart below with the description of each of the grades of reflex responses.

Grading of Reflex Responses

Grade	Description
0	
1	
2	
3	
4	

Instructions: A cranial nerve examination is an essential part of every complete neurologic examination. Fill in the chart below with the missing answers.

Test Response

Nerve	Test	Normal	Abnormal
I. Olfactory	Volatile substance	Blink	No response
II. Optic	Menace Pupillary light reflex	Direct, consensual responses present	
III. Oculomotor	Pupillary light reflex Observe eye following an object	Direct, consensual responses present Normal eye movement	
IV. Trochlear	Observe		Muscle atrophy
	Palpate temporalis		No blink
	Corneal reflex		No blink
	Palpebral reflex		
V. Trigeminal	Observe ability to chew	Normal jaw movement	
	Palpate masseter muscle	Normal muscle tone	
	Pupillary light reflex		No direct or consensual response present
VI. Abducens	Observe	Normal eye position	
VII. Facial	Observe		
	Corneal reflex	Eye blink	
	Palpebral reflex		No blink
	Menace	Eye blink	
VIII. Acoustic	Hand clap	Startle response	
	Move head horizontally, vertically	Normal nystagmus	
IX. Glossopharyngeal	Gag reflex	Swallow	No response
X. Vagus	Gag reflex	Swallow	
	Oculocardiac reflex	Bradycardia	
	Laryngeal reflex	Cough	
XI. Accessory	Palpate neck muscles	Normal muscle tone	
XII. Hypoglossal	Tongue stretch		No response

EXERCISE 7.9 CASE STUDY: HISTORY AND PHYSICAL EXAMINATION FINDINGS

A 16-year-old, spayed female Burmese cat named Coco presents with vomiting of 4 days' duration. Coco's vaccinations are current and she is strictly an indoor cat. This is Coco's first visit to your hospital. The doctor has asked you to take a history, perform an initial physical examination, and give her the results so that a decision can be made regarding next steps. You ask all the standard questions required at your clinic, including each of the following.

1. Briefly explain why each question is important.

   a. Are there any other cats in the house?

   _____

   _____

   b. Can you describe the vomitus?

   _____

   _____

   c. When does she vomit?

   _____

   _____

   d. What, when, and how often do you feed her?

   _____

   _____

   e. When was the last time she was normal?

   _____

   _____

   f. Do you keep the windows open at home?

   _____

   _____

   g. Has there been a change in her appetite or water consumption?

   _____

   _____

   h. What toys does she play with?

   _____

   _____

63

Coco is quiet and depressed but purrs as you begin your physical examination. The pertinent physical findings are as follows:

- Body temperature of 97.5° F
- Heart rate of 260 beats per minute
- Poor pulse quality
- Pale, dry mucous membranes
- Normal respiratory effort
- No abnormal lung sounds noted
- Prolonged capillary refill time
- Body condition score of 4/9
- Prolonged response to the "skin pinch" test
- Cool extremities
- Severe halitosis
- Poor dentition
- Vomit stains under chin and sternum
- Oral ulcerations along gingiva

2. Which of these physical findings suggest poor perfusion? Why?

_____

_____

_____

3. Which physical findings suggest dehydration?

_____

_____

_____

4. Is this an emergency case that needs immediate attention? Why or why not?

_____

_____

_____

5. Coco is tachycardic with a heart rate of 260 beats per minute. What physical findings could be linked to the tachycardia?

_____

_____

_____

6. The owner inquires about her halitosis and tells you that it was noticed several months ago. What other physical examination findings listed previously are possibly linked to the bad breath?

_____

_____

_____

8 Preventive Health Programs

When you have completed this chapter, you will be able to:

1. Pronounce, define, and spell all of the key terms in this chapter.
2. Compare and contrast the issues and information discussed during wellness visits at various life stages of a dog or cat (puppy/kitten, adult, senior/geriatric) and discuss the importance of grooming.
3. Do the following regarding immunity in cats and dogs:
   - Differentiate between active and passive immunity, and discuss why it is necessary to administer a series of vaccinations to young puppies and kittens.
   - Differentiate between noninfectious and infectious types of vaccines, and explain the purpose of adjuvants.
   - Describe the storage, handling, reconstitution, and dosing of animal vaccines.
   - List the recommended administration locations for various canine and feline vaccinations.
   - Distinguish between core and noncore vaccines, and explain what is meant by duration of immunity.
   - Identify core and noncore vaccines that are used for dogs and cats.
   - Describe potential adverse vaccine events and how to deal with various adverse events should they occur.
4. Explain the importance of discussing potential canine and feline parasitic infections with owners, and describe general preventive measures that can be taken.
5. Describe a routine preventive health program for horses, including physical examination, vaccinations, prevention of parasitic infections, dental and hoof care, and nutrition.
6. Describe vaccines and other preventive measures that can be used during various life stages of pigs, cattle, sheep, and goats.

EXERCISE 8.1 TERMS AND DEFINITIONS: PREVENTATIVE HEALTH PROGRAMS

Instructions: Define each term in your own words.

1. Active immunity

   _____

   _____

2. Biosecurity

   _____

   _____

3. Anaphylaxis

   _____

   _____

4. Toxoid

   _____

   _____

5. Adjuvant

   _____

   _____

6. Passive immunity

   _____

   _____

7. Congenital

   _____

   _____

8. Fomite

   _____

   _____

9. Colostrum

   _____

   _____

10. Antitoxin

    _____

    _____

EXERCISE 8.2 MATCHING: ABBREVIATIONS RELATED TO PREVENTIVE HEALTH PROGRAMS FOR DOGS AND CATS

Instructions: Match each term in column A with its corresponding definition in column B by writing the appropriate letter in the space provided.

Column A

1. _____ T$_4$
2. _____ FVRCP
3. _____ FeLV
4. _____ FHV-1
5. _____ FCV
6. _____ FPV
7. _____ FIV
8. _____ CDV
9. _____ CAV-2
10. _____ CPV-2
11. _____ DA$_2$PP

Column B

A. Highly contagious virus in dogs that produces vomiting, diarrhea, leukopenia, and fever.

B. Combination vaccine for cats, including herpesvirus, calicivirus, and panleukopenia.

C. Lentivirus that causes immunosuppression in cats.

D. Retrovirus that causes immunosuppression, anemia, and lymphoma in cats.

E. Upper respiratory disease in cats that causes oral ulcerations.

F. Combination vaccine for dogs, including distemper, parvovirus, adenovirus type 2, and parainfluenza.

G. Serum hormone that may be high in senior cats and low in senior dogs.

H. Herpesvirus that causes sneezing, ocular, and nasal discharge and fever.

I. Paramyxovirus that causes fever, respiratory disease, vomiting, diarrhea, anorexia, dehydration, seizures, ataxia, and paresis in dogs.

J. Parvovirus in cats that causes leukopenia, fever, lethargy, anorexia, dehydration, vomiting, and diarrhea.

K. One of the causes of canine infectious tracheobronchitis that gives cross-immunity for infectious canine hepatitis.

EXERCISE 8.3 FILL-IN-THE-BLANK: COMPREHENSIVE

Instructions: Fill in each of the spaces provided with the missing word or words that complete the sentence.

1. Preventive health programs are especially important in situations where animals are housed _____.

2. Puppies and kittens are vaccinated every 3 to 4 weeks until they are 16 weeks old to stimulate an _____ immune response once _____ immunity declines.

3. Vaccines should be injected within _____ _____ of reconstitution.

4. Vaccines recommended for all animals to protect against highly contagious pathogens are called _____ vaccines.

5. _____ vaccines are recommended for animals at high risk to develop disease.

6. _____ of _____ is the length of time an animal is considered to be immune from developing disease after exposure to a pathogen.

7. Kittens that are infected with feline panleukopenia can develop _____ _____ in utero or shortly after birth.

8. The trivalent vaccine for equine encephalomyelitis protects against _____, _____, and _____ viruses.

9. Heavy parasite loads in horses lead to decreased _____ and _____ performance plus weight loss and colic.

10. Fecal examinations in horses that show ova after deworming indicate that _____ has developed to the agent, and egg counts of _____ eggs per gram before deworming indicate that treatment intervals are too long.

11. To minimize the risk that disease will spread, _____ pigs should be worked with before _____ pigs.

12. Swine operations do not routinely deworm because pigs are not housed _____.

13. A virus that causes reproductive failure, respiratory disease, and chronic infections in pigs is called porcine _____ and _____ syndrome virus.

14. Beef calves are weaned at about _____ months of age by removing the calf from the dam, whereas dairy calves are raised away from their dams, so weaning is a _____ adjustment and not as stressful.

15. Cattle vaccinated against brucellosis are identified with a(n) _____ ear tag and tattoo in the _____ ear.

16. Cattle vaccines are administered in the _____ region to preserve _____ quality.

17. Deficiency of _____ causes white muscle disease in lambs.

18. To dehorn goats at a young age, the horn bud is destroyed by a _____ _____ instrument.

EXERCISE 8.4 TRUE OR FALSE: COMPREHENSIVE

Instructions: Read the following statements and write "T" for true or "F" for false in the blanks provided. If a statement is false, correct the statement to make it true.

1. _____ Neutering eliminates intermale aggression, separation anxiety, enlargement of the prostate, and testicular cancer.

2. _____ Serum thyroxine levels are frequently measured in senior pets to rule out hyperthyroidism in dogs and hypothyroidism in cats.

3. _____ Dogs that regularly swim are prone to excessive nail growth and will need more frequent nail trims.

4. _____ Active immunity can only be stimulated by an antigen injected in the form of a vaccine.

5. _____ Foals that fail to ingest colostrum at birth are vaccinated with core vaccines within 24 hours of birth.

6. _____ Immune competence is when an animal is capable of mounting an active immune response in the face of declining maternal antibody levels.

7. _____ Noninfectious vaccines are more likely to cause hypersensitivity reactions than infectious vaccines.

8. _____ Administering an intranasal vaccine subcutaneously or intramuscularly may cause serious side effects.

9. _____ Sites for canine vaccination are not standardized, but the rabies vaccination is frequently administered in the left hind leg and the DA$_2$PP in the left front leg, in keeping with feline recommendations.

10. _____ Cats will test positive on the antibody-based FeLV screening test after vaccination.

11. _____ Minor side effects to vaccines include lethargy, soreness at injection site, and decreased appetite.

12. _____ Conditions that may be adverse reactions to vaccination include immune-mediated thrombocytopenia, immune-mediated hemolytic anemia, and thyroiditis.

13. _____ *Clostridium tetani* causes muscular weakness, and horses should be vaccinated for it annually.

14. _____ Wolf teeth are removed under general anesthesia at 6 months of age in the horse to avoid problems with the bit when the training regime begins.

15. _____ Thrush occurs on the sole of the horse foot as a result of a moist environment and dirt accumulation allowing bacterial growth.

16. _____ Preventive medicine is important in livestock species to maintain herd productivity.

17. _____ Kids and lambs born to unvaccinated does and ewes are vaccinated at 6 and 10 weeks of age.

18. _____ The barber pole worm causes anemia in sheep by attaching to their abomasums, and this parasitism is a major issue in small ruminants.

19. _____ Horses are wormed for bots and tapeworms in the spring with either moxidectin or ivermectin, with praziquantel.

20. _____ Core vaccination in cattle protects them from leptospirosis, campylobacteriosis, rotavirus, and coronavirus.

EXERCISE 8.5 MULTIPLE CHOICE: COMPREHENSIVE

Instructions: Circle the one correct answer for each of the following questions.

1. Spaying before the second heat cycle in cats and dogs decreases
   a. Aggression
   b. Vaccine-induced sarcoma
   c. Lymphoma
   d. Mammary carcinoma

2. Older dogs may require more frequent nail trims because of decreased exercise associated with
   a. Kidney disease
   b. Cognitive dysfunction
   c. Degenerative joint disease
   d. Hyperthyroidism

3. Passive immunity in puppies and kittens primarily occurs
   a. When antibodies pass to the offspring in utero via the placenta
   b. By vaccination within 24 hours of birth
   c. By ingestion of colostrum within 24 hours of birth
   d. With intravenous infusion of antibody-rich plasma at birth

4. To maximize the chance of successful treatment in the event that a vaccine-induced sarcoma develops, it is now recommended that feline vaccines be administered
   a. Distal to the shoulder or hip
   b. Proximal to the shoulder or hip
   c. In the intrascapular region
   d. Intranasally

5. Core vaccines for the cat are
   a. Feline leukemia, panleukopenia, calicivirus, and rabies
   b. Feline leukemia, feline immunodeficiency virus, panleukopenia, and rabies
   c. Feline viral rhinotracheitis, calicivirus, panleukopenia, and rabies
   d. Feline viral rhinotracheitis, *Chlamydophila felis*, panleukopenia, and rabies

6. Core vaccines in the dog protect against
   a. Parvovirus, adenovirus-2, leptospirosis, and rabies
   b. Distemper, parvovirus, *Bordetella*, and rabies
   c. Distemper, parvovirus, leptospirosis, and rabies
   d. Parvovirus, distemper, adenovirus-2, and rabies

7. Many of the core feline combination and canine combination vaccines are administered every
   a. Year
   b. 2 years
   c. 3 years
   d. 5 years

8. Cats should test negative before vaccination against
   a. Feline immunodeficiency virus
   b. Feline panleukopenia
   c. *Chlamydophila felis*
   d. Calicivirus

9. Which noncore feline vaccination is recommended for multicat households with a past history of bacterial upper respiratory infections?
   a. Feline leukemia
   b. Feline immunodeficiency virus
   c. *Chlamydophila felis*
   d. *Giardia*

10. A disease process in dogs that manifests as a dry, honking cough and that is transmitted dog to dog through respiratory secretions is caused by
    a. Canine distemper virus
    b. Canine coronavirus
    c. *Bordetella bronchiseptica*
    d. Canine parvovirus

11. Veterinary assistance should be sought if, following vaccination, the animal exhibits
    a. Mild fever and decreased appetite
    b. Soreness at the injection site
    c. Sneezing after an intranasal vaccine
    d. Facial swelling and difficulty breathing

12. For most core vaccines, the recommended length of time between initial and booster vaccines during the initial vaccine series in dogs, cats, livestock, and horses is generally
    a. 2 weeks
    b. 4 weeks
    c. 6 weeks
    d. 8 weeks

13. Foals born to unvaccinated mares are routinely vaccinated at which age?
    a. 1 to 2 months
    b. 3 to 4 months
    c. 5 to 6 months
    d. 7 to 8 months

14. Head tossing, excessive chewing of the bit, and bucking in the horse can be signs of
    a. Tick infestation
    b. Internal parasitism
    c. Nutritional deficiency
    d. Dental issues

15. Young horses and horses with dental issues should have dental exams
    a. Every 6 months
    b. Once a year
    c. Every 2 years
    d. Every 3 years

16. Upper cheek teeth in the horse can be removed by driving the tooth root into the oral cavity from the
    a. Frontal sinus
    b. Nasal sinus
    c. Maxillary sinus
    d. Orbit

17. To maintain proper balance and avoid problems with lameness in the horse, hooves should be trimmed
    a. Every 2 to 4 weeks
    b. Every 4 to 6 weeks
    c. Every 6 to 8 weeks
    d. Every 8 to 10 weeks

18. Thrush is treated by frequent cleaning of the sole of the foot and application of
    a. Copper- or iodine-based solutions
    b. Moxidectin or ivermectin
    c. Praziquantel
    d. Fenbendazole or oxibendazole

19. Anemia is prevented in piglets with supplementation of
    a. Selenium
    b. Magnesium
    c. Iron
    d. Calcium

20. Piglet tails are docked to prevent
    a. Chewing by other piglets
    b. Fecal contamination
    c. Maggot infestation
    d. Increased price of meat

21. Before entering the breeding herd, pigs are vaccinated for
    a. Parvovirus, erysipelas, and leptospirosis
    b. Parvovirus, brucellosis, and pseudorabies
    c. Leptospirosis, pseudorabies, and brucellosis
    d. Brucellosis, pseudorabies, and erysipelas

22. To prevent disease transmission, newly acquired pigs are not introduced to the rest of the herd for
    a. 10 days
    b. 14 days
    c. 21 days
    d. 30 days

23. Passive immunity blocks active immune response in calves that are vaccinated when younger than
    a. 3 months of age
    b. 4 months of age
    c. 5 months of age
    d. 6 months of age

24. Bovine leukosis virus in cattle causes
    a. Cancer
    b. Reproductive failure
    c. Respiratory disease
    d. Corkscrew hooves

25. Dairy cows are vaccinated against mastitis caused by
    a. *Clostridium perfringens*
    b. *Escherichia coli*
    c. *Streptococcus equi*
    d. *Campylobacter fetus*

26. Dairy cows should have their hooves trimmed
    a. Every 3 months
    b. Every 6 months
    c. At least once a year
    d. Every 2 years

27. During the first few weeks of life, either tail docking or castration in sheep can be performed by
    a. Using a hot metal instrument to burn tissue off
    b. Applying a tight elastic band around the tail or to the scrotum
    c. Surgical removal
    d. Using an emasculatome

28. Diarrhea in sheep and goats is caused by single-celled parasites called
    a. *Leptospira pomona*
    b. *Clostridium perfringens* type C and D
    c. *Haemonchus contortus*
    d. *Coccidia*

29. Sheep and goats can be rapidly screened for anemia by checking the
    a. Conjunctiva
    b. Red blood cell count
    c. Mouth
    d. Capillary refill time

30. Core vaccination in sheep and goats protects against
    a. *Rabies*
    b. *Haemonchus contortus*
    c. *Clostridium perfringens* and *Clostridium tetani*
    d. *Contagious ecthyma*

EXERCISE 8.6 WORD SEARCH: PREVENTIVE HEALTH PROGRAMS FOR HORSES AND LIVESTOCK

Instructions: Find the words that are identified by the clues given below. The words may be located horizontally, vertically, or diagonally, and may be reversed.

```
S R S C O T P I R A I X O N I L I A L S N
A T E I P E B R U C E L L O S I S I C I U
A Z R V L O Z L C I M R E A R R L O E T Q
L M N A E I E R R G T C I S E R K O L I N
M E S E N F H S A A Y E S R R X R O S L S
N S K R U G E J O H N E S D I S E A S E A
I S I S I L L S O R U S R T B U N J I Y O
S O E L A N F E R R P R S P R T S B O M T
U R A N U S B N S O N F T D H T A T D O E
R E C A E T E O I M H T Z R I R P I T L Z
I M R S I S O I R E T C A B O L Y P M A C
V O V I I I I B B H N X A D N C Y E E H L
E U E O U E S S E A R I U M R M M E R P O
L T F U V T T I S R R E U H O R I S Y E S
I H S U H U U S U U S L A Q O T N D S C T
N E L S I S O R I P S O T P E L O A I N R
T N S T T U Y A O R M V B V S H T P P E I
S I T I V I T C N U J N O C O T A R E K D
E Q U I N E H E R P E S V I R U S S L E I
W E I R X V L A U S R P I I A E I A A N U
R O L R A R P S U P R R L G A I S A S R M
```

Strangles	Campylobacteriosis	EquineHerpesVirus
PotomacHorseFever	Brucellosis	Pseudorabies
JohnesDisease	Leptospirosis	EquineInfluenza
PurpuraHemorrhagica	Clostridium	Botulism
Rabies	WestNileVirus	Anthrax
Encephalomyelitis	Erysipelas	Keratoconjunctivitis
SoreMouth		

72

EXERCISE 8.7 CASE STUDY: FELINE PREVENTIVE HEALTH

Lily, a calico, female, domestic shorthair cat of unknown age presents for a checkup and vaccinations. According to the client, Ms. Rose, she found Lily wandering the neighborhood and decided to bring her into her home. As the veterinary technician, you take Ms. Rose and Lily back to an examination room and obtain the following information about Lily.

Weight and Vital Signs: Weight: 4 lbs; Heart Rate: 180 bpm; Respiratory Rate: 32 bpm; Temperature: 101.8° F.

Recent History: Lily has been in the neighborhood for about 4 weeks, since the neighbor on the corner moved away. Ms. Rose believes the neighbor who moved left Lily behind. Ms. Rose has been feeding Lily for the last 2 weeks, and she appears to eat well but not gain weight. She has no information as to urinations or bowel movements, as Lily is outside. She has decided to bring her inside with her two indoor cats, Petunia and Violet. She is concerned about Lily's introduction into the home and wants to make sure her other cats are not exposed to any diseases. She is also concerned that Lily may not acclimate to being an indoor-only cat, since she has lived outdoors for a while.

Physical Examination Findings: Lily's adult canine teeth are erupted, indicating she is 6 months old. Lily is thin, and black specks are noticed in her hair coat. The rest of her physical examination findings are unremarkable. A spay scar cannot be palpated on the ventral midline. It is expected that she may not be spayed.

Instructions: Answer the following questions based on the case with regard to the best preventive health program for Lily and Ms. Rose, considering the home and the environmental situation.

1. Because Lily has been an outdoor cat with no known vaccination history, what are the first diagnostic tests Lily should receive based on current recommendations?

   _____

   _____

   _____

2a. How could you explain the black specks in Lily's hair coat? What external parasite might they indicate?

   _____

   _____

   _____

2b. What is a commonly recommended treatment protocol that could be used for Lily to treat this parasite, including both eggs and adults?

   _____

   _____

   _____

   _____

   _____

2c. How could Petunia and Violet be protected from this problem?

   _____

   _____

   _____

   _____

   _____

   _____

3a. Assuming the diagnostics in #1 are negative, discuss the core vaccinations Lily should receive, including the site of injection for each.

_____

_____

_____

_____

_____

_____

3b. How often should each vaccine be boostered, assuming Lily will be living exclusively indoors?

_____

_____

_____

_____

_____

_____

4a. Describe potential adverse effects to the vaccines that you will have Ms. Rose monitor for.

_____

_____

_____

4b. Which of the adverse effects listed previously warrants immediate notification of the veterinary practice if it occurs?

_____

_____

_____

5. If Lily exhibits any of the more serious side effects, what steps might the veterinarian take to minimize the likelihood of these effects in the future?

_____

_____

_____

_____

_____

_____

6a. If Lily develops a lump at the site of a vaccine injection, what are some possible reasons for this?

_____

_____

_____

_____

_____

_____

6b. Explain this to Ms. Rose using language she can understand.

_____

_____

_____

_____

_____

_____

_____

_____

6c. What might be done by the attending veterinarian to differentiate these causes?

_____

_____

_____

7. Discuss a surgical procedure that would keep Lily from having an unwanted pregnancy and describe the other health benefits this procedure provides.

_____

_____

_____

_____

_____

_____

_____

8a. If after surgery Lily will not stay indoors, discuss the noncore vaccines she should receive, including the recommended injection site for each.

_____

_____

_____

_____

_____

_____

8b. How often should each vaccine be boostered?

_____

_____

_____

8c. How might this change in Lily's activity affect the vaccines given to Violet and Petunia?

_____

_____

_____

_____

_____

_____

9 Companion Animal Nutrition

LEARNING OBJECTIVES

When you have completed this chapter, you will be able to:

1. Pronounce, define, and spell all the key terms in this chapter.
2. List the macronutrients and micronutrients found in pet food. Explain what building-block molecules compose these nutrients, if any.
3. Compare and contrast the concepts of energy units, energy partitioning, metabolizable energy measurement, Atwater factors, energy density, and measurements of energy expenditure.
4. Discuss the requirements for protein, fat, carbohydrates, fiber, vitamins, and minerals in the diet of dogs and cats.
5. Explain various aspects regarding commercial pet food, including the following:
   - Describe which marketing language bears little nutritional significance, and explain how veterinary therapeutic diets may be used appropriately and inappropriately.
   - Explain how pet food manufacturing is regulated in the United States and identify the government agencies and organizations involved in the regulation of pet food.
   - List the components of pet food labels, and explain how the information provided in each component should be interpreted.
6. Compare and contrast the reasons why clients might feed home-cooked diets to their pets.
7. Describe feeding protocols for healthy dogs and cats at each stage of life, including pregnant and lactating females.
8. Do the following related to clinical nutrition:
   - Explain the principles of clinical nutrition.
   - Describe methods of providing therapeutic enteral and parenteral nutrition.
   - Describe a safe and effective weight-loss program for dogs and cats.

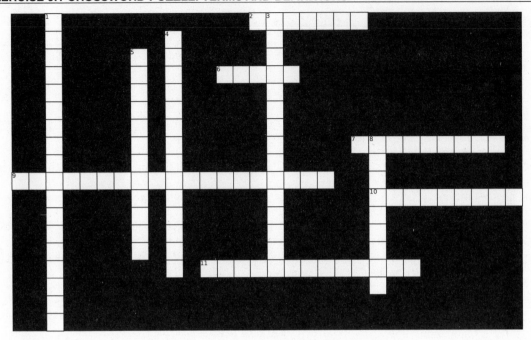

Across

2 Unit of Energy.
6 Any fat or oil or related compound that is insoluble in water but soluble in nonpolar solvents.
7 The building blocks of fat. (2 words)
9 Energy available to the animal after energy from feces, urine, and combustible gases has been subtracted from gross energy. Used to express the energy content of foods and commercial diets.
10 Substances that provide nourishment for growth and maintenance of life.
11 The number of calories provided in foods.

Down

1 Evaluated periodically to assess weight gain or loss. (3 words)
3 The name of a type of nutritional support that should be started withing 3 days of the onset of anorexia in stable, ill patients. (2 words)
4 Assigned energy values of the macronutrients. (2 words)
5 Description of the taste, texture, aroma, and other characteristics of pet food.
8 The building blocks of proteins. (2 words)

EXERCISE 9.2 MATCHING #1: KEY TERMS

Instructions: Match each key term in column A with its corresponding definition in column B by writing the appropriate letter in the space provided.

Column A

1. _____ Calorie
2. _____ Nutrient
3. _____ Energy density
4. _____ Amino acids
5. _____ Metabolizable (maintenance) energy requirement
6. _____ Palatability
7. _____ Atwater factors
8. _____ Assisted feeding
9. _____ Resting energy requirement
10. _____ Fatty acid
11. _____ Metabolizable energy
12. _____ Body condition score
13. _____ Lipid
14. _____ Kilojoule

Column B

A. Something essential that a plant or animal obtains from the environment for growth and maintenance of life.

B. The small molecules that are the building blocks of proteins.

C. Molecules that provide and store energy, make up cell membrane structure, and act as signaling agents and hormones.

D. A component of triglycerides that may be synthesized by the body or required in the diet of an animal.

E. A measure of energy defined as the energy needed to move a 1 kilogram weight 1 meter by 1 Newton.

F. The energy needed to increase the temperature of 1 gram (g) of water from 14.5° C to 15.5° C.

G. Result of subtracting the energy lost in urine and gases produced by the body from the digestible energy (DE) of a food or diet.

H. The estimated energy (caloric) content assigned to the three macronutrients.

I. The kcal per unit of a food ingredient or pet food.

J. A widely used estimate of energy expenditure by a normal animal at rest.

K. An estimated daily energy requirement for a healthy animal with daily activity and exercise.

L. A method used regularly to assess the weight gain or weight loss of an animal.

M. Refers to the tasty and acceptable properties of a dog food.

N. Providing nutritional support to a sick, injured, or hospitalized pet.

EXERCISE 9.3 MATCHING #2: ENERGY PARTITIONING

Instructions: Match each abbreviation in column A with its corresponding description in column B by writing the appropriate letter in the space provided.

Column A

1. _____ kcal
2. _____ kJ
3. _____ ME
4. _____ RER
5. _____ MER
6. _____ DE
7. _____ GE
8. _____ NE
9. _____ EE
10. _____ BCS

Column B

A. Used to estimate how much to feed an overweight dog or cat or a hospitalized patient.

B. Energy burned for normal body functions and increased energy demands, such as exercise.

C. The energy from a diet available after digestion and absorption of nutrients.

D. Equal to kcal/0.239.

E. The total potential energy available in a food or diet provided to an animal.

F. The standard measurement for energy that is also referred to as "calories" to an animal owner.

G. The energy available to an animal after some energy from the diet is lost in the feces.

H. Energy (kcal) available from pet foods for the animal to use for normal body functions, such as digestion.

I. Used to estimate how much to feed a healthy, active dog or cat. This measurement may be altered by level of activity or reproductive status of the animal.

J. An assessment to assist in monitoring adequacies of daily food intake.

EXERCISE 9.4 MATCHING #3: PET FOOD LABELS

Instructions: A client presents a bag of food to you with the following information. Help the client understand this information by matching each piece of information with the section of the food label that it is listed in from column B by writing the appropriate letter in the space provided.

Column A

1. _____ Purina Dog Chow
2. _____ Crude protein 42% (minimum)
3. _____ Chicken, brewers rice, corn gluten meal
4. _____ Adult maintenance
5. _____ Feed 1–1½ cups per 5–10 lb dog
6. _____ 3 lbs (1.36 kg)
7. _____ Best before Jun 30 2013

Column B

A. Net weight

B. Guaranteed analysis

C. Feeding directions

D. Ingredient statement

E. Information panel and freshness date

F. Principal display panel

G. Statement of nutritional adequacy

Instructions: Read the following statements and write "T" for true or "F" for false in the blanks provided. If a statement is false, correct the statement to make it true.

1. _____ Nutrients are most commonly listed in kilogram (kg) units on a pet food label.

2. _____ Many animals will consume more water than is necessary for daily functions, with the excess being excreted in the feces.

3. _____ Animals and humans are composed of approximately 30% water by weight.

4. _____ Proteins are made from amino acids and stored in the muscle.

5. _____ Essential fatty acids, including linoleic acid, are required in the diets of dogs and cats.

6. _____ Carbohydrates are broken down into glycogen and stored in the pancreas as glucose.

7. _____ Cats and guinea pigs require vitamin C in their diets.

8. _____ Vitamin requirements in the diet vary between different species of animals.

9. _____ The expressions "as-fed," "dry matter," and "metabolizable energy" refer to measurements of a nutrient in a diet and are interchangeable with each other.

10. _____ "AAFCO-approved" pet foods contain high-quality ingredients and are formulated for feeding during all life stages.

11. _____ Raw meat diets are balanced and appropriate to feed animals during any life stage.

12. _____ Neonatal puppies should never be tube fed as there is a great risk for aspiration.

13. _____ At weaning age, puppies can be offered a gruel-type diet that consists of canned food blended with water.

14. _____ Spayed or neutered animals often have higher energy needs than intact animals.

15. _____ Cats, in general, have higher protein requirements than dogs.

16. _____ Adult, intact cats tend to lose their appetite inhibition and easily gain weight.

17. _____ High "ash" diets have been proven to cause lower urinary tract disease in cats.

18. _____ A sick, hospitalized patient should not be fed in order to allow the GI tract to "rest."

19. _____ TPN, total parenteral nutrition, is administered through a central intravenous catheter because of the high osmolality of the solution.

20. _____ Force feeding or syringe feeding a sick animal is the best method for providing enteral nutrition.

EXERCISE 9.6 MULTIPLE CHOICE: COMPREHENSIVE

Instructions: Circle the one correct answer to each of the following questions.

1. All of the following components are legally required on a pet food label except
   a. Ingredient statement
   b. Net weight
   c. Freshness date
   d. Feeding directions

2. The nutrients that supply energy to an animal include
   a. Vitamins, carbohydrates, and fats
   b. Fats, protein, and minerals
   c. Protein, carbohydrates, and fats
   d. Carbohydrates, vitamins, and minerals

3. Each of the following is a major function of proteins except
   a. Providing structure to organs and tissues
   b. Acting as enzymes for certain reactions
   c. Regulating water balance
   d. Carrying oxygen to tissues

4. Fatty acids
   a. Are short, saturated molecules
   b. Are building blocks of triglycerides
   c. Are all nonessential and do not need to be supplied in the diet
   d. Are only utilized by fat cells

5. Carbohydrates in the diet
   a. Are broken down into glucose in the intestinal tract
   b. Are stored in liver and muscle as glycogen
   c. Do not provide energy to the animal
   d. A and B

6. Which of the following items is optional in a guaranteed analysis on a pet food label?
   a. Crude protein
   b. Moisture
   c. Calcium
   d. Crude fiber

7. Fiber is often a component of dog or cat foods and
   a. Is an essential nutrient
   b. Comes from protein found in animal tissues
   c. Is broken down by the body into glucose
   d. Resists digestion in the gastrointestinal tract

8. An adult dog weighing 25 kg should be offered _____ (amount) of protein per day in the diet.
   a. 30 g
   b. 40 g
   c. 50 g
   d. 60 g

9. Anemia is caused by a deficiency of
   a. Fat
   b. Carbohydrate
   c. Protein
   d. Calcium

10. Dogs and cats have minimum dietary requirements for all of the following nutrients except
    a. Protein
    b. Fat
    c. Carbohydrate
    d. Vitamins and minerals

11. The essential nutrients required in the diet of cats include all of the following except
    a. Taurine
    b. Arachidonic acid
    c. Vitamin C
    d. Calcium

12. Raw meat diet recipes
    a. Contain adequate levels of calcium and phosphorus to support growth
    b. Are safe for people to handle and for animals to eat
    c. Rarely cause GI upset, as the ingredients do not contain preservatives
    d. May include bones, which can obstruct or perforate the GI tract

13. Consider this scenario: An outbreak of *Salmonella* has been traced to a facility that manufactures several brands of dog food. These contaminated products will be recalled through a mandate by the
    a. AAFCO
    b. USDA
    c. FDA-CVM
    d. FTC

14. AAFCO, an important organization in the pet food industry,
    a. Is a government agency that ensures the safety of all pet food ingredients and products
    b. Publishes the *Nutrient Requirements of Dogs and Cats* with guidelines for formulating dog and cat foods
    c. Establishes protocols for animal feeding tests with various pet food products
    d. Performs feeding tests on dogs and cats using a variety of products in a laboratory setting

15. A diet deficient in protein will result in
    a. Dull, dry hair coat
    b. Reduced fecal production
    c. Weight gain
    d. Increased activity level

16. When caring for a neonatal puppy or kitten, one should
    a. Measure the body weight weekly to assess adequate nutritional intake
    b. Microwave the milk replacer to 120° F before feeding
    c. Use a commercial milk replacer instead of cow's milk when needed
    d. Watch for voluntary urination and defecation following feeding

17. During the growth phase, puppies will require
    a. The same amount of energy on a dry-matter basis as an adult dog
    b. Higher levels of calcium and phosphorus than an adult dog
    c. Higher levels of EPA and DHA than an adult dog
    d. Lower levels of protein than an adult dog

18. The owner of a 5-month-old, intact male Labrador wants to know how much to feed his dog per day. The most appropriate recommendation is
    a. Feed the dog *ad libitum* until he reaches 12 months of age.
    b. Calculate the RER for this dog, and feed that amount per day.
    c. Use the feeding instructions on the dog food bag, and monitor BCS frequently.
    d. Feed the dog 4 cups of food.

19. "Fluffy," a sedentary, 5-year-old, spayed female mixed-breed dog weighs 25 kg. Her calculated RER (kcal/day) would be
    a. 534
    b. 662
    c. 783
    d. 897

20. "Chance," a 3-kg, active, 7-month-old, male, domestic shorthair feline, would require approximately how much energy supplied by the diet (kcal/day)?
    a. 160 to 320 kcal/day
    b. 320 to 480 kcal/day
    c. 480 to 640 kcal/day
    d. 640 to 800 kcal/day

21. Predisposing factors for obesity in pets include all of the following except
    a. High fat content in the diet
    b. Overfeeding
    c. High fiber content in the diet
    d. Sedentary lifestyle

22. Kittens during the growth stage need to be routinely monitored for all of the following except
    a. Excessive weight gain
    b. Developmental orthopedic disease
    c. Water intake
    d. Overeating

23. Fiber in a feline diet
    a. Is an essential nutrient required by the species
    b. Is useful for thin animals to improve weight gain
    c. Can improve GI function and prevent hairballs
    d. Reduces fecal quantity

24. Adult cats
    a. Require taurine as an essential amino acid
    b. Should be fed free-choice
    c. Are often sedentary and do not need more than RER
    d. All of the above
    e. A and C

25. Short-term enteral nutrition (for 3 weeks or less) can best be provided by placing a
    a. Central IV catheter into the jugular vein
    b. G-tube percutaneously into the stomach
    c. N-E tube through the nasal passage into the distal esophagus
    d. J-tube surgically into the intestine

26. Parenteral nutrition is administered
    a. In a peripheral vein because the osmolality of these formulations is high
    b. To patients that may be vomiting and at risk for aspiration
    c. To provide nutritional support for any hospitalized patient
    d. Via a nasoesophageal or esophagostomy tube

27. When administering TPN, the patient requires 24-hour monitoring by all members of the veterinary team. Complications that need immediate attention include all of the following except
    a. Alterations in laboratory values such as glucose or potassium
    b. Redness at the IV catheter site
    c. Serum or plasma that is a clear, straw color
    d. A blockage in the TPN administration line

28. To measure the body condition score of an animal, you will
    a. Put the animal on a scale and record its weight in kilograms
    b. Measure the circumference of the animal's chest, just behind the elbow
    c. Use calipers to measure the thickness of a skin fold
    d. Feel along the rib cage and check for a waist and abdominal tuck

29. An ideal body condition score (BCS) is 5/9. If an animal has a BCS of 7/9, approximately which percentage of body weight should this animal lose to reach ideal condition?
    a. 10% to 15%
    b. 20% to 30%
    c. 30% to 45%
    d. Greater than 45%

30. An appropriate weight loss plan for a canine should
    a. Include vigorous exercise and induce weight loss of 5% per week
    b. Include a 20% reduction in the amount of the current diet being fed
    c. Transition the animal to an all-purpose diet once ideal weight is achieved
    d. Occur with the use of an energy-restricted diet with weight loss at 1% to 2% per week

EXERCISE 9.7 FILL-IN-THE-BLANK: COMPREHENSIVE

Instructions: Fill in each of the spaces with the missing word or words that complete the sentence.

1. Macronutrients consist of _____, _____, and _____ and are used by the body to produce _____.

2. _____ is an important nutrient that contributes to 50% to 70% of an animal's body weight. Deficiencies of this nutrient lead to a state of _____ in the body.

3. Proteins are composed of amino acids but may also be bound to other molecules such as _____ and _____ .

4. Proteins can be _____ from amino acids, but not _____, and therefore must be consumed in the diet.

5. Essential fatty acids are required in the diets of animals that cannot synthesize them. _____ _____ and _____ _____ are fatty acids essential to both dogs and cats.

6. Carbohydrates in the diet can be broken down into _____, which is used for _____ and is stored in the form of _____ .

7. _____ are organic molecules used for certain metabolic processes in the body and are considered micronutrients. These nutrients are required in the diets of dogs and cats in different amounts.

8. Minerals are _____ molecules supplied in the diet that may result in disease if the levels are _____ or _____ .

9. Soluble fiber is an example of a complex carbohydrate that may be present in an animal diet. The term *soluble* means that the carbohydrate can be _____ by bacteria in the _____ intestine.

10. _____ is/are a category of dietary supplements that may delay or prevent oxidative processes in the body and have potential health benefits.

11. Feline diets have a higher _____ density than canine diets.

12. A home-cooked diet may be beneficial to an animal with a food _____ or _____, as the ingredients can be limited.

13. Raw meat diets predispose growing animals to _____ disorders.

14. A nutrient that has a lower digestibility will need to be fed in _____ amounts.

15. The nutrient requirements of dogs and cats are based on _____ and _____ publications (*names of two organizations*).

EXERCISE 9.8 CASE STUDY #1: WEIGHT LOSS

"Suzie," a 5-year-old, spayed, female mixed-breed dog, presents to your clinic, as the owners are concerned about her excessive weight gain over a 4-month period. After obtaining a good history, it is learned that there is a toddler in the family and the recent addition of a new baby. The feeding of Suzie has become inconsistent, as the new baby is quite a distraction, and exercise is limited to short walks around the neighborhood. Suzie spends much of her time indoors, following the toddler around and cleaning up the messes from dropped food. On physical examination, Suzie weighs 65 lbs with a BCS of 8/9. All other examination findings were unremarkable. CBC, chemistry, and thyroid hormone levels were also unremarkable.

1. Discuss a logical approach to beginning a weight-loss program for Suzie.

_____

_____

_____

_____

_____

_____

2. What factors from Suzie's history may be affecting and/or increasing her energy intake?

_____

_____

_____

3. Because it is difficult to measure Suzie's actual energy intake, you will use her RER at her current body weight to start her weight-loss program. Estimate her RER in the space that follows.

_____

4. By what percentage can her intake be reduced safely? How many kcal/day should she then receive on her new weight-loss plan?

_____ kcal/day

5. Should her normal maintenance diet be used in her weight-loss plan? Why or why not?

_____

_____

_____

_____

_____

_____

6. How many pounds per week would be appropriate for Suzie to lose?

_____ pounds/week

7. If an ideal weight for Suzie is 45 lbs, how many weeks can her owner expect it to take for the weight loss to occur?

_____ weeks

EXERCISE 9.9 CASE STUDY #2: HOSPITALIZED PATIENT

"Stubby," an 8-year-old, neutered, male, domestic shorthair cat, presents to your clinic with a 3-day history of anorexia and acute vomiting. Physical examination revealed a string foreign body under his tongue, a painful abdomen, approximately 7% dehydration, and a current body weight of 5 kg. Abdominal radiography supports the presence of an intestinal foreign body. Stubby is stabilized with intravenous fluids and taken to surgery for removal of the foreign body. The plan is to provide some nutritional support to Stubby, as he has been anorexic for more than 72 hours.

1. What routes could be used to provide nutrition to this patient?

_____

_____

_____

2. Discuss the factors that should be considered to determine the appropriate route for this patient.

_____

_____

_____

It was decided at the time of surgery to place a 5-French jejunostomy tube (J-tube). The plan is to begin providing nutritional support using an infusion pump and administering EnteralCare MLP slowly at 33% RER on day 1, 66% RER on day 2, and 100% RER on day 3. This diet has an energy density of 1.20 kcal/mL.

3. Calculate the RER for Stubby at his current body weight of 5 kg (11 lbs).

_____ kcal/day

4. Calculate the infusion pump setting to administer EnteralCare MLP on day 1, day 2, and day 3.
   Day 1: _____ mL/hour
   Day 2: _____ mL/hour
   Day 3: _____ mL/hour

5. What are some potential complications of having this J-tube placed?

   _____

   _____

   _____

6. What parameters need to be monitored closely while Stubby is receiving enteral nutrition?

   _____

   _____

   _____

7. What is an important complication that can occur when reintroducing food to an anorexic or starved animal? What findings are seen with this condition?

   _____

   _____

   _____

8. Stubby is bright and alert 3 days after surgery and is looking for food in his cage. Is he ready to have the tube removed and be sent home?

   _____

   _____

   _____

10 Large Animal Nutrition

LEARNING OBJECTIVES

When you have completed this chapter, you will be able to:
1. Pronounce, define, and spell all the key terms in this chapter.
2. Do the following regarding nutrients:
   - Explain the relationship between nutrition, productivity, and profitability in livestock production.
   - List the building block molecules that make up proteins, fats, and carbohydrates.
   - List two ways in which carbohydrates are digested in horses.
   - List the energy-producing and non–energy-producing components of food.
   - List the variables affecting energy requirements of livestock.
   - Differentiate between microminerals and macrominerals, and give examples of each.
   - Explain the importance of water in metabolic reactions.
3. Describe the two commonly used feeding systems for dairy cattle.
4. Compare and contrast the special considerations and protocols employed when feeding dairy cattle, beef cattle, sheep, and swine. Also do the following:
   - State the importance of water and list the factors affecting water intake of livestock.
   - Describe how the nutritional requirements of each of these species are affected by the animal's stage of life and by its energy expenditure (maintenance, growth, finishing, lactation, work, or wool production).
   - List advantages and disadvantages of pasture feeding of livestock.
5. Do the following regarding nutrition in horses:
   - Explain the importance of grass and hays in the equine diet.
   - Describe how pregnancy and lactation alter a mare's nutritional requirements.
   - List steps taken to provide appropriate nutrition to foals and young, growing horses.
   - Describe how-work levels are classified in working horses and how these levels affect water, energy, and mineral requirements.
   - Describe general guidelines for feeding sick and postoperative horses.

EXERCISE 10.1 MATCHING #1: TERMS AND DEFINITIONS

Instructions: Match each term in column A with its corresponding definition in column B by writing the appropriate letter in the space provided.

Column A

1. _____ Amino acids
2. _____ Biologic value
3. _____ Concentrates
4. _____ Digestible energy
5. _____ Digestion
6. _____ Forage
7. _____ Gross energy
8. _____ Maintenance nutrient requirements (MNRs)
9. _____ Metabolizable energy (ME)
10. _____ Net energy (NE)
11. _____ Protein efficiency ratio
12. _____ Total digestible nutrients (TDNs)

Column B

A. Subtraction of the energy lost in the feces from the consumed GE.

B. The number of grams of body weight gain per unit of protein consumed.

C. Percentage of true absorbed protein that is available for productive body functions.

D. A general measure of the nutritive value of a feed.

E. The building blocks of proteins.

F. The actual portion of energy available to the animal for use in maintaining body tissues or during pregnancy or lactation.

G. The process of protein, carbohydrate, and fat breakdown into absorbable nutrients.

H. The total energy potentially available in a feed consumed by an animal.

I. Grains or high-starch compounds.

J. The levels of nutrients needed to sustain body weight without gain or loss.

K. Grass, legumes, and hays.

L. Energy available to the animal after energy from feces, urine, and combustible gases has been subtracted from gross energy.

EXERCISE 10.2 MATCHING #2: BREEDS OF SHEEP

Instructions: Indicate whether each breed in column A is a wool breed, meat breed, or combination breed by writing the appropriate letter in the space provided. Note that each response can be used more than once.

Column A

1. _____ Cheviot
2. _____ Columbia
3. _____ Debouillet
4. _____ Dorset
5. _____ Hampshire
6. _____ Leicester
7. _____ Merino
8. _____ Oxford
9. _____ Polypay
10. _____ Rambouillet
11. _____ Southdown
12. _____ Shropshire
13. _____ Suffolk
14. _____ Targhee
15. _____ Texel
16. _____ Tunis

Column B

A. Wool

B. Meat

C. Combination

Instructions: Match each equine body condition score in column A with its corresponding description in column B by writing the appropriate letter in the space provided.

Column A

1. _____ Poor
2. _____ Very thin
3. _____ Thin
4. _____ Moderately thin
5. _____ Moderate
6. _____ Moderately fleshy
7. _____ Fleshy
8. _____ Fat
9. _____ Extremely fat

Column B

A. Fat built about halfway on spinous processes; transverse processes cannot be felt. Slight fat cover over the ribs. Spinous processes and ribs easily discernible. Tailhead prominent, but individual vertebrae cannot be visually identified. Tuber coxae appear rounded, but easily discernible. Tuber ischii not distinguishable. Withers, shoulders, and neck accentuated.

B. May have crease down back. Individual ribs can be felt, but noticeable filling between ribs with fat. Fat around tailhead is soft. Fat deposited along withers, behind shoulders, and along neck.

C. Animal extremely emaciated. Spinous processes, ribs, tailhead, tuber coxae, and ischii projecting prominently. Bone structure of withers, shoulders, and neck easily noticeable. No fatty tissue can be felt.

D. Obvious crease down back. Patchy fat appearing over ribs. Bulging fat around tailhead, around withers, behind shoulders, and along neck. Fat along inner thighs may rub together. Flank filled with fat.

E. Negative crease along back. Faint outline of ribs discernible. Tailhead prominence depends on conformation; fat can be felt around it. Tuber coxae not discernible. Withers, shoulders, and neck not obviously thin.

F. Back level. Ribs cannot be visually distinguished but can easily be felt. Fat around tailhead beginning to feel spongy. Withers appear rounded over spinous processes. Shoulders and neck blend smoothly into body.

G. Animal emaciated. Slight fat covering over base of spinous processes; transverse processes of lumbar vertebrae feel rounded. Spinous processes, ribs, tailhead, tuber coxae, and ischii prominent. Withers, shoulders, and neck structures faintly discernible.

H. Crease down back. Difficult to feel ribs. Fat around tailhead very soft. Area behind shoulder filled with fat. Noticeable thickening of neck. Fat deposited along inner thighs.

I. May have crease down back. Fat over ribs feels spongy. Fat around tailhead feels soft. Fat beginning to be deposited along side of the withers, behind the shoulders, and along the sides of the neck.

EXERCISE 10.4 TRUE OR FALSE: COMPREHENSIVE

Instructions: Read the following statements and write "T" for true or "F" for false in the blanks provided. If a statement is false, correct the statement to make it true.

1. _____ Most livestock producers will need the help of a veterinary technician to formulate proper diets for their herds.

2. _____ It is not the alfalfa hay, corn, or oats that are used by cells, but the amino acids, simple sugars, fatty acids, minerals, and vitamins.

3. _____ Combining different types of proteins has no effect on the biologic value.

4. _____ The measurement called "total digestible nutrients" is a useful measurement of energy available to the animal for use in maintaining body tissues.

5. _____ Ruminants have the ability to break down fiber content to be used as energy, and this allows them to utilize feed that other animals cannot use.

6. _____ Lactating dairy cattle cannot consume enough forage to meet their nutritional requirements and thus are supplemented with concentrated feeds.

7. _____ It is important to restrict protein during lactation so that the milk produced is not too protein concentrated.

8. _____ The calf benefits the most from colostrum within the first 24 hours of life.

9. _____ Colostrum should not be frozen, as this causes it to lose all efficacy.

10. _____ Beef cows need little to no feed supplementation from grain if they are fed high-quality forage or pasture.

11. _____ Finishing cattle are fed high-fiber diets to increase weight gain and improve the carcass characteristics.

12. _____ Young cattle require a higher percentage of protein than older cattle.

13. _____ Cow's milk works well as milk replacement for lambs.

14. _____ Lambs older than 2 months can be vaccinated for enterotoxemia.

15. _____ A sow must have 5 to 7 litters per year for the swine producer to realize a profit.

16. _____ A lactating sow should be fed 4 to 5 lb of the base ration plus 1 additional pound for every pig she is nursing.

17. _____ When feeding swine, the producer should be more concerned about the amino acid levels of the feed than about the protein content.

18. _____ Horses should not have access to salt, as an overdose can lead to toxicity.

19. _____ Protein should be restricted in lactating mares or the foal will grow too quickly.

20. _____ Growing horses should not be fed above energy requirements, as this increases the risk of developmental orthopedic disease.

21. _____ Exercising horses require additional protein for muscle development and repair.

EXERCISE 10.5 MULTIPLE CHOICE: COMPREHENSIVE

Instructions: Circle the one correct answer to each of the following questions.

1. Protein is made up of _____ that are linked in a chain.
   a. Fatty acids
   b. Minerals
   c. Amino acids
   d. Simple sugars

2. Amino acids consist of
   a. Nitrogen, carbon, oxygen, and sulfur
   b. Nitrogen, hydrogen, oxygen, and sulfur
   c. Helium, carbon, oxygen, and sulfur
   d. Nitrogen, carbon, oxygen, and selenium

3. Fat has _____ times more energy per gram than protein or carbohydrates.
   a. 0.225
   b. 2.55
   c. 22.5
   d. 2.25

4. What is the primary energy source used in livestock rations?
   a. Proteins
   b. Fat
   c. Carbohydrates
   d. Minerals

5. What two measures of feed energy value are used most widely in equine nutrition?
   a. DE and TDN
   b. DE and ME
   c. GE and TDN
   d. TDN and ME

6. What measure of feed energy value is used most widely in beef, dairy, and sheep nutrition?
   a. NE
   b. CE
   c. DE
   d. ME

7. What measure of feed energy value is used in swine and poultry nutrition?
   a. NE
   b. CE
   c. DE
   d. ME

8. What nutrient is the cheapest and most abundant?
   a. Carbohydrate
   b. Water
   c. Protein
   d. Vitamins and minerals

9. Water makes up what percent of an animal's body at maturity?
   a. 35% to 50%
   b. 45% to 60%
   c. 65% to 70%
   d. 65% to 85%

10. What factor most determines the productivity of lactating dairy cattle?
    a. Water intake
    b. Vitamins and minerals
    c. Feeding
    d. Environment

11. Carbohydrates constitute which percentage of energy on a dry-matter basis for forage and grain?
    a. 20% to 50%
    b. 30% to 60%
    c. 40% to 70%
    d. 50% to 80%

12. Newborn calves require colostrum in the first _____ hours after they are born.
    a. 72
    b. 48
    c. 36
    d. 24

13. Feeding represents almost _____ of the cost of beef production.
    a. 75%
    b. 50%
    c. 25%
    d. 10%

14. A finished steer will be _____ year(s) old and weigh more than _____ pounds.
    a. 6 months to 1; 500
    b. 6 months to 1; 1000
    c. 1 to 2; 500
    d. 1 to 2; 1000

15. Sheep are more susceptible to toxicity from this mineral than other species.
    a. Zinc
    b. Copper
    c. Iron
    d. Magnesium

16. Milk replacement for lambs should contain _____ fat.
    a. 5% to 10%
    b. 15% to 20%
    c. 25% to 30%
    d. 40% to 55%

17. What percentage of the cost of raising swine is the cost of feed?
    a. 60% to 70%
    b. 50% to 60%
    c. 40% to 50%
    d. 30% to 40%

18. Forage should be at least _____% of a horse's diet.
    a. 40
    b. 50
    c. 60
    d. 70

19. Which nutrient is the most important in a horse's diet?
    a. Roughage
    b. Carbohydrates
    c. Protein
    d. Water

20. The body score of a mare at breeding should be
    a. 3 to 4
    b. 4 to 5
    c. 5 to 6
    d. 6 to 7

EXERCISE 10.6 CASE STUDY #1: IRON-DEFICIENCY ANEMIA IN PIGS

Your client's daughter is thinking about farrowing pigs as a part of an FFA project. Your client has heard that baby pigs need extra iron. She asks why this is the case and then asks you to explain some things she can do to prevent iron-deficiency anemia in baby pigs.

1. Please respond to this client's query.

_____

_____

_____

_____

_____

_____

_____

_____

EXERCISE 10.7 CASE STUDY #2: COLIC IN A HORSE

Mrs. Ratcliff's favorite gelding, Red, was admitted to the clinic as an emergency several days previously for colic. Red had surgery and has been recovering well. Mrs. Ratcliff came to see Red today and was very upset about the tube sticking out of Red's nose. She wanted to know why the hay and grain she had sent up with her farm manager was *not* being used for Red. "He will only eat the best!" she declares.

1. The barn attendant brings her to you for an explanation. What do you tell her?

_____

_____

_____

_____

_____

_____

_____

_____

_____

_____

_____

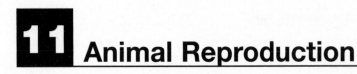

11 Animal Reproduction

LEARNING OBJECTIVES

When you have completed this chapter, you will be able to:
1. Pronounce, define, and spell all of the key terms in this chapter.
2. Do the following regarding reproduction:
   - Locate the anatomic parts of the reproductive system, including endocrine organs in the cranium.
   - Describe hormonal changes that occur during the estrous cycle and pregnancy.
   - Compare and contrast the processes of oogenesis and spermatogenesis.
   - Explain the process of fertilization and embryo development, including the anatomic locations of these events.
3. Compare and contrast canine, feline, and equine estrous cycles, gestation, and parturition. Also do the following:
   - Describe the collection process and interpretation of canine vaginal cells, and state the importance of vaginal cytologic examination in breeding dogs.
4. Compare and contrast the bovine, ovicaprine, and camelid estrous cycles, gestation, and parturition.
5. Identify and put in order the important aspects of a breeding soundness examination in a male and female.

EXERCISE 11.1 CROSSWORD PUZZLE: TERMS AND DEFINITIONS

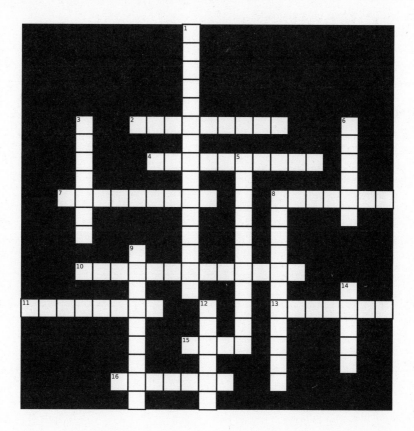

Across

2 The term used to describe parturition in the camelid species.
4 The estrous cycle of the mare is divided into the _____ phase and the luteal phase.
7 The tail of the spermatid is referred to as a _____.
8 The term used to describe the life stage at which a given species is capable of reproduction.
10 When semen is frozen in liquid nitrogen for preservation, it is said to be _____.
11 The term for the delivery of fetuses in the canine species.
13 The word used to describe a system that utilizes actual physical contact of the stallion and the mare to help determine the presence of physiologic estrus in the mares that do not exhibit signs of heat.
15 The term for the male of the canine species.
16 This word, when used as an adjective, relates to the "kind" of cycle.

Down

1 The name of the thick tunic that covers the ovary in the mare. (2 words)
3 The term for the oviductal entry into the uterus.
6 The placentation type of the bitch indicating a narrow band of attachment of the chorioallantoic membrane to the endometrium.
5 The term used for male species if one or both testes have not descended into the scrotum.
8 The equine species is a seasonally _____ animal, thereby influenced greatly by increasing amounts of light in the spring of the year.
9 The breeding _____ examination is performed on all male species before they are used for breeding.
14 The term for the female of the canine species.
12 The noun that describes the period of time the female is in "heat" or sexually receptive.

Chapter **11** Animal Reproduction

EXERCISE 11.2 TERMS AND DEFINITIONS

Instructions: Define each term in your own words.

1. Ovulation: _____

    _____

2. Ampulla (in the female): _____

    _____

3. Fertilization: _____

    _____

4. Isthmus: _____

    _____

5. Puberty (in the female): _____

    _____

6. Anestrus: _____

    _____

7. Mare: _____

    _____

8. Stallion: _____

    _____

9. Foaling: _____

    _____

10. Gelding: _____

    _____

11. Ovariectomized mare: _____

    _____

12. Foal heat: _____

    _____

13. Queening: _____

14. Ewe: _____

_____

15. Wether: _____

_____

16. Ewe lambs: _____

_____

17. Ram lambs: _____

_____

18. Doe: _____

_____

19. Buck: _____

_____

20. Kids: _____

_____

21. Heifer: _____

_____

22. Cow: _____

_____

23. Bull: _____

_____

24. Steer: _____

_____

25. Calf: _____

_____

26. Cria: _____

_____

Instructions: Match each definition in column A with its corresponding term in column B by writing the appropriate letter in the space provided.

Column A

1. _____ The study of reproduction in animals.

2. _____ Cells that cover the ovum upon being released from the follicle.

3. _____ Multiple fathers of a given litter.

4. _____ When a pregnant dam ovulates and conceives again while pregnant.

5. _____ The type of placenta found in the human and rodent.

6. _____ Physical and biochemical cell membrane changes of the sperm, allowing for fertilization.

7. _____ The type of placenta present in the horse, swine, ruminant, dog, and cat.

8. _____ The term for uterine lining where the placenta attaches.

9. _____ The term for a bitch if the uterus and gonads have been removed.

10. _____ The hormone that influences early development of the follicle and estrogen production in the canine species.

11. _____ A rapid rise in LH at the start of estrus.

12. _____ The process that occurs during proestrus in the canine species, characterized by enlargement and neovascularization of the endometrium resulting in the leakage of blood through the vessel walls.

13. _____ Bitches in physiologic estrus may never show signs of _____ heat.

14. _____ To cause regress.

15. _____ The term for a young mare that usually implies she is younger than 3 years of age.

16. _____ The term used for a newborn equine species.

17. _____ When relating to the equine species, the onset of estrus is initiated by

production and release of _____.

Column B

A. Capacitation

B. LH surge

C. Filly

D. Cumulus

E. Standing

F. Spayed

G. Superfecundation

H. GnRH

I. Theriogenology

J. Hemochorial

K. Diapedesis

L. Endometrium

M. Superfetation

N. Foal

O. FSH

P. Lyse

Q. Epitheliochorial

EXERCISE 11.4 MATCHING #2: TERMS AND DEFINITIONS

Instructions: Match each definition in column A with its corresponding term in column B by writing the appropriate letter in the space provided.

Column A

1. _____ The presence of a CL under the influence of progesterone in the equine species will occur during this phase of the estrous cycle.

2. _____ The gland that is effected by the use of artificial lighting to induce early estrus in the mare.

3. _____ A thick covering on the ovary preventing ovulation anywhere except at the ovulation fossa.

4. _____ The substance produced within a mare after the fetal membrane embeds itself in the endometrium.

5. _____ The substance commonly used to induce parturition.

6. _____ The membrane expected to rupture during stage II of parturition in the equine.

7. _____ Used for correcting abnormalities of the vulva.

8. _____ The term used for the female of the feline species.

9. _____ Increases during estrus and decreases after ovulation in the feline.

10. _____ The type of placentation noted in the feline.

11. _____ The term used for the delivery of fetuses in the sheep.

12. _____ The process of feeding a higher level of nutrition to a ewe with a low-body condition score prior to breeding to increase the number of oocytes.

13. _____ The term used for the birthing process in the goat.

14. _____ The term used for the birthing process in the bovine.

15. _____ The device that utilizes a dye packet to detect mounting when breeding cows.

16. _____ The female component of the embryo that originates from the follicle of the ovary.

17. _____ The structure similar in appearance to a mushroom that protrudes from the endometrium in pregnant cows.

18. _____ The first secretion of a cow's udder, which is important for calves to consume by means of nursing.

19. _____ An example of a polyestrous species.

20. _____ The device typically used to count sperm for determining concentration levels.

Column B

A. Zonary

B. Camelids

C. Chorioallantoic

D. Heat detector patches

E. Pineal

F. Caruncle

G. Equine chorionic gonadotropin

H. Flushing

I. Hemocytometer

J. Queen

K. Kidding

L. Lambing

M. Diestrus

N. Estrogen

O. Calving

P. Colostrum

Q. Tunica albuginea

R. Caslick's surgery

S. Oxytocin

T. Oocyte

EXERCISE 11.5 ORDERING: BREEDING SOUNDNESS EXAMINATION IN THE MALE

Instructions: Place the eight parts of the breeding soundness examination in the proper order (from first to last) by placing the appropriate letter in the space provided.

Column A

1. _____
2. _____
3. _____
4. _____
5. _____
6. _____
7. _____
8. _____

Column B

A. Examination of sperm motility.

B. A detailed examination of the external and internal genitalia.

C. Other tests as necessary.

D. Identification of the patient (ideally through a microchip, tattoo, or brand).

E. Examination of sperm morphology.

F. A thorough history focusing on the reproductive system.

G. Determination of a sperm count.

H. Semen collection.

EXERCISE 11.6 TRUE OR FALSE: COMPREHENSIVE

Instructions: Read the following statements and write "T" for true or "F" for false in the blanks provided. If a statement is false, correct the statement to make it true.

1. _____ Although the follicle matures as ovulation approaches, the ovum within only matures following ovulation.

2. _____ When an oocyte is released from an ovarian follicle, it is covered with cumulus cells.

3. _____ Regression of the corpus luteum is accompanied by a rapid drop in progesterone.

4. _____ Superfetation is a normal occurrence.

5. _____ When animals are bred naturally, semen deposited at the beginning of a heat will still be capable of fertilizing the oocyte after ovulation.

6. _____ The general body temperature is higher than that of the testes.

7. _____ The production of sperm is cyclical.

8. _____ Capacitation is a process by which an ovum is made ready for fertilization.

9. _____ The castrated male canine is referred to as a neutered male.

10. _____ The canine estrous cycle does not include the stage of anestrus.

11. _____ During canine estrus, the bitch may play with the male in the beginning of "courtship" to establish a friendly behavioral relationship.

12. _____ The ova in the bitch can be fertilized at the time of ovulation.

13. _____ Parturition in the bitch occurs during the diestrus period of the estrous cycle.

14. _____ Parturition takes place in the bitch within approximately 24 hours after the CL is no longer functional.

15. _____ Progesterone and luteinizing hormone levels can be used to predict when a bitch should be bred.

16. _____ Once thawed, frozen semen has a short life span.

17. _____ Frozen semen can be potentially stored for thousands of years in liquid nitrogen.

18. _____ When using fresh semen, canine insemination should be performed 2 to 3 times to ensure fertilization takes place.

19. _____ Vaginal cytology is used for predicting insemination time in the bitch after progesterone assay concentrations have reached greater than 10 ng/mL.

20. _____ Radiography is used to determine the number of pups in utero, their size, and their position.

21. _____ The drop in body temperature that occurs in the canine before stage II of whelping is related to a decrease in estrogen.

22. _____ During whelping it is normal to see a blackish-green vaginal discharge.

23. _____ A female feline that has had its gonads removed is referred to as ovariectomized or spayed.

24. _____ The queen is a seasonally polyestrous animal.

25. _____ The anatomy of the reproductive tract of the queen is similar to that of the bitch.

26. _____ The queen is an induced ovulator.

27. _____ The queen is one of many animals capable of assisting itself with dystocia.

28. _____ Increased vocalization during estrus in the queen is a normal occurrence.

29. _____ Vulvar discharge in the queen should occur during the estrus stage of the heat cycle.

30. _____ Prostaglandin $F_2\alpha$ has the ability to induce abortion in the queen and in the bitch.

31. _____ Transuterine migration of fertilized eggs occurs in all multiparous species.

32. _____ Ultrasonographic imaging starting at approximately day 15 postbreeding is an excellent resource for diagnosing pregnancy in the queen.

33. _____ Failure to deliver fetuses within 2 to 3 hours of parturition will result in poor survival rates in the queen.

34. _____ The uterine size will take weeks to reduce to a normal size after stage III parturition has occurred in the queen.

35. _____ Dystocia is a common occurrence in the queen.

36. _____ A newborn foal is not referred to as a yearling until after 12 months of age.

37. _____ It is common to call ovariectomized mares "spayed."

38. _____ When a filly reaches puberty, the reproductive tract is mature.

39. _____ Signs of estrus in the filly may appear before puberty is reached.

40. _____ Although twin ovulations occur about 18% of the time, the live birth of equine twins is rare.

41. _____ It is not uncommon for mares to show signs of heat without being in physiologic estrus.

42. _____ The length of heat in the mare may vary from fewer than 2 to 9 days.

43. _____ Mares will always exhibit signs of heat during physiologic estrus.

44. _____ Some mares will exhibit signs of estrus even when not in physiologic estrus.

45. _____ Twin ovulation is very rare in the equine.

46. _____ The equine ovum requires no additional time for maturation once released, allowing fertilization to occur immediately if the sperm are present.

47. _____ The CL is fully functional within approximately 5 days postovulation in the equine.

48. _____ At 30 days postovulation, progesterone concentration in the equine begins to decrease.

49. _____ Foals born on December 31st are considered 1 year old the next day.

50. _____ Artificial lighting is not of significance when it pertains to the estrus cycle in mares.

51. _____ Examination of the anatomical conformation of the vulva in the mare is a very important part of a reproductive tract evaluation.

52. _____ The use of surgical scrub to prepare for vaginal examination of the mare is highly recommended to reduce contamination during the procedure.

53. _____ The cervix and vaginal wall should be easily visible once the vaginal speculum has entered the vagina during examination of the mare.

54. _____ A "deep" intrauterine insemination technique is the usual method for performing artificial insemination in the mare.

55. _____ Equine chorionic gonadotropin is also known as pregnant mare serum gonadotropin.

56. _____ After the second trimester of equine pregnancy, the progesterone hormone will decrease and no longer be responsible for maintaining pregnancy in the mare.

57. _____ The most accurate method of diagnosing pregnancy in the equine is palpation of the reproductive tract via rectal examination.

58. _____ The age of puberty in bovines depends on breed and level of nutrition.

59. _____ The desired age at first calving in the bovine is 4 years.

60. _____ The cow is a seasonally polyestrous animal.

61. _____ A sign of estrus in the cow may include the presence of clear mucous vulvar discharge.

62. _____ The approximate estrous cycle length of a cow is 21 days.

63. _____ The cow has an average of 75 to 120 uterine caruncles, which are irreplaceable once damaged or destroyed.

64. _____ Pregnancy in the cow is primarily determined with the use of ultrasonographic examination.

65. _____ Sheep are seasonally polyestrous animals.

66. _____ The onset of puberty in sheep is solely influenced by body weight.

67. _____ The primary breeding season is September through December in the ovine species.

68. _____ The flushing of ewes with a body condition score above 2.5 is highly recommended.

69. _____ The ewe will only seek out the ram while in estrus.

70. _____ The semen deposited during breeding by the ram at the beginning of a ewe's heat cycle will still have the capability to fertilize oocytes during ovulation.

71. _____ A yearling ram is capable of servicing (breeding) up to 10 to 15 naturally cycling ewes under appropriate pasture conditions.

72. _____ The estrus cycle in sheep is 36 hours.

73. _____ Abortion rates for sheep are generally low.

74. _____ Pregnancy determination may be performed via ultrasonographic rectal examination in the ewe at 25 days into gestation.

75. _____ Infectious causes of abortion in sheep and goats include leptospirosis, toxoplasmosis, and *Chlamydophila abortus*.

76. _____ Mating that has occurred in the absence of a mature follicle in camelids will not result in ovulation.

77. _____ Camelid species are induced ovulators.

78. _____ Pregnancies in camelids occur predominately in the left horn.

79. _____ The size of the testes or the scrotum is important information to obtain during the breeding soundness examination of a male animal.

80. _____ The horse is the only domestic species in which the penis is cleansed prior to the collection of semen.

81. _____ The sperm of most species move rapidly forward in a straight line.

82. _____ The head of a sperm cell is characterized as rounded, not flat.

83. _____ During a breeding soundness examination, the motility of sperm is assessed before the morphologic examination is performed.

84. _____ Uterine cultures are more easily obtained on smaller animals.

85. _____ The uterine lumen is sterile in all species.

86. _____ The mare and cow are the only species in which endometrial biopsies may be obtained through the vaginal lumen.

87. _____ Cultures of the reproductive tract of the bitch should be obtained by the use of a conventional culture swab.

Instructions: Circle the one correct answer to each of the following questions.

1. Prior to placentation, which of the following comprise the maternal and fetal layers?
   a. Endothelium
   b. Mesoderm
   c. Epithelium
   d. All of the above

2. Antibody protection of the newborn at birth is solely dependent upon which of the following?
   a. A diffuse placenta
   b. The chorionic epithelium remaining in contact with the maternal component
   c. Maternal layers remaining intact
   d. Colostrum consumption after birth

3. Within the testis, developing sperm cells are surrounded by
   a. Sertoli cells
   b. A layer of mucous
   c. Interstitial cells
   d. Primordial germ cells

4. The hormone that acts on Sertoli cells to increase primordial sperm cell division and release more sperm cells is
   a. Testosterone
   b. FSH
   c. GnRH
   d. LH

5. After sperm cells are released, they attain motility and the ability to fertilize in the
   a. Seminiferous tubules
   b. Epididymis
   c. Tunica albuginea
   d. Female reproductive tract

6. The length of time required from the initiation of sperm development until formation of a mature sperm cell is approximately
   a. 25 days
   b. 30 days
   c. 55 days
   d. 60 days

7. The age at which puberty is reached in the bitch is approximately
   a. 4 to 6 months
   b. 7 to 12 months
   c. 6 to 24 months
   d. 24 to 42 months

8. Once mature, in the bitch, ova remain fertilizable for
   a. 12 hours
   b. 36 hours
   c. 24 hours
   d. 3 days

9. Which of the following choices represents the proper order of the canine estrous cycle?
   a. Proestrus, estrus, diestrus, anestrus
   b. Estrus, diestrus, proestrus, and anestrus
   c. Estrus, proestrus, anestrus, and diestrus
   d. Anestrus, estrus, proestrus and diestrus

10. The approximate length of the canine estrous cycle is
    a. 2 months
    b. 4 months
    c. 6 months
    d. 8 months

11. The proestrus and estrus stages of the bitch will each last approximately
    a. 3 days
    b. 5 days
    c. 7 days
    d. 9 days

12. In most canine breeds, anestrus will last approximately
    a. 2 months
    b. 4 months
    c. 6 months
    d. 8 months

13. The release of ova from the ovaries in the bitch will occur at approximately _____ days following the LH spike:
    a. 1
    b. 2
    c. 4
    d. 5

14. Once released and mature, the ova of the bitch will remain fertilizable for
    a. 3 days
    b. 6 days
    c. 9 days
    d. 12 days

15. During the natural breeding process of the canine species, the male and female will be "locked together" for up to _____ minutes.
    a. 15
    b. 30
    c. 45
    d. 50

16. The period of least reproductive activity in the bitch will occur during
    a. Estrus
    b. Proestrus
    c. Diestrus
    d. Anestrus

17. The BSE in males is designed to assess
    a. Semen quality
    b. Attitude
    c. Disposition
    d. All of the above

18. Because of its short life span, once frozen semen has thawed, fertilization should occur within
    a. 6 hours
    b. 8 hours
    c. 12 hours
    d. 15 hours

19. Examination for pregnancy in the bitch by palpation is possible in most bitches between _____ and _____ days of gestation.
    a. 12, 25
    b. 15, 38
    c. 21, 30
    d. 30, 36

20. In the bitch, the length of gestation from the point of fertilization is approximately
    a. 48 days
    b. 60 days
    c. 72 days
    d. 84 days

21. A drop in body temperature to 99° F in a near-term pregnant bitch signals that whelping is imminent. This change generally occurs about_____ hours before stage II.
    a. 8
    b. 12
    c. 24
    d. 48

22. Young female felines should have an estrus cycle by
    a. 6 months of age
    b. 12 months of age
    c. 18 months of age
    d. 24 months of age

23. The approximate weight at which the queen will reach puberty is
    a. 3 to 4 pounds
    b. 5 to 6 pounds
    c. 6.5 to 7 pounds
    d. 7.5 to 8 pounds

24. The average estrous cycle length in the queen is
    a. 2 to 15 days
    b. 4 to 30 days
    c. 10 to 25 days
    d. 14 to 19 days

25. The estrus stage in the queen will last approximately
    a. 5 days
    b. 10 days
    c. 15 days
    d. 30 days

26. Less than _____ of all queens will ovulate with a single mating.
    a. 15%
    b. 25%
    c. 35%
    d. 50%

27. The average duration of pregnancy in the queen following breeding is
    a. 55 days
    b. 63 days
    c. 75 days
    d. 82 days

28. What stage of parturition in the queen is characterized by lactational secretion, increased fetal movements, and relaxation around the perineal area?
    a. Stage I
    b. Stage II
    c. Stage III

29. What is the only commonly seen animal in a veterinary practice that can assist itself with a dystocia?
    a. Feline
    b. Canine
    c. Equine
    d. Porcine

30. The speed of movement of sperm is reflected in
    a. The size of the individual sperm cells
    b. The quantity of sperm cells
    c. The rotation of the sperm cells
    d. The age of the sperm sample

31. The approximate age range at which the estrous cycle is initiated in the filly is
    a. 6 to 12 months
    b. 12 to 24 months
    c. 24 to 48 months
    d. 48 to 60 months

32. The peak of estrous activity in the equine species occurs near which of the following dates?
    a. June 21st
    b. August 21st
    c. December 21st
    d. May 21st

33. The average length of heat in the mare is
    a. 5 days
    b. 6 days
    c. 7 days
    d. 9 days

34. The average length of the estrous cycle in the equine is
    a. 16 days
    b. 21 days
    c. 24 days
    d. 36 days

35. Which behavior is not related to estrus in the equine?
    a. Frequent urination
    b. Raised tail
    c. Frequent opening and closing of the vulva exposing the clitoris
    d. Increased tendency to kick

36. As their reproductive tract is not yet mature, fillies that are younger than 2 years old can have an abortion rate as high as
    a. 5%
    b. 25%
    c. 50%
    d. 85%

37. Sperm of the equine species usually have a high fertilizing life span of
    a. 12 hours
    b. 24 hours
    c. 48 hours
    d. 72 hours

38. Postovulation insemination performed in the equine species is highly successful when performed within
    a. 6 hours
    b. 8 hours
    c. 12 hours
    d. 16 hours

39. In the equine species, the approximate natural breeding season is
    a. January 1st to June 1st
    b. April 1st to September 1st
    c. July 1st to December 1st
    d. October 1st to March 1st

40. To ensure survival, once the chorioallantoic membrane ruptures during stage II parturition in the equine, the fetus must be outside of the birth canal

    within _____ minutes.
    a. 20
    b. 45
    c. 60
    d. 70

41. The desired age for first calving in the cow is approximately
    a. 2 years of age
    b. 3 years of age
    c. 4 years of age
    d. 7 years of age

42. Pregnancy must occur at which of the following ages in order for a first calving to occur at the desired time?
    a. 10 months
    b. 15 months
    c. 20 months
    d. 24 months

43. The estrous cycle length of the cow is approximately
    a. 18 days
    b. 21 days
    c. 24 days
    d. 32 days

44. Ovulation in the cow will occur about _____ hours after the end of standing heat.
    a. 4 to 6
    b. 6 to 8
    c. 8 to 12
    d. 12 to 16

45. The gestation length of the cow is approximately
    a. 256 to 259 days
    b. 265 to 269 days
    c. 279 to 283 days
    d. 341 to 345 days

46. The length of the estrous cycle in the ewe is approximately
    a. 10 days
    b. 13 days
    c. 17 days
    d. 19 days

47. The estrous cycle length in the goat is
    a. 21 days
    b. 28 days
    c. 32 days
    d. 34 days

48. The estrus stage of the goat estrous cycle lasts approximately
    a. 1 to 2 days
    b. 3 to 4 days
    c. 5 to 6 days
    d. 7 to 10 days

49. The female camelid will reach puberty at the approximate age of
    a. 6 to 10 months
    b. 10 to 12 months
    c. 12 to 18 months
    d. 18 to 24 months

50. The average length of estrus in a camelid is between
    a. 1 and 4 days
    b. 1 and 7 days
    c. 2 and 8 days
    d. 3 and 15 days

51. The approximate pregnancy length of the camelid is
    a. 290 to 310 days
    b. 310 to 330 days
    c. 340 to 350 days
    d. 350 to 370 days

52. In the camelid, ovulation and fertility will return postpartum at approximately
    a. 5 days
    b. 10 days
    c. 15 days
    d. 20 days

EXERCISE 11.8 FILL-IN-THE-BLANK: COMPREHENSIVE

Instructions: Fill in each of the spaces provided with the missing word or words that complete the sentence.

1. After ovulation, the empty follicular sac fills with clotted blood, forming a _____ _____.

2. The _____ contains half the genetic material of the future offspring and the _____ contains the other half.

3. Fertilization occurs near the junction of the _____ and the _____ of the oviduct.

4. The estrous cycle is determined by the functional interrelationship of the _____ gland, hypothalamus, _____ gland, gonads, and _____.

5. The _____ gland is particularly important to reproduction. Both this and the hypothalamus are part of the _____ system, which is part of the brain that regulates _____ and _____ functions.

6. During estrus, the uterine tone is turgid and feels tightly coiled when palpated due to increasing levels of _____.

7. The ectoderm or outer layer will develop into the hair, skin, and _____ system.

8. In the male, testosterone is produced by the _____ cells of the testis.

9. The testis is covered by a capsule known as the _____ _____.

10. The word _____ refers to an animal in which one or both testes are not in the scrotum.

11. Production of testosterone is initiated by the release of the _____-_____ hormone from the hypothalamus and the subsequent release of the _____ hormone from the anterior pituitary.

12. In the male, the changes in blood flow that initiate an erection are mediated by the _____ branch of the autonomic nervous system. In contrast, ejaculation is mediated by the _____ branch of the autonomic nervous system.

13. The female canine that has had the _____ removed is referred to as an ovariectomized bitch.

14. The canine estrous cycle consists of _____, _____, _____, and anestrus.

15. The beginning of proestrus in the bitch is indicated by the commencement of a _____ vulvar discharge.

16. During proestrus in the bitch, the endometrium becomes highly _____ and the vessels reach the surface and leak blood through the vessel walls.

17. One of the most commonly used clinical tests to determine the reproductive stage and health of the bitch is _____ _____.

18. Radiographic diagnosis in the feline is possible from day _____ to term but is most useful around _____ days.

19. Uterine involution following whelping or in the nonpregnant bitch is not complete until approximately 120 days following _____.

20. The queen is an induced ovulator, although spontaneous ovulation may occur if triggered by the proper _____ or _____ cues.

21. The foal may also be called a _____ following separation from its mother or reaching 2 to 3 months of age.

22. Ovulation can be induced in the equine when a nearly mature follicle is present by the administration of _____ or _____.

23. The findings on genital palpation of a mare in heat include a decrease in _____ tone, relaxation of the _____, and an increase in size of the follicles present.

24. Secondary CLs maintain the _____ in the mare until day 100 and then are no longer required.

25. Equine chorionic gonadotropin is produced by the _____ cups.

26. Foal heat occurs between 2 and 18 days following _____ and can be a fertile heat in many mares.

27. The cow has year-round estrous cycles with minimal seasonal influence and therefore is considered to be _____.

28. In the ruminant, ovulation occurs from anywhere on the surface of the _____.

29. The _____ reflex is a mechanism whereby the dilation of the cervical lumen stimulates a neural response that increases _____ release, which further dilates the cervix.

30. Cows may be in _____ or _____ recumbency at the time of delivery.

31. Rams that have been _____ are frequently used as part of an artificial breeding program.

32. The ewe's pregnancy is maintained by the production of progesterone from the _____ after the initial beginning of the CL production of progesterone.

33. Mating of camelids occurs in a _____ recumbent position.

34. The placenta of the camelid should be passed within 6 hours, and if retained, the patient should be treated with _____ .

35. Although spermatogenesis is completed in the testis, the spermatozoa must pass through the _____ for maturation to occur.

36. Scrotal circumference is primarily used to evaluate the size of the testes or the scrotum in _____ .

37. The _____ gland is the only accessory sex gland present in the dog.

38. Any vaginal examination or diagnostic technique in the mare should be preceded by a thorough cleansing of the _____ area.

39. The _____ is the portion of the uterus most involved with pregnancy maintenance.

EXERCISE 11.9 CASE STUDY: PARTURITION

Ms. Allen, a longtime client, calls your hospital asking for advice. She has several feral cats living under her porch. Although she has worked with a local humane organization to have all of the cats trapped, neutered, and released, a new female (who she named "Emily") showed up a few weeks ago.

Emily is tame enough that Ms. Allen was able to coax her into the garage and was even able to handle her a little bit. Emily seems very healthy but appears to be pregnant. Ms. Allen is calling today to make an appointment to bring her in for a checkup, pregnancy check, and any other care she might need, but would like some information concerning what to expect when the kittens are born (assuming Emily is pregnant, as Ms. Allen suspects).

1. Answer her question by describing the series of events that takes place during parturition in the queen, starting from stage I to birth of the kittens, as well as the likelihood of dystocia in the queen.

_____

_____

_____

_____

_____

_____

_____

_____

EXERCISE 11.10 WORD SEARCH: TERMS

Instructions: Find the words that are defined by the clues given below. The words may be located horizontally, vertically, or diagonally and may be reversed.

```
N G A I N I C H P T E P O T L
K E N I T P I R C O M O R B S
S E T I L N T R G E S S R H B
P V R T T L S O P R E T P T R
Z I U A O A A D M T T P P I R
E T M C A S L I C K S A R T I
G C C C E P B L A R E R I U O
U U S M E I O T I C T T L U T
A D T E O I H S R C S U A M N
R O T E P C P N I N S M O R O
D R T O O T O S E R T O L I P
E P T L A I R T E M O D N E I
D E Z I M O T C E I R A V O C
E R T I V I G M O C R R E N S
O T S C K H T C I O C L T A L
```

Colt
Reproductive
Caslicks
Kittens
Ovariectomized
Sertoli
Postpartum
Meiotic
Testes
Oscillating
Guarded
Endometrial

Chapter **11** **Animal Reproduction**

12 Hematology and Cytology

LEARNING OBJECTIVES

When you have completed this chapter, you will be able to:

1. Pronounce, define, and spell all the key terms in this chapter.
2. Describe proper collection techniques, handling of blood samples, and components of a complete blood count (CBC).
3. Describe advantages, disadvantages, and capabilities of automated hematology analyzers.
4. Do the following regarding blood counts:
   - Compare and contrast procedures used to determine red blood cell (RBC) mass (packed cell volume [PCV], hematocrit [HCT], hemoglobin, and red blood cell [RBC] count), and discuss the causes and significance of abnormal values.
   - Describe methods used to calculate RBC indices and red cell distribution width (RDW), and discuss the causes and significance of abnormal values.
   - Describe methods used to determine plasma protein concentration, and discuss the causes and significance of abnormal values.
   - Describe methods used to determine the white blood cell (WBC) count and the platelet count.
5. Do the following regarding blood smears:
   - Describe the technique used to prepare a stained blood smear, list factors that influence the quality of the smear, and discuss the process used to evaluate a blood smear.
   - Describe normal and abnormal morphology of RBCs, WBCs, and platelets in each species as they appear on a blood smear.
   - Discuss the causes and significance of RBC, WBC, and platelet abnormalities commonly observed on a blood smear.
   - Describe the procedure used to perform a differential WBC count, and calculate absolute values.
6. Do the following regarding coagulation testing:
   - Explain normal primary and secondary hemostasis, including intrinsic, extrinsic, and common pathways.
   - Discuss bleeding time, activated clotting time (ACT), activated partial thromboplastin time (APTT), and prothrombin time (PT) and the uses and significance of each.
   - Discuss tests used to evaluate fibrinolysis, including fibrin(ogen) degradation products (FDPs), D-dimer tests, and fibrinogen tests.
7. Do the following regarding cytology:
   - Explain uses for and limitations of cytology.
   - Describe procedures used to evaluate the cytology of solid tissue masses, enlarged organs, thoracic and abdominal effusions, and synovial fluid.
   - Discuss procedures used to submit cytology samples to a reference laboratory.
   - Describe collection and preparation of otic cytology samples, and identify common findings on normal and abnormal otic cytology preparations.

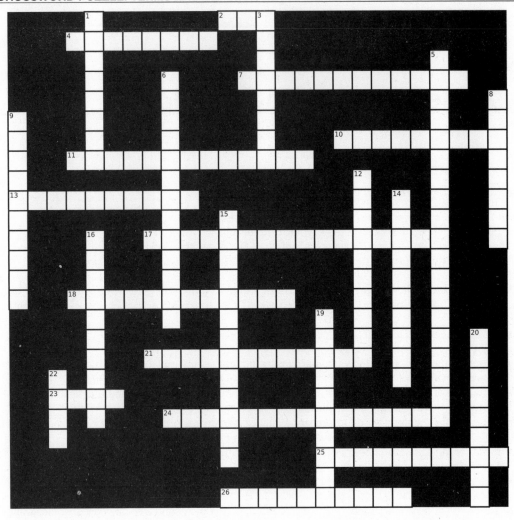

Across

2 A test that gives information about the numbers and types of circulating cells.
4 Stacking of red blood cells.
7 Vacuolization, Döhle bodies, and cytoplasmic basophilia in neutrophils. (2 words)
10 Nonnucleated fragments of cytoplasm released from megakaryocytes.
11 A nucleated red blood cell.
13 Falsely decreased in patients with red blood cell agglutination.
17 Percentage of RBCs in a specific volume of blood. (3 words)
18 Large in some poodles, very small in goats, and oval in camels. (3 words)
21 Variation in cell size.
23 A test that evaluates the intrinsic pathway of the coagulation cascade.
24 The term "leukopenia" means decreased numbers of these. (3 words)
25 The most abundant granulocyte in rabbits.
26 In most species, this is approximately equal to the PCV divided by 3.

Down

1 Becomes a macrophage in the tissues.
3 Used to evaluate exfoliated tissue cells.
5 MCV, MCHC, and MCH. (4 words)
6 This change in RBC distribution occurs in patients with immune-mediated hemolytic anemia (IHA).
8 Normally very few in circulation, but may be the most abundant leukocyte in some species of turtles.
9 The predominant circulating white blood cell in cattle, sheep, and goats.
12 Evaluated by the PT and ACT.
14 May contain Döhle bodies.
15 Counted to differentiate regenerative from nonregenerative anemia.
16 A red blood cell that has lost a portion of its membrane.
19 In cats, this cell contains numerous small, rod-shaped granules.
20 An increased number of circulating bands. (2 words)
22 An immature neutrophil.

EXERCISE 12.2 MATCHING #1: ABBREVIATIONS RELATED TO HEMATOLOGY AND COAGULATION

Instructions: Match each abbreviation related to hematology and coagulation in column A with its corresponding description in column B by writing the appropriate letter in the space provided.

Column A

1. _____ MCV
2. _____ MCHC
3. _____ FDP
4. _____ PT
5. _____ MCH
6. _____ RDW
7. _____ HCT
8. _____ APTT

Column B

A. An indicator of variation in red cell size.

B. The average amount of hemoglobin in each RBC.

C. The average amount of hemoglobin in a specific volume of blood.

D. Evaluates the extrinsic and common pathways of the coagulation cascade.

E. Evaluates the intrinsic and common pathways of the coagulation cascade.

F. A measure of fibrinolysis.

G. A measure of red blood cell mass.

H. The average size of the RBCs.

EXERCISE 12.3 MATCHING #2: NUCLEATED CELLS SEEN ON A BLOOD SMEAR EXAM

Instructions: Match each cell type in column A with its corresponding description in column B by writing the appropriate letter in the space provided.

Column A

1. _____ Neutrophils
2. _____ Band neutrophils
3. _____ Pelger-Huet anomaly
4. _____ Eosinophils
5. _____ Basophils
6. _____ Lymphocytes
7. _____ Reactive lymphocytes
8. _____ Neoplastic lymphocytes
9. _____ Monocytes
10. _____ Mast cells

Column B

A. Have more intensely basophilic cytoplasm and may have a perinuclear clear area.

B. The predominant circulating white blood cell in dogs, cats, and horses.

C. Have a twisted or irregular nucleus in dogs.

D. Contain numerous purple granules and a round nucleus.

E. Are also called "stabs."

F. Up to 50% may be intermediate to large size in cows.

G. These cells have prominent nucleoli.

H. A congenital or acquired defect most often seen in dogs.

I. Have abundant gray-blue cytoplasm, possibly with clear vacuoles.

J. Contain numerous, large, brightly staining granules in horses.

EXERCISE 12.4 MATCHING #3: HEMOSTASIS

Instructions: Match each term related to hemostasis in column A with its corresponding description in column B by writing the appropriate letter in the space provided.

Column A

1. _____ Activated clotting time (ACT)
2. _____ Blood smear
3. _____ Coagulation cascade
4. _____ D-Dimers
5. _____ Fibrin degradation products (FDP)
6. _____ Fibrinolysis
7. _____ Hemocytometer
8. _____ Plasmin
9. _____ Prothrombin time (PT)
10. _____ Refractometer

Column B

A. Activates secondary hemostasis.

B. Evaluates the extrinsic and common pathways.

C. Products of fibrin proteolysis that are considered to be reflective of active degradation of clots.

D. A device used in the measurement of plasma protein concentration.

E. This test requires use of a special tube that contains diatomaceous earth.

F. Evaluated by measuring FDPs.

G. Form when fibrin undergoes proteolysis by plasmin.

H. Used to evaluate platelet morphology.

I. Causes proteolysis of fibrin.

J. A device that can be used to manually count white blood cells.

EXERCISE 12.5 MATCHING #4: ABNORMAL BODY CAVITY FLUIDS AND ASSOCIATED CAUSES

Instructions: Normal thoracic and abdominal fluid is clear and colorless in small animals but may have a yellow tint in large animals. Disease states can cause a number of color changes that give clues as to the nature of the problem. Match each description of the appearance of abnormal body fluids in column A with the common associated causes in column B by writing the appropriate letter in the space provided.

Column A

1. _____ Red or pink
2. _____ White or tan
3. _____ Brown
4. _____ Green
5. _____ Yellow

Column B

A. Hemolysis and icterus, previous hemorrhage, or ruptured bladder.

B. Previous hemorrhage or leakage of bowel contents.

C. Ruptured bile duct.

D. Internal hemorrhage.

E. Lipid or high numbers of cells.

EXERCISE 12.6 PHOTO QUIZ: PHOTOGRAPHS OF RED BLOOD CELLS WITH SHAPE CHANGES

Instructions: Match each red blood cell circled with the letter corresponding to the morphologic change.

Names

A. Acanthocyte

B. Eccentrocyte

C. Echinocyte

D. Cell with a Heinz body

E. Keratocyte

F. Apple stem cell

G. Schistocytes

H. Spherocyte

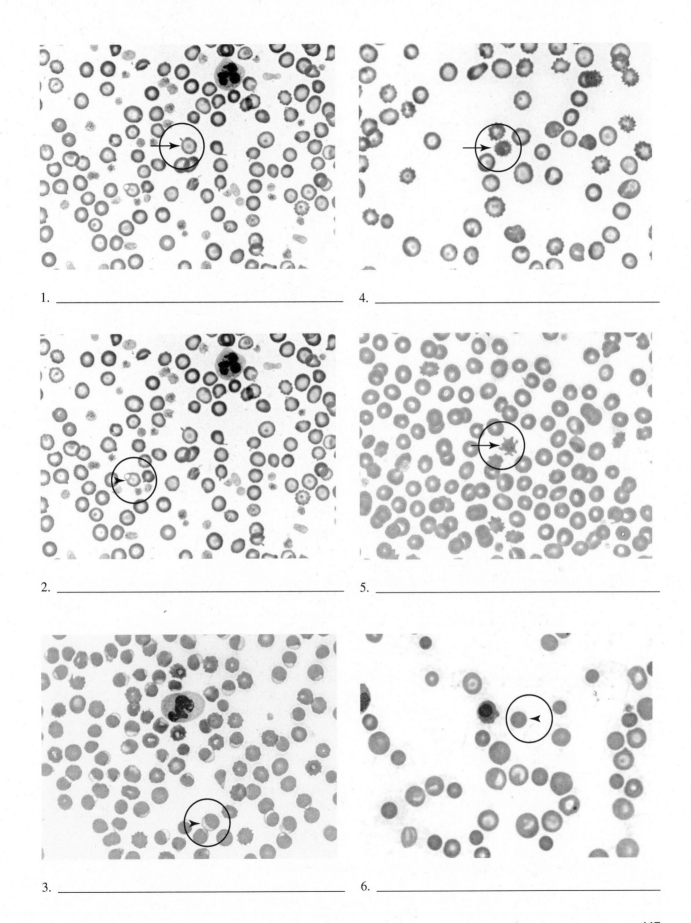

1. _____

4. _____

2. _____

5. _____

3. _____

6. _____

Chapter **12** **Hematology and Cytology**

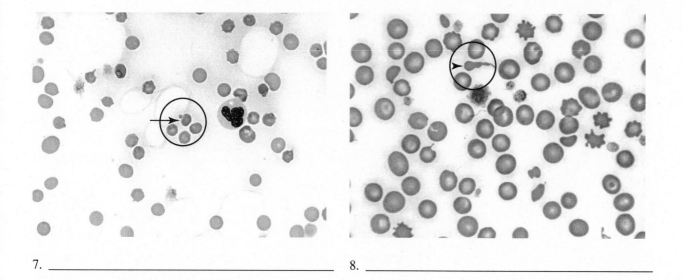

7. _____ 8. _____

EXERCISE 12.7 TRUE OR FALSE: COMPREHENSIVE

Instructions: Read the following statements and write "T" for true or "F" for false in the blanks provided. If a statement is false, correct the statement to make it true.

1. _____ A longer period of time for centrifugation may be required for blood samples from sheep and goats because their RBCs are smaller than those of dogs and cats.

2. _____ A PCV is determined by a mathematical calculation.

3. _____ A hematology analyzer utilizing impedance methodology uses an electrical current to count blood cells and determine their size.

4. _____ WBCs are heavier than both RBCs and blood plasma and thus are found on the bottom of a micro-hematocrit tube following centrifugation.

5. _____ Changes in the hemoglobin concentration are generally proportional to changes in the WBC count.

6. _____ An increased red cell distribution width (RDW) indicates anisocytosis.

7. _____ Platelet clumps occur most commonly in dogs.

8. _____ Ideally, a blood smear should be stained within 24 hours.

9. _____ The substage condenser of the microscope should be in a relatively high position when evaluating a blood smear or cytology prep.

10. _____ Target cells, when noted on a blood smear, are usually seen in animals with hemangiosarcoma or heart-worm disease.

11. _____ Echinocytes are most often seen in animals with lymphoma (cancer of the lymph nodes).

12. _____ Almost all RBCs often look like spherocytes near the feathered edge.

13. _____ The presence of any metarubricytes on a blood smear is abnormal.

14. _____ In normal animals, up to 10% of the RBCs are polychromatophils.

118

15. _____ The blood parasite *Anaplasma marginale* is easily mistaken for stain precipitate.

16. _____ A metamyelocyte is an immature neutrophil sometimes released into the circulation in the face of intense inflammatory reactions.

17. _____ A neutrophil has a higher nuclear-to-cytoplasmic ratio than a lymphocyte.

18. _____ When performing a differential cell count, broken cells should not be counted.

19. _____ Plasma samples for APTT and PT testing should be kept frozen until arrival at the reference lab.

20. _____ The mucin clot test is used to evaluate blood coagulation.

EXERCISE 12.8 MULTIPLE CHOICE: COMPREHENSIVE

Instructions: Circle the one correct answer to each of the following questions.

1. Citrate is the anticoagulant contained in a
   a. Lavender-top tube
   b. Red-top tube
   c. Green-top tube
   d. Blue-top tube

2. Which one of the following tests does not indicate the oxygen carrying capacity of blood?
   a. RBC count
   b. HCT
   c. PDW
   d. PCV

3. Automated hematology analyzers determine the HCT by
   a. Direct measurement
   b. Multiplying the MCV count by the RBC
   c. Dividing the PCV by the RBC count
   d. Dividing the PCV by 3

4. MCV is often increased in patients with
   a. Inflammation
   b. Chronic renal failure
   c. Primary bone marrow disease
   d. Blood loss

5. Red blood cells in an animal with a decreased MCHC are called
   a. Hypochromic
   b. Microcytic
   c. Normochromic
   d. Macrocytic

6. Plasma is often clear and light yellow in
   a. Horses and cats
   b. Dogs and cows
   c. Cats and dogs
   d. Cows and horses

7. Rouleaux formation is most common in
   a. Horses and cats
   b. Dogs and cows
   c. Cats and dogs
   d. Cows and horses

8. Agglutination refers to irregular, variable-sized clumps of RBCs that occur most commonly in animals with
   a. Liver disease
   b. Immune-mediated hemolytic anemia
   c. Lead poisoning
   d. Blood loss

9. In which species do platelets not tend to stain as well on a blood smear as in other species?
   a. Dogs
   b. Cats
   c. Horses
   d. Cattle

10. Macroplatelets may be normal in cats and
    a. Akitas
    b. Cavalier King Charles Spaniels
    c. Greyhounds
    d. Poodles

11. The central pallor in RBCs is most prominent in the normal RBCs of
    a. Dogs
    b. Cats
    c. Horses
    d. Cattle

12. Anisocytosis tends to be most prevalent in _____ and least prevalent in _____.
    a. Dogs; horses
    b. Horses; cats
    c. Cats; cows
    d. Cows; dogs

13. Animals with immune-mediated hemolytic anemia often have _____ on the blood smear.
    a. Spherocytes
    b. Apple-stem cells
    c. Eccentrocytes
    d. Heinz bodies

14. Howell-Jolly bodies are often increased in patients with
    a. Liver disease
    b. Bone marrow suppression
    c. Iron-deficiency anemia
    d. Regenerative anemia

15. A reticulocyte count is used to determine
    a. Whether an anemia is regenerative or nonregenerative
    b. Whether an anemia will get better or not
    c. The severity of an anemia
    d. Whether an anemia is longstanding

16. Segmented neutrophils have a segmented nucleus with an average of
    a. 2 to 3 lobes
    b. 3 to 5 lobes
    c. 4 to 6 lobes
    d. 5 to 7 lobes

17. This in-house coagulation test may be used to detect abnormal platelet function.
    a. Activated clotting time
    b. Prothrombin time
    c. Bleeding time
    d. Activated partial thromboplastin time

18. This value is calculated as the TP of an unheated plasma sample minus the TP of a heated sample.
    a. Fibrinogen
    b. D-dimers
    c. PT
    d. FDPs

19. Cytologic examination of tissue masses enables evaluation of
    a. Surgical margins
    b. Vascular invasion
    c. Morphology of isolated cells
    d. Association of abnormal cells with normal tissues

20. When preparing thoracic or abdominal effusion samples for cytologic examination, direct smears are often made, but some samples require concentration of the cells. Which of the following fluids is most likely to require cell concentration?
    a. Bloody fluid
    b. Fluid with a high cell count
    c. Clear fluid
    d. Turbid fluid

EXERCISE 12.9 FILL-IN-THE-BLANK: COMPREHENSIVE

Instructions: Fill in each of the spaces provided with the missing word or words that complete the sentence.

1. EDTA prevents blood clotting by binding _____.

2. Serum protein is usually a little lower than plasma protein, because there is no _____ in it.

3. The presence of increased numbers of circulating nucleated red blood cells may occur with a markedly regenerative anemia. When this occurs in the absence of anemia and is accompanied by basophilic stippling, it may indicate _____ _____.

4. A blood smear may be too thick if, when preparing the smear, the drop of blood is too _____, the spreader slide is pushed too _____, or the angle of the spreader slide is too _____.

5. The three areas of the blood smear, in order from nearest the drop to furthest away, are the _____, the _____ _____, and the _____ _____.

6. Regarding the shape of nuclei of WBC, the nucleus of a neutrophil is segmented with three to five lobes, whereas the nucleus of a monocyte is round, _____, _____, or _____ in shape, and the nucleus of a lymphocyte is generally _____ in shape.

7. The RBCs of birds and reptiles differ from those of mammals in that they contain a _____ and are _____ in shape.

8. Automatic cell counters may erroneously count nRBCs as WBCs. This error will cause the WBC count to be falsely _____. A WBC count that includes nRBCs should be referred to as a total _____ cell count.

9. The differential WBC count is performed by identifying and counting a minimum of _____ cells consecutively encountered in the monolayer.

10. A state in which the number of bands exceeds the number of segmented neutrophils is referred to as a _____ left shift.

11. Primary hemostasis refers to formation of the _____ _____ _____.

12. Blood for a platelet count should be drawn in a tube containing _____ anticoagulant.

13. To determine viscosity of joint fluid, place a wooden applicator stick in the fluid and slowly withdraw it. If viscosity is normal, a strand _____ to _____ cm long should form.

EXERCISE 12.10 CASE STUDY: IMMUNE-MEDIATED HEMOLYTIC ANEMIA (IHA) AND THROMBOCYTOPENIA (ITP)

Signalment: 6-year-old, spayed female Collie

History: Acute onset of severe lethargy

Physical Examination: Pale, icteric mucous membranes; tachypnea; enlarged spleen

Please examine the following CBC results *(taken from case presentation 12.1 in the text)* and answer the questions below:

CBC	Patient		Reference Interval
Plasma protein (g/dL)	7.6	H	5.7 – 7.2
Plasma appeared clear and moderately yellow.			
HCT (%)	17	L	36 – 54
RBCs ($\times 10^{12}$/L)	2.2	L	4.9 – 8.2
MCV (fl)	80	H	64 – 75
MCHC (g/dL)	29.1	L	32.9 – 35.2
RDW	19.1	H	13.4 – 17.0
Reticulocytes ($\times 10^9$/L)	477.5	H	<60

RBC Morphology: There is marked agglutination that did not disperse with saline. Moderate anisocytosis, marked polychromasia, and numerous spherocytes are observed. Numbers of Howell-Jolly bodies and nRBCs are increased.

Platelets ($\times 10^9$/L)	94	L	106 – 424
WBCs ($\times 10^9$/L)	34.6	H	4.1 – 15.2
nRBCs ($\times 10^9$/L)	10.9	H	0
Band neutrophils ($\times 10^9$/L)	8.2	H	0 – 0.1
Segmented neutrophils ($\times 10^9$/L)	28.2	H	3.0 – 10.4
Lymphocytes ($\times 10^9$/L)	1.8		1.0 – 4.6
Monocytes ($\times 10^9$/L)	7.3	H	0.0 – 1.2
Eosinophils ($\times 10^9$/L)	0		0 – 1.2

WBC Morphology: Moderate numbers of Döhle bodies and moderate cytoplasmic basophilia and vacuolation are interpreted as toxic change.

1. What blood collection tube would you select for this blood draw, and what anticoagulant (if any) does this tube contain?

   Test   **Tube top color**   **Anticoagulant (N/A if none)**

   CBC and platelet count   _____   _____

2. The hemoglobin concentration of any patient is usually proportional to the PCV or hematocrit. Using the technique for estimating hemoglobin you learned in this chapter, please estimate this patient's hemoglobin concentration in g/dL.

   Hemoglobin = _____ g/dL

3a. Are this patient's RBCs normal in size?

   _____

3b. How do you know this by looking at the CBC?

   _____

4. What is the term used to describe RBCs that are too large?

   _____

5. Polychromasia is marked on the blood smear examination. What does this mean?

   _____

6. How are polychromatophils recognized on a blood smear?

   _____

   _____

7. On the blood smear, there were also about 5 platelets/100× field. This correlates to an estimated platelet count of

   _____ platelets/µL.

8. This patient had increased nRBCs. When performing a manual cell count, the presence of many nRBCs will falsely increase the total WBC count because nRBCs cannot be differentiated from other nucleated cells. However, the WBC count can be mathematically corrected.

   Assume that a patient you were performing a CBC on had a total WBC count of 23,000 cells/µL, and 35 nRBCs were noted while performing the differential cell count. Using the formula you learned in this chapter, correct this patient's WBC count.

   Corrected WBC count: _____ cells/µL

9. This patient also had markedly increased numbers of reticulocytes (477.5×10^9/L). What is the significance of this increase?

   _____

   _____

10. Calculate absolute values by considering the following scenario: You have performed a manual white blood cell count and a 100-cell differential on a patient. The results are as follows:

Total WBC count: 25,000 cell/μL
2% band neutrophils
55% segmented neutrophils
35% lymphocytes
5% monocytes
3% eosinophils

Calculate the absolute numbers of each cell.

Band neutrophils: _____ cells/μL

Segmented neutrophils: _____ cells/μL

Lymphocytes: _____ cells/μL

Monocytes: _____ cells/μL

Eosinophils: _____ cells/μL

13 Clinical Chemistry, Serology, and Urinalysis

When you have completed this chapter, you will be able to:

1. Pronounce, define, and spell all the Key Terms in this chapter.
2. Do the following regarding clinical chemistry:
   - Explain the purpose of the clinical chemistry profile, and list the preanalytic and analytic factors that can affect clinical chemistry testing.
   - Compare and contrast the use of chemistry analyzers in veterinary and human medicine.
   - Define a calibrator and a control, and describe how they are used in quality control.
3. Describe the general principles of serologic testing, and discuss the most common methods of serologic testing.
4. Do the following regarding urinalysis:
   - Describe proper collection techniques and handling of urine samples.
   - List and describe methods for the physical and biochemical evaluation of urine.
   - Describe the preparation of urine for microscopic evaluation, list the cellular elements that can be found in the urine sediment, and identify the three most common urine crystals.

EXERCISE 13.1 CROSSWORD PUZZLE: TERMS

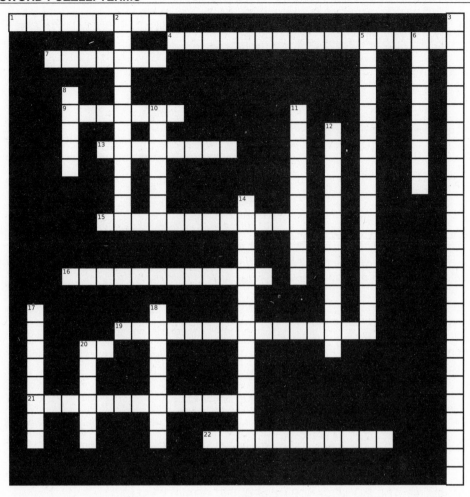

Across

1　Destruction of RBCs that may result from improper handling of the blood.
4　A graph with a chronological record of control test results. (2 words)
7　Material that contains a known quantity of the analyte that is being tested.
9　The presence of circulating triglycerides.
13　Increased blood urea nitrogen (BUN) and serum creatinine (SC).
15　A urine specific gravity between 1.008 and 1.012.
16　May be associated with a risk for urolithiasis.
19　A measure of the ability of the kidney to concentrate urine. (2 words)
20　This will increase in a urine sample over time due to loss of CO_2.
21　Measures the bending of light as it passes through a solution.
22　Increased number of casts in urine.

Down

2　Chemicals in the liquid portion of clotted blood that are released from damaged cells, and used to detect liver damage, muscle damage, or cholestasis. (2 words)
3　Detailed step-by-step description for performing a test and operating an instrument. (3 words)
5　A method of measuring chemistries based on light transmission through a liquid.
6　This term is used to describe a urine sample with a pH of 8.
8　The snap test uses this technology to detect antigens. (acronym)
10　Caused by increased serum bilirubin.
11　A standardized material that contains a known amount of reference material.
12　The preferred urine collection method for bacterial culture.
14　Procedures necessary to produce accurate and reliable results. (2 words)
17　This term means increased hydrogen ions in the urine.
18　The detection of antigens by using antibodies.
20　Increased numbers of leukocytes in the urine.

EXERCISE 13.2 MATCHING #1: THE APPEARANCE OF NORMAL AND ABNORMAL BLOOD SERUM

Instructions: Match each description of the appearance of blood serum in column A with its associated significance in column B by writing the appropriate letter in the space provided.

Column A

1. _____ Milky
2. _____ Red
3. _____ Clear and colorless
4. _____ Light yellow
5. _____ Pink, milky
6. _____ Orange

Column B

A. Normal in large animals.

B. Normal in small animals.

C. Concurrent hemolysis and lipemia.

D. From rough transfer of the blood to the collection tube.

E. Bilirubin in the serum.

F. Increased serum triglycerides (lipemia).

EXERCISE 13.3 MATCHING #2: ELISA SEROLOGY ASSAY

Instructions: Match each item associated with the ELISA test designed to test for patient antigens in column A with its corresponding description in column B by writing the appropriate letter in the space provided.

Column A

1. _____ Antibody
2. _____ Patient sample
3. _____ Enzyme-labeled antigen/antibody complex
4. _____ Unbound antigen and enzyme-labeled antibody
5. _____ Colorless chemical substrate
6. _____ Antigen of interest

Column B

A. Captured by the matrix-bound antibody.

B. Acted on by the enzyme in the enzyme-labeled antibody.

C. Bound to a solid matrix.

D. In the patient sample.

E. Mixed with reagent containing an enzyme-labeled antibody.

F. Washed away during a washing step.

EXERCISE 13.4 MATCHING #3: THE SIGNIFICANCE OF SPECIFIC GRAVITY VALUES

Instructions: Match each specific gravity in column A with its corresponding description of the significance of each value in column B by writing the appropriate letter in the space provided.

Column A

1. _____ 1.000
2. _____ 1.005
3. _____ 1.010
4. _____ 1.025
5. _____ 1.030
6. _____ 1.035

Column B

A. Indicates normal kidney function in a dehydrated cat.

B. The SG should be at or above this level if a dog is dehydrated.

C. Indicates kidneys are able to dilute the urine.

D. The SG of distilled water.

E. A minimal SG level expected in a dehydrated cow.

F. Indicates the urine is neither being concentrated nor diluted by the kidneys.

EXERCISE 13.5 MATCHING #4: CHEMICAL EVALUATION OF URINE

Instructions: Match each chemical constituent found on urine chemistry reagent strips in column A with the corresponding statement that applies to each in column B by writing the appropriate letter in the space provided.

Column A

1. _____ pH
2. _____ Protein
3. _____ Glucose
4. _____ Ketones
5. _____ Bilirubin
6. _____ Blood

Column B

A. Male dogs may have small amounts in concentrated urine, but not cats.

B. May be false negative when the urine is exposed to formaldehyde.

C. May change from positive to negative if the urine is centrifuged.

D. May increase as a result of loss of carbon dioxide as urine stands.

E. May appear in the urine as a consequence of glomerular disease.

F. May be present in the urine in animals with starvation.

EXERCISE 13.6 MATCHING #5: CONSTITUENTS OF A ROUTINE CHEMISTRY PANEL

Instructions: Match each constituent of a routine chemistry panel in column A with the corresponding statement in column B by writing the appropriate letter in the space provided.

Column A

1. _____ Glucose
2. _____ Electrolytes
3. _____ Creatinine
4. _____ Alanine aminotransferase
5. _____ Sorbitol dehydrogenase
6. _____ Creatine kinase
7. _____ Alkaline phosphatase
8. _____ Immunoglobulins
9. _____ Aspartate aminotransferase

Column B

A. May increase in patients with impaired kidney function.

B. Increased levels indicate hepatocellular damage in large animals.

C. Increased levels indicate either hepatocellular or muscle damage.

D. Increases in the presence of inflammation.

E. May decrease if the clot is left in contact with the serum for more than 1 hour.

F. Increased levels indicate hepatocellular damage in small animals.

G. Increased levels indicate muscle damage.

H. Play(s) a role in regulating water balance and acid–base status.

I. Increased from cholestasis or induced by corticosteroids.

EXERCISE 13.7 PHOTO QUIZ: PHOTOGRAPHS OF URINE CRYSTALS

Instructions: Match each urine crystal (indicated by the arrow) with the name corresponding to the crystal type.

Names

A. Ammonium biurate

B. Calcium carbonate

C. Bilirubin

D. Struvite

E. Calcium oxalate dihydrate

F. Cystine

G. Calcium oxalate monohydrate

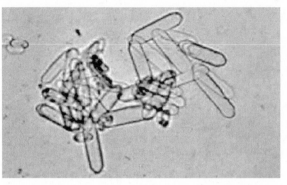

1. _____

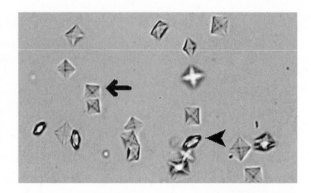

5. _____

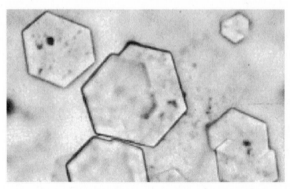

2. _____

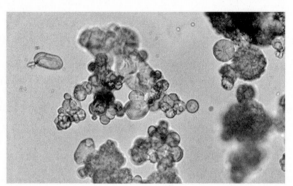

6. _____

3. _____

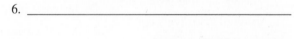

7. _____

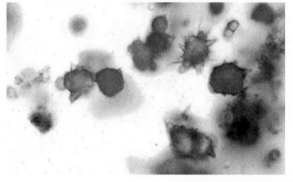

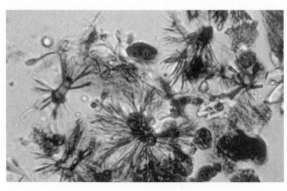

4. _____

EXERCISE 13.8 TRUE OR FALSE: COMPREHENSIVE

Instructions: Read the following statements and write "T" for true or "F" for false in the blanks provided. If a statement is false, correct the statement to make it true.

1. _____ The function of organs such as the liver can be measured using a routine chemistry panel.

2. _____ Increased serum bilirubin specifically indicates cholestatic disease.

3. _____ Serum calcium concentration may not accurately reflect total body content of calcium.

4. _____ Fasting is required in all domestic species prior to sample collection for a chemistry panel.

5. _____ The breed and age of a patient may affect what is considered a normal amount of each analyte in the blood.

6. _____ A disadvantage of dry reagent chemistry systems is that they are more sensitive to interference by lipemia, hemolysis, and icterus than liquid reagent systems.

7. _____ Point-of-care chemistry instruments, like the iSTAT (Abaxis, Union City, CA), that use single-use, self-contained cartridges do not require in-house calibration.

8. _____ It takes approximately 1 to 3 weeks for a patient to develop an antibody response to an active infection.

9. _____ If a patient is actively infected with a pathogen, the antibody titer is expected to double over a period of 2 to 3 weeks.

10. _____ ELISA serologic tests can be used to test for either antigens or antibodies.

11. _____ A urine container must be tightly capped to prevent loss of protein.

12. _____ Catheterization is the preferred way of obtaining urine samples for bacterial culture.

13. _____ Specific gravity is an indicator of the concentrating ability of the kidney.

14. _____ If the kidneys are healthy, urine will be diluted in a dehydrated patient or concentrated when the patient is overhydrated.

15. _____ The presence of urease-positive bacteria in urine can cause the urine pH to decrease.

16. _____ Normal urine should not contain glucose.

17. _____ Interpretation of the significance of blood in the urine is affected by the method of collection.

18. _____ Transitional epithelial cells are larger than other cells seen in urine.

19. _____ Urinary casts form in the glomeruli of the kidneys.

20. _____ Urinary crystals may form in response to changes in the diet.

Instructions: Circle the one correct answer to each of the following questions.

1. Which of the following constituents of a routine chemistry panel is a calculated value?
   a. Alanine aminotransferase (ALT)
   b. Albumin
   c. Anion gap
   d. Potassium

2. Increased serum creatinine (SC) indicates azotemia and can be caused by impaired kidney function or dehydration. To differentiate these causes, the SC must be interpreted along with
   a. Albumin
   b. Urine specific gravity (SG)
   c. Blood urea nitrogen (BUN)
   d. Alanine aminotransferase (ALT)

3. Each of the following is a serum electrolyte except
   a. Chloride
   b. Bicarbonate
   c. Creatinine
   d. Phosphorus

4. The serum protein normally present in the highest concentrations is
   a. Albumin
   b. Globulin
   c. Fibrinogen
   d. Prothrombin

5. To avoid serum lipemia, dogs and cats should be
   a. Fed
   b. Fasted for 4 hours
   c. Fasted for 8 hours
   d. Fasted for 12 hours

6. With the exception of birds and other small pets, when sending blood to an outside lab, serum samples should be collected in a tube containing
   a. Sodium citrate anticoagulant
   b. EDTA anticoagulant
   c. No anticoagulant
   d. Lithium heparin anticoagulant

7. In reference to quality control, an SOP is a
   a. Sample of the material used to calibrate the machine
   b. Graph used to track control results
   c. Step-by-step description for performing a test
   d. Measure of test result trends

8. Controls must be run routinely as an integral part of good quality control. In small and large labs, they should be run at least
   a. Twice a day
   b. Daily
   c. Once every other day
   d. Once a week

9. When running controls, an acceptable variation is within ±2 standard deviations of the mean. This means that the control may be slightly out of the acceptable range less than
   a. 2% of the time
   b. 5% of the time
   c. Two times out of 10
   d. Every other time it is run

10. Over time, control results may gradually progress toward the upper or lower acceptable limits. This would most likely happen if
    a. The wrong reagent is being used
    b. The technician's technique for performing the test is incorrect
    c. An instrument component is deteriorating
    d. The samples are not being processed properly

11. Serology is not commonly used to test for
    a. Drugs
    b. Hormones
    c. Infectious agents
    d. Enzymes

12. A single positive serologic test for antibodies to a pathogen indicates that the patient
    a. Is actively infected by the pathogen
    b. Has been exposed to the pathogen either currently or in the past
    c. Has never been exposed to the pathogen
    d. Is sick from exposure to the pathogen

13. Which of the following is *not* an example of a serologic test?
    a. IRMA
    b. GGT
    c. ELISA
    d. AGID

14. Exposure of urine to UV light may cause deterioration of
    a. Ketones
    b. Protein
    c. Bilirubin
    d. Glucose

15. Urine samples least likely to be contaminated with squamous epithelial cells are those collected by
    a. Midstream void
    b. Urinary catheter
    c. Manual compression
    d. Cystcentesis

16. The presence of hematuria, hemoglobinuria, or myoglobinuria in urine may cause it to be
    a. Yellow-brown in color
    b. Amber in color
    c. Light yellow in color
    d. Reddish-brown in color

17. Normal urine should be clear in the common domestic species of animals, except for
    a. Dogs
    b. Cats
    c. Cattle
    d. Horses

18. Reagent test pads that do not work in animals and so should not be used are the
    a. Ketone and leukocyte pads
    b. Leukocyte and specific gravity pads
    c. Specific gravity and bilirubin pads
    d. Bilirubin and ketone pads

19. The protein pad on a reagent strip is most sensitive to
    a. Globulins
    b. Myoglobin
    c. Albumin
    d. Mucoproteins

20. Squamous epithelial cells come from the
    a. Kidney tubules
    b. Renal pelvis and ureters
    c. Bladder
    d. Urethra, vagina, and prepuce

21. Which of the following kind of cells may appear in clusters or rafts in a urine sample?
    a. RBCs
    b. WBCs
    c. Transitional cells
    d. Squamous cells

22. Which urinary casts are normal in very low numbers (1 or fewer/LPF)?
    a. Waxy and hyaline
    b. Hyaline and granular
    c. Granular and cellular
    d. Cellular and waxy

23. Which crystal is not expected in the urine of normal dogs and cats?
    a. Hippuric acid-like calcium oxalate monohydrate
    b. Struvite
    c. Calcium phosphate
    d. Calcium oxalate dihydrate

24. Normal horses have which of the following urinary crystals in their urine?
    a. Calcium oxylate monohydrate
    b. Struvite
    c. Calcium phosphate
    d. Calcium carbonate

EXERCISE 13.10 FILL-IN-THE-BLANK: COMPREHENSIVE

Instructions: Fill in each of the spaces provided with the missing word or words that complete the sentence.

1. Corticosteroids can induce increases in the cholestatic serum enzyme _____ _____, especially in dogs.

2. Hypoalbuminemia (decreased albumin) can cause a decrease in blood _____ because this electrolyte binds to albumin in the blood.

3. Inflammatory diseases and some lymphoid cancers may cause the blood protein _____ to increase.

4. Use of an incorrect needle size for blood collection, or excessive pressure on the syringe, can result in _____.

5. When preparing a serum sample for a chemistry profile, the blood should be allowed to clot for _____ to _____ minutes at _____ temperature, then centrifuged for _____ minutes at _____ to _____ g.

6. A SNAP test is a serologic screening test, designed to detect infectious agents, that uses _____ technology.

7. Urine should be at _____ temperature when analyzed and should be examined within _____ hour(s) of collection.

8. Collection of urine by _____ _____ may damage or even rupture a fragile, diseased bladder.

9. A special urine collection technique for acquiring samples from bladder masses is _____ _____.

10. Urine that is colored red or reddish-brown indicates the presence of _____, _____, or _____ in the urine.

11. When using a medical refractometer to determine the urine SG in a cat, a conversion scale must be used, because the actual SG of cat urine is _____ than the reading on the scale.

12. Uncentrifuged urine should be used for biochemical testing unless the urine is _____.

13. The protein pad on a reagent strip may be false _____ when the urine is alkaline.

14. Glycosuria occurs when blood glucose level exceeds the _____ _____.

15. The blood pad on the reagent test strip is sometimes alternatively labeled _____.

16. When preparing urine samples for microscopic examination, _____ to _____ mL of urine should be centrifuged in a conical centrifuge tube at _____ to _____ rpm for _____ minutes. The supernatant should be removed by pipetting or decanting, until only _____ mL of supernatant is left with the pellet.

17. Squamous cells in urine sediment are _____ in shape and of no clinical significance.

18. Ammonium biurate crystals may be observed in the urine of _____ (a dog breed).

EXERCISE 13.11 CASE STUDY: PRESURGICAL PANEL ON A YOUNG DOG

Signalment: 10-month-old, mixed-breed male dog
History: A presurgical chemistry panel was run prior to orthopedic surgery for hip dysplasia.
Examine the following presurgical chemistry panel *(modified from the case presentation in the text)* and answer the following questions:

	Units	Sample 2		Reference Interval
BUN	mg/dL	13		5–20
Creatinine	mg/dL	0.9		0.6–1.6
Phosphorus	mg/dL	6.4		3.2–8.1
Calcium	mg/dL	11.5		9.3–11.6
Sodium	mEq/L	152		143–153
Potassium	mEq/L	4.7		4.2–5.4
Chloride	mEq/L	111		109–120
Anion gap	mEq/L	21		15–25
Osmolality (calculated)	mOsm/kg	303		285–304
Bicarbonate	mmol/L	25		16–25
ALT	IU/L	25		10–55
AST	IU/L	28		12–40
ALP	IU/L	35		15–120
CK	IU/L	131		50–400
Cholesterol	mg/dL	166		80–315
Total bilirubin	mg/dL	0.4		0.1–0.4
Total protein	g/dL	5.4		5.1–7.1
Albumin	g/dL	3.6		2.9–4.2
Globulin	g/dL	1.8	L	2.2–2.9
A:G ratio		2.0		0.8–2.2
Glucose	mg/dL	112		77–126

A:G, albumin-to-globulin; ALP, alkaline phosphatase; ALT, alanine aminotransferase; AST, aspartate aminotransferase; BUN, blood urea nitrogen; CK, creatine kinase.

1a. What are the two main constituents of total serum protein?

    i. _____

    ii. _____

1b. How are albumin and globulins measured?

_____

_____

1c. What disease condition(s) typically cause both albumin and globulins to decrease?

_____

1d. What disease condition(s) can cause hypoalbuminemia with normal globulins?

_____

_____

1e. What disease condition(s) typically cause both albumin and globulins to increase?

_____

1f. What disease condition(s) can cause globulins to increase with no increase in albumin?

_____

2. Which analytes indicate increased nitrogenous wastes in the blood?

_____

_____

3. Which analyte is generally increased in patients with diabetes mellitus and is used to diagnose this condition?

_____

_____

4a. Which analytes are enzymes that indicate hepatocellular damage in small animals?

_____

_____

4b. Why does aspartate aminotransferase (AST) have to be interpreted along with creatine kinase (CK) to accurately screen for hepatocellular damage?

_____

_____

4c. What other enzyme is measured to screen for hepatocellular damage in large animals?

_____

5. Which of the analytes are electrolytes?

_____

_____

6a. What is cholestatic disease?

_____

6b. Which analytes indicate cholestatic disease?

_____

_____

6c. Which analyte is not specific for cholestasis because it can also be increased by hemolysis?

_____

_____

14 Parasitology

LEARNING OBJECTIVES

When you have completed this chapter, you will be able to:

1. Pronounce, define, and spell all the key terms in this chapter.
2. Identify the common name, affected species, key clinical signs, methods of diagnosis, life cycle, zoonotic potential, treatment, prevention, and control of the trematodes (flukes) of zoonotic importance.
3. Identify the common name, affected species, key clinical signs, methods of diagnosis, life cycle, zoonotic potential, treatment, prevention, and control of the cestodes (tapeworms) and metacestodes (larval tapeworms) of zoonotic importance.
4. Identify the common name, affected species, key clinical signs, methods of diagnosis, life cycle, zoonotic potential, treatment, prevention, and control of the nematodes (roundworms) of zoonotic importance. Also do the following regarding nematodes:
   - Describe the origin and clinical signs of *visceral larva migrans, ocular larva migrans, neurologic larva migrans,* and *cutaneous larva migrans,* including risk factors for and methods of preventing these zoonotic diseases.
   - Identify the common name, affected species, key clinical signs, methods of diagnosis, life cycle, zoonotic potential, treatment, prevention, and control of *Dirofilaria immitis* (heartworm).
5. Identify the common name, affected species, key clinical signs, methods of diagnosis, life cycle, zoonotic potential, treatment, prevention, and control of the arthropods of zoonotic importance.
6. Identify the common name, affected species, key clinical signs, methods of diagnosis, life cycle, zoonotic potential, treatment, prevention, and control of the protozoans of zoonotic importance.
7. Identify the common name, affected species, key clinical signs, methods of diagnosis, life cycle, zoonotic potential, treatment, prevention, and control of the pentastomes (snake parasites) of zoonotic importance.
8. Do the following regarding collection and examination of fecal samples for the diagnosis of endoparasitism:
   - Describe the principles of collection, storage, and examination of fecal samples, including safety precautions that must be observed.
   - Describe indications for and procedures used to examine feces by direct fecal smear, fecal flotation, and sedimentation.
9. Do the following additional tasks regarding diagnosis of endoparasitism:
   - List the special procedures used to detect the coccidian parasites *Giardia, Cryptosporidium* spp., and *Cystoisospora* spp.
   - Describe how necropsy findings are used to diagnose parasitism after death.
   - Explain how samples are prepared and shipped to an outside laboratory for diagnosis of parasitism.
   - Explain how the Baermann technique is used to detect nematode larvae in feces and tissues.
   - Compare and contrast the blood examination and concentration techniques used to diagnose *Dirofilaria immitis.*

136

Chapter **14** Parasitology

Copyright © 2018, Elsevier Inc. All Rights Reserved.

EXERCISE 14.1 CROSSWORD PUZZLE: TERMS AND DEFINITIONS

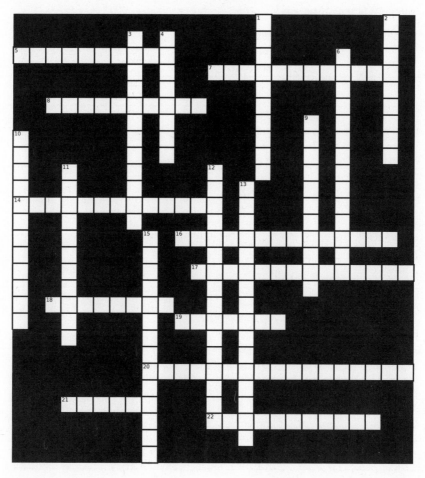

Across

5 A slowly replicating stage of development of the parasite *Toxoplasma gondii.*

7 A parasite that lives on the exterior of another organism.

8 A segment that comprises the body of a cestode.

14 A host in which a parasite does not undergo further development, but in which it remains encysted. (2 words)

16 A word used to describe a living organism that contains complete functioning sets of both male and female reproductive organs.

17 The host that harbors the adult, sexual, or mature stages of a parasite. (2 words)

18 A soft, moist, adhesive mass that is usually heated, spread on cloth, and applied to warm, moisten, or stimulate an aching or inflamed part of the body.

19 A parasite that is either a mite or a tick.

20 The type of roundworm larval migration that occurs in puppies younger than 3 months old where the larvae eventually reach the lungs, are coughed up and swallowed, and end up maturing in the host's small intestines. (2 words)

21 Pregnant; carrying fertilized eggs or a fetus.

22 A fast-growing developmental stage that occurs in cysts in the life cycle of *Giardia.*

Down

1 A state of arrested development of a parasite larva.

2 A life cycle that utilizes a first and second intermediate host along with a definitive host.

3 The motile, prelarval stage of filarial parasites.

4 A roundworm.

6 An object that is not a parasite but one that can be mistaken for a parasite; an example would be pollen grain because it is similar in size, shape, and color to a parasite egg.

9 A disease caused by the ingestion and harboring of the plerocercoid stage of the zipper tapeworm.

10 A parasite that lives inside another organism.

11 Any host organism from which a parasite cannot escape to continue its life cycle. (2 words)

12 The host that harbors the immature, asexual, or larval stages of a parasite. (2 words)

13 The type of roundworm larval migration that occurs in puppies older than 3 months of age where the second stage larvae encyst extraintestinally in the host's body. (2 words)

15 A parasite egg that contains an operculum—a "lid" or "door" that can be found on some parasite eggs—through which the larvae escapes. (2 words)

EXERCISE 14.2 DEFINING KEY TERMS

Instructions: Define each term in your own words.

1. Heterogonic life cycle

   _____

   _____

2. One-host tick

   _____

   _____

3. Unilocular hydatid cyst

   _____

   _____

4. Three-host tick

   _____

   _____

5. Visceral larva migrans

   _____

   _____

6. Multilocular hydatid cyst

   _____

   _____

7. Homogonic life cycle

   _____

   _____

8. Many-host tick

   _____

   _____

9. Ocular larva migrans

   _____

   _____

10. Two-host tick

_____

_____

EXERCISE 14.3 MATCHING #1: TERMS AND DEFINITIONS

Instructions: Match each term in column A with its corresponding definition in column B by writing the appropriate letter in the space provided.

Column A

1. _____ Oocyst
2. _____ Merozoite
3. _____ Schistosome
4. _____ Cestode
5. _____ Acariasis
6. _____ Tachyzoite
7. _____ Parthenogenesis
8. _____ Brood capsule
9. _____ Hexacanth embryo
10. _____ Neurologic larva migrans
11. _____ Cutaneous larva migrans

Column B

A. A fast-growing developmental stage that occurs in cysts in the life cycle of _Toxoplasma gondii_.

B. A blood fluke.

C. A skin disease in humans caused by the larvae of hookworm parasites that leave migratory tracks in the skin.

D. A protozoan cell that arises from the multiple fission (schizogony) of parent sporozoans and may enter either the asexual or sexual phase of the life cycle.

E. Tapeworm eggs that are usually produced by taeniid-type tapeworms.

F. A disease, usually of the skin, caused by infestation with mites.

G. A condition caused by the migration of the larval stage of _Baylisascaris procyonis_ through the brain and spinal cord of avian or mammalian paratenic hosts, including humans.

H. The parasitic stage produced by the sporozoites of _Cryptosporidium parvum_.

I. The adult stage of a tapeworm.

J. A type of nonsexual reproduction in which an organism develops from an unfertilized ovum.

K. A structure that is formed from the germinal membrane of a hydatid cyst.

EXERCISE 14.4 MATCHING #2: TERMS AND DEFINITIONS

Instructions: Match each term in column A with its corresponding definition in column B by writing the appropriate letter in the space provided.

Column A

1. _____ Egg packet
2. _____ Aberrant parasite
3. _____ Otoacariasis
4. _____ Protozoan
5. _____ Simian
6. _____ Metacercaria
7. _____ Procercoid
8. _____ Germinal membrane
9. _____ Pseudotapeworms
10. _____ Miracidium

Column B

A. The infective stage of a digenic fluke.

B. A single-cell organism.

C. The innermost lining of a hydatid cyst.

D. A parasite found in a location in which it does not normally live.

E. Pertaining to or resembling an ape or a monkey.

F. The ciliated, motile stage that emerges from the operculated egg of a digenetic fluke.

G. The developmental stage in the life cycle of a pseudotapeworm that parasitizes the first intermediate host.

H. These members of the order *Cotyloidea* include *Spirometra mansonoides*.

I. What is typically passed in the feces in an animal infected with *Dipylidium caninum* when a gravid proglottid is ruptured during defecation.

J. Infestation of the ear with mites.

EXERCISE 14.5 MATCHING #3: TERMS AND DEFINITIONS

Instructions: Match each term in column A with its corresponding definition in column B by writing the appropriate letter in the space provided.

Column A

1. _____ Cercaria
2. _____ Dioecious
3. _____ Gynecophoric canal
4. _____ Plerocercoid
5. _____ Metacestode
6. _____ Schistosome cercarial dermatitis
7. _____ Cyst
8. _____ Arthropod
9. _____ Trematode
10. _____ Cysticercoid

Column B

A. The infective developmental stage that parasitizes the second intermediate host in the life cycle of a pseudotapeworm.

B. The noninfective stage of *Giardia* that is resistant to both heat and cold and to drying out.

C. A fluke.

D. The larval stage of a tapeworm.

E. The infective stage of the tapeworm.

F. Denoting species in which male and female genitals do not occur in the same individual; sexually distinct.

G. A ventral groove running the length of male schistosome flukes, into which the thread-like female worm fits.

H. Sometimes referred to as swimmer's itch.

I. The free-swimming trematode larva that emerges from its host snail.

J. Any animals of the phylum that includes insects, crustaceans, arachnids, and myriapods.

EXERCISE 14.6 PHOTO QUIZ: PHOTOGRAPHS OF PARASITES

Instructions: Match each parasite with its corresponding name.

Names

A. *Paragonimus kellicotti* egg

B. *Dipylidium caninum* proglottids

C. Adult *Otodectes cyanotis* mite

D. Adult *Cheyletiella parasitivorax* mite

E. *Toxoplasma gondii* oocyst

F. Adult *Sarcoptes scabei* mite

G. *Toxascaris leonina* egg

H. *Spirometra mansonoides* egg

I. *Trichuris vulpis* egg

J. Adult *Demodex canis* mite

K. *Dipylidium caninum* egg packet

L. *Giardia* cyst

M. *Ancylostoma caninum* egg

N. Oocysts of *Cryptosporidium parvum*

O. Typical Taeniid-type egg

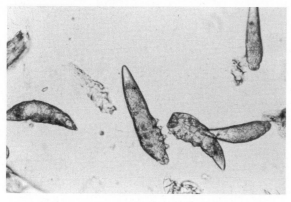

1. _____

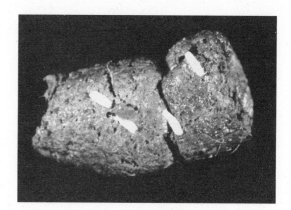

3. _____

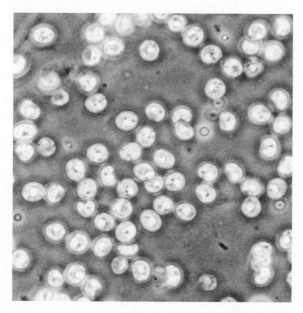

2. _____

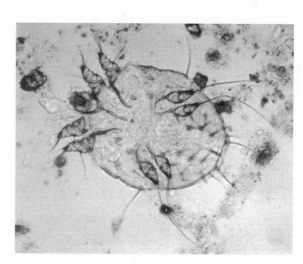

4. _____

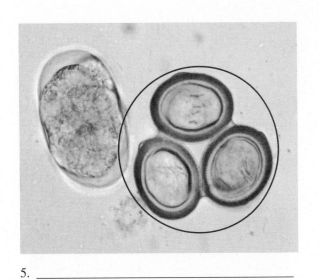

5. _____

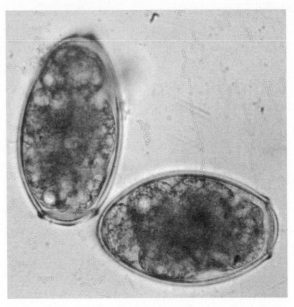

7. _____

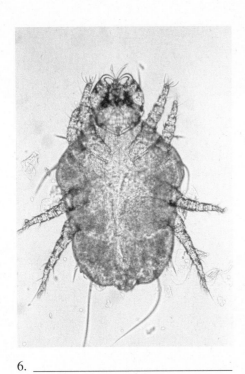

6. _____

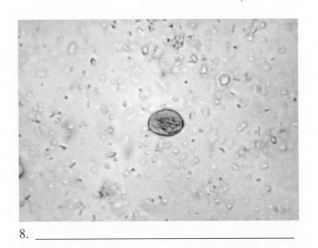

8. _____

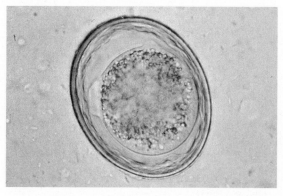

9. _____

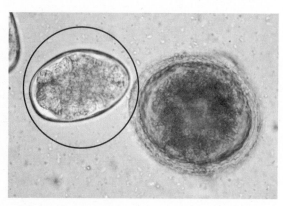

12. _____

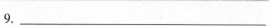

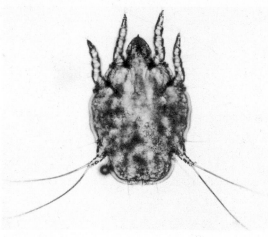

10. _____

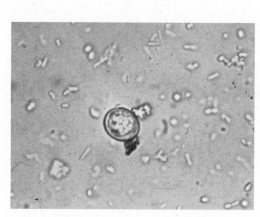

13. _____

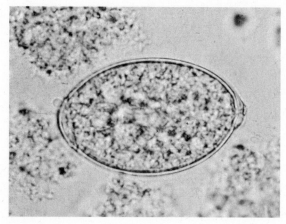

11. _____

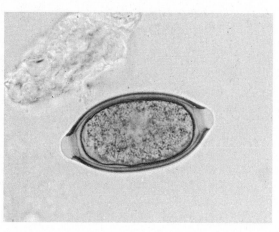

14. _____

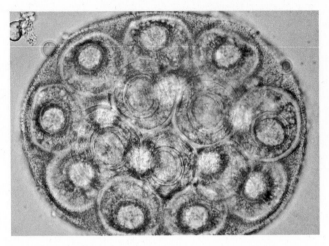

15. _____

EXERCISE 14.7 TRUE OR FALSE: COMPREHENSIVE

Instructions: Read the following statements and write "T" for true or "F" for false in the blanks provided. If a statement is false, correct the statement to make it true.

1. _____ Parasite infections are not found in all species of animal.

2. _____ Human infection with *Paragonimus kellicotti* is a rare occurrence.

3. _____ The eggs of *Paragonimus kellicotti* usually exit the host in coughed up sputum.

4. _____ Humans become infected with *Schistosome cercarial dermatitis* when the cercarial stage penetrates their skin.

5. _____ The intermediate host for *Dipylidium caninum* is the mosquito.

6. _____ When dogs and cats are infected with *Echinococcus granulosus* or *Echinococcus multilocularis*, they are often asymptomatic.

7. _____ Humans are considered the definitive host for both *Echinococcus granulosus* and *Echinococcus multilocularis*.

8. _____ *Spirometra mansonoides* eggs are usually voided in the external environment via gravid proglottids passed in the feces.

9. _____ When the eggs of *Toxocara canis* are passed in the feces, they are immediately infective.

10. _____ Puppies can be infected with *Toxocara canis* while nursing.

11. _____ If a dog ingests a paratenic host infected with *Toxocara canis*, somatic migration will take place in the dog.

12. _____ *Baylisascaris procyonis* usually causes clinical disease in dogs and cats.

13. _____ Hookworms can be a cause of anemia in young puppies.

14. _____ Humans are typically infected with hookworms via ingestion of infective larvae.

15. _____ The eggs of *Trichuris vulpis* can survive in the environment for years.

16. _____ Intestinal threadworms are best diagnosed using fecal flotation.

144

17. _____ Heartworm microfilariae that are circulating in a dog's peripheral blood will eventually mature to adult heartworms.

18. _____ Most species of mammals have their own variety of *Sarcoptes scabei*.

19. _____ Lesions associated with *Cheyletiella* are usually moist and inflamed in appearance.

20. _____ The parasite *Demodex canis* usually lives in the hair follicles of animals it infests.

21. _____ Chiggers typically burrow into the skin of infested hosts.

22. _____ *Giardia* is capable of infecting many different species of animals, including humans.

23. _____ The feline is the only animal that can serve as the intermediate host for *Toxoplasma gondii*.

24. _____ *Toxoplasma gondii* infection is typically diagnosed by fecal flotation.

25. _____ A healthy host will usually be able to fight off a *Cryptosporidium* infection on its own.

26. _____ A good way for veterinary practices to save money is to reuse vials and filters used to perform fecal flotations.

EXERCISE 14.8 MULTIPLE CHOICE: COMPREHENSIVE

Instructions: Circle the one correct answer to each of the following questions.

1. Once an infected dog produces a *Paragonimus kellicotti* egg, what must happen before the life cycle can advance?
   a. The egg must be ingested by another intermediate host
   b. The egg must penetrate the skin of another animal
   c. The egg must go through parthenogenesis
   d. The egg must come into contact with water

2. *Paragonimus kellicotti* is also known by the common name
   a. Whipworm
   b. Lung fluke
   c. Blood fluke
   d. Intestinal threadworm

3. The life cycle of *Paragonimus kellicotti* utilizes

   _____ intermediate host(s).
   a. 0
   b. 1
   c. 2
   d. 3

4. An accurate and economical way to diagnose a *Paragonimus kellicotti* infection is to perform a
   a. Fecal flotation
   b. Fecal sedimentation
   c. Direct smear
   d. Baermann technique

5. The primary definitive host for *Schistosome cercarial dermatitis* is
   a. Humans younger than the age of 12 years
   b. Aquatic, migratory birds
   c. Raccoons
   d. Aquatic crustaceans

6. If an owner is reporting that his or her dog is dragging its anus across the floor on a frequent basis, this could be a sign of
   a. Hookworm infection
   b. Whipworm infection
   c. Tapeworm infection
   d. Roundworm infection

7. A client has just dropped off a fresh fecal sample on which you find several proglottids. Upon examining these proglottids under the microscope, you notice there is a pair of genital pores, which leads you to

   believe that these are _____ proglottids.
   a. *Multiceps*
   b. *Echinococcus*
   c. *Taenia*
   d. *Dipylidium*

8. One of the best ways to prevent *Echinococcus granulosus* infection in dogs is to
   a. Prevent them from ingesting rodents
   b. Prevent them from ingesting sheep viscera
   c. Prevent them from ingesting crayfish
   d. Use a monthly flea preventative

Chapter **14** **Parasitology**

9. The typical life cycle of *Spirometra mansonoides* utilizes _____ intermediate host(s).
   a. 0
   b. 1
   c. 2
   d. 3

10. Typically, if a dog younger than 3 months of age ingests a *Toxocara canis* egg containing the second-stage larva, the larva will go through
    a. Tracheal migration
    b. Somatic migration
    c. Visceral migration
    d. Ocular migration

11. The best way to diagnose ascarid infections in dogs and cats is
    a. Direct smear
    b. Fecal flotation
    c. Fecal sedimentation
    d. Baermann technique

12. Neurologic larval migrans is a condition that can occur when a paratenic host ingests the larval stage of
    a. *Toxocara canis*
    b. *Baylisascaris procyonis*
    c. *Echinococcus multilocularis*
    d. *Ancylostoma caninum*

13. There are two main ways a dog can become infected with *Ancylostoma caninum*. One way is ingestion of infective larvae, and the other is
    a. Coitus
    b. Inhalation
    c. Ingestion of an intermediate host
    d. Skin penetration

14. Whipworm is the common name for which one of the following parasites?
    a. *Trichuris vulpis*
    b. *Spirometra mansonoides*
    c. *Paragonimus kellicotti*
    d. *Uncinaria stenocephala*

15. From the time a dog ingests a whipworm egg containing the second-stage larva to the time that the larva is a mature, egg-producing adult is approximately
    a. 9 weeks
    b. 10 weeks
    c. 11 weeks
    d. 12 weeks

16. One of the unique aspects of intestinal threadworms is that
    a. The adult worms can live in the lungs or intestines of the host
    b. The eggs are immediately infective when passed in feces
    c. Only the females are parasitic
    d. Only the males are parasitic

17. In dogs and cats, adult heartworms are typically found in the
    a. Pulmonary veins and left ventricle
    b. Pulmonary arteries and right ventricle
    c. Aorta and vena cava
    d. Left and right ventricles

18. The intermediate host that is utilized during the life cycle of *Dirofilaria immitis* is the
    a. Fly
    b. Tick
    c. Mosquito
    d. Flea

19. The extreme pruritus associated with a *Sarcoptes scabei* infestation is caused by the mite
    a. Chewing on the host's skin debris
    b. Piercing the host's skin with its proboscis
    c. Cementing eggs to hair shafts on the host's skin
    d. Tunneling into the host's epidermis

20. With the *Trombicula* species, only the _____ stage of the life cycle is parasitic.
    a. Pupal
    b. Larval
    c. Nymph
    d. Adult

21. For an animal or human to become infected with *Cryptosporidium*, a(n) _____ must be ingested.
    a. Oocyst
    b. Merozoite
    c. Sporozoite
    d. Egg

22. Adult *pentastomes* are always associated with the
    a. Lymph nodes
    b. Gastrointestinal tract
    c. Urogenital tract
    d. Respiratory tract

23. When asking a client to bring in a fecal sample from his or her dog, the client should be instructed to bring approximately _____ of feces in to be examined.
    a. 1 teaspoon
    b. 2 teaspoons
    c. 1 tablespoon
    d. 2 tablespoons

24. When using a microscope to examine fecal specimens, the _____ objective is the one that is most commonly used.
    a. 4×
    b. 10×
    c. 40×
    d. 100×

25. Which one of the following flotation solutions corrodes lab equipment and can severely distort parasite eggs?
    a. Sugar solution
    b. Zinc sulfate solution
    c. Sodium nitrate solution
    d. Saturated sodium chloride solution

26. Fecal sedimentation is typically performed when _____ eggs are suspected, as they are too heavy to float in flotation solution.
    a. Hookworm
    b. Roundworm
    c. Fluke
    d. Protozoan

27. Sometimes parasite larvae are recovered from feces or tissues instead of eggs. The procedure that allows for the recovery of parasite larvae is the
    a. McMaster technique
    b. Baermann technique
    c. Acid-fast technique
    d. Modified Knott technique

EXERCISE 14.9 CASE STUDY: PARASITE INFECTION IN A PUPPY

A client who has just obtained a new 10-week-old Golden Retriever puppy contacts the practice at which you are working as a credentialed veterinary technician. The breeder gave the puppy some dewormer when it was 6 weeks old, but the puppy has not yet been to a veterinarian to be examined. The owner indicates to you that the puppy is having some vomiting and diarrhea and also seems to have a "pot-bellied" appearance. You tell the owner that it would be a good idea to bring the puppy in to be examined by the DVM and that the owner should bring a stool sample to be examined for parasites. Answer the following series of questions about dealing with this owner and his puppy.

1. What information should you give the owner over the phone about obtaining a fecal sample from his puppy that will result in the most accurate diagnosis?

   _____

   _____

   _____

   _____

   _____

   _____

2. Unfortunately, the owner arrived at the clinic and forgot to bring in a stool sample. What are two possible ways that a fecal sample could be collected at the clinic?

   a. _____

   b. _____

3. Prior to performing any diagnostic tests on the stool sample, what type of examination should be completed and what should be recorded and reported to the veterinarian?

_____

_____

_____

4. You have decided to use a concentration method to examine the feces for the presence of parasite eggs. What are the two biggest advantages of using a concentration method?

a. _____

b. _____

5. The clinic at which you work uses sodium nitrate as its fecal flotation solution. What is a disadvantage of using sodium nitrate?

_____

_____

6. When looking at the fecal sample under the microscope, you see eggs that look like the one on the right side in the picture below. Identify the genus and species of the parasite that produced this egg.

_____

7. When you inform the owner that his Golden Retriever puppy has intestinal parasites, the owner is confused because the puppy was dewormed once when it was 6 weeks old. What should you tell the owner?

_____

_____

_____

8. The owner then tells you that there are small children in the home and asks if the children are at risk of becoming infected with *Toxocara canis*. What should you tell the owner?

_____

_____

_____

_____

_____

_____

_____

_____

15 Clinical Microbiology

LEARNING OBJECTIVES

When you have completed this chapter, you will be able to:
1. Pronounce, define, and spell all the key terms in this chapter.
2. Identify circumstances under which dangerous microorganisms (including those classified as "select") should not be cultured in a private practice setting.
3. Do the following regarding the collection of samples:
   - Describe factors that must be considered to ensure that quality specimens are obtained for bacterial culture.
   - List the indigenous flora and pathogens commonly recovered from specific anatomic sites, describing methods used to collect representative samples.
   - Describe the special collection and handling procedures used to culture samples from tissues, urine, the respiratory tract, blood, joints, milk, and feces.
   - Describe the procedure for the California mastitis test.
   - Identify appropriate transport media and conditions that must be met for safe transport of culture samples to an outside laboratory.
4. Do the following regarding sample processing:
   - Identify primary stains used to prepare samples for direct microscopic examination and specific organisms identified by each.
   - Describe the procedure for preparing and staining a sample with Gram stain, acid-fast stain, or modified acid-fast stain, including the appearance of positive and negative reactions for each.
5. Do the following regarding bacterial culture and identification:
   - Describe the principles of bacterial culture, including options for safe disposal of microbiological laboratory waste and basic equipment required to perform routine microbiological cultures.
   - Describe the differences between nutrient, enrichment, selective, and differential media, identifying commonly used plate and tube media in each category.
   - Describe the information derived from the results of biochemical testing with (1) triple sugar iron agar slant, (2) lysine iron agar slant, (3) Christensen's urea agar slant, (4) motility media, (5) indole test media, and (6) citrate test media.
   - Describe the procedures used to inoculate a culture plate for isolation and tube media for biochemical testing.
   - Identify media used for primary isolation of bacterial pathogens and conditions required for incubation of aerobic and anaerobic bacteria.
   - Explain how examination of growth on a culture plate is used to identify pathogens and guide clinical decisions.
   - Describe the roles that catalase, oxidase, and coagulase biochemical tests, as well as hemolysis patterns, play in preliminary grouping of Gram-positive and Gram-negative bacteria.
   - Describe the procedure used to perform, interpret, and report results of a quantified urine culture.
6. List common bacterial flora and pathogens; identify the classification of each and associated diseases caused by each agent.
7. Do the following regarding antimicrobial susceptibility testing:
   - Explain the reasons for susceptibility testing and the guidelines set by the Clinical and Laboratory Standards Institute (CLSI) for performing and interpreting antimicrobial susceptibility tests.
   - Describe the procedures for and principles of interpretation of the broth dilution test and the disc diffusion test.
8. Describe the principles of quality control testing and quality assurance.
9. Do the following regarding fungal culture (mycology):
   - Describe the methods used to collect dermatophytes, inoculate dermatophyte test medium and Sabouraud dextrose agar, and interpret culture results.
   - List common pathogenic yeasts and dimorphic fungi and associated diseases caused by each agent.
10. Do the following regarding the molecular detection of pathogens:
    - List the methods commonly used to detect viral pathogens in patient samples.
    - Explain principles underlying each of the following methods: enzyme-linked immunosorbent assay (ELISA) testing, virus isolation, electron microscopy, and immunohistochemical staining.

150

- Explain the difference between monoclonal and polyclonal antibodies in terms of their use in detecting viral pathogens.
- Explain the uses and principles of the polymerase chain reaction (PCR) test and deoxyribonucleic acid (DNA) sequencing.
11. Do the following regarding nosocomial infections:
- Explain why an understanding of the nature of nosocomial infections is crucial to a veterinary technician's ability to provide high-quality patient care.
- List the agents commonly associated with nosocomial infections, factors that predispose a patient to these infections, and methods used to control and prevent them.

EXERCISE 15.1 CROSSWORD PUZZLE: TERMS AND DEFINITIONS

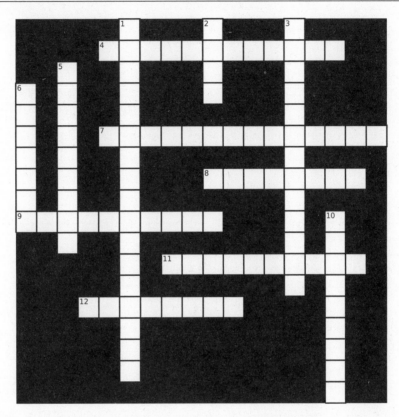

Across
4 Media that detects and discriminates between two organisms based on the results of a biochemical reaction.
7 The antimicrobial _____ test is used to determine whether an antimicrobial agent will kill or inhibit growth of a particular organism.
8 A stain that distinguishes bacteria that have mycolic acid incorporated in their cell walls.
9 Culture medium used to enhance the growth of specific bacteria.
11 Antibodies that recognize a single antigen.
12 Biochemical test used to differentiate *Staphyloccocus* spp. from *Streptococcus* spp.

Down
1 The lowest concentration of antimicrobial required to slow bacterial growth. (2 words)
2 Stain used to differentiate bacteria based on the composition of their cell wall.
3 Another name for the Kirby-Bauer susceptibility test. (2 words)
5 Medium that maintains bacteria in original concentrations without encouraging growth or causing death of the bacteria.
6 Biochemical test used to differentiate and identify Gram-negative bacteria.
10 Biochemical test used to differentiate pathogenic *Streptococcus* spp. and nonpathogenic *Streptococcus* spp.

Chapter **15 Clinical Microbiology**

EXERCISE 15.2 TERMS AND DEFINITIONS: INFECTIOUS AGENTS

Instructions: Define each term in your own words.

1. Abscess _____

   _____

2. Aerobe _____

   _____

3. Anaerobe _____

   _____

4. Dermatophyte _____

   _____

5. Fastidious _____

   _____

6. Hemolysis _____

   _____

7. Indigenous flora _____

   _____

8. Nosocomial infection _____

   _____

9. Opportunistic infection _____

   _____

10. Yeast _____

    _____

Instructions: Match each media in column A with its corresponding description in column B by writing the appropriate letter in the space provided.

Column A

1. _____ Blood agar plate

2. _____ Indole test media

3. _____ Hektoen enteric agar

4. _____ Selenite or tetrathionate broth

5. _____ Lysine iron agar slant

6. _____ Brucella blood agar plate

7. _____ Salt mannitol agar

8. _____ Motility media

9. _____ MacConkey agar plate

10. _____ Christensen urea agar slant

11. _____ Citrate test media

12. _____ Triple sugar iron agar slant

Column B

A. For direct isolation of *Salmonella* spp. from feces.

B. For determining whether an organism has and is able to use flagella.

C. This media is used for the primary isolation of organisms and for subculture of organisms.

D. Primary isolation medium for selection of Gram-negative organisms.

E. For determining the ability of organisms to utilize glucose, sucrose, and lactose, and to produce hydrogen sulfide.

F. Media used to enrich samples for the detection of *Salmonella* spp.

G. The results of this test are determined by observing for a purple or port-wine color in the slant and a purple color in the butt.

H. When this biochemical test is positive, the media turns blue, whereas a negative reaction leaves the media green.

I. Primarily used to differentiate species of *Staphylococcus* based on fermentation.

J. These plates provide a rich media for the culture of anaerobic organisms.

K. When this biochemical test is positive, a red color forms within seconds of the addition of the Kovac reagent.

L. A tube medium used to determine whether an organism produces urease.

EXERCISE 15.4 MATCHING #2: GRAM-POSITIVE ORGANISMS

Instructions: Match each Gram-positive organism in column A with the disease that it causes in column B by writing the appropriate letter in the space provided.

Column A

1. _____ *Erysipelothrix rhusiopathiae*

2. _____ *Corynebacterium pseudotuberculosis*

3. _____ *Arcanobacterium pyogenes*

4. _____ *Actinomyces* spp.

5. _____ *Rhodococcus equi*

6. _____ *Bacillus anthracis*

7. _____ *Streptococcus* spp.

8. _____ *Corynebacterium renale*

9. _____ *Staphylococcus pseudointermedius*

10. _____ *Listeria monocytogenes*

Column B

A. A cause of bony lesions of the head and neck of ruminants.

B. A cause of septicemia in neonatal animals, abortion, and encephalitis in ruminants.

C. The cause of anthrax. Classified as a select agent.

D. A cause of the serious zoonosis, necrotizing fasciitis.

E. A cause of pneumonia in foals.

F. Pleomorphic Gram-positive rod. A cause of pyelonephritis in cattle.

G. The cause of caseous lymphadenitis in sheep and goats.

H. A cause of disease in swine, turkeys, and marine mammals, including diamond skin disease.

I. Catalase-positive cocci that are normal inhabitants of the skin of dogs.

J. A Gram-positive rod that is an inhabitant of the skin and mucous membranes of cattle and other ruminants.

EXERCISE 15.5 MATCHING #3: GRAM-NEGATIVE ORGANISMS

Instructions: Match each Gram-negative organism in column A with its corresponding description in column B by writing the appropriate letter in the space provided.

Column A

1. _____ *Escherichia coli*

2. _____ *Proteus* spp.

3. _____ *Actinobacillus* spp.

4. _____ *Bordetella bronchiseptica*

5. _____ *Pasteurella multocida*

6. _____ *Brucella abortus*

7. _____ *Aeromonas* spp.

8. _____ *Salmonella* spp.

Column B

A. A bacterial select agent that is a cause of abortion and reproductive failure in ruminants.

B. An important cause of diarrhea and septicemia in a variety of animal species and commonly isolated from feces of reptiles and amphibians.

C. A cause of infections in aquatic animals, including fish and amphibians.

D. An oxidase-positive, short, fat rod that causes a rapidly progressing cellulitis in people who have been bitten by cats.

E. The causative agent of canine tracheobronchitis.

F. An opportunistic urinary pathogen that swarms on culture plates.

G. Typically grown on MacConkey agar. Often isolated from foals with septicemia or joint infections.

H. An oxidase-negative member of the family Enterobacteriaceae and a cause of opportunistic infections of the urine and wounds.

EXERCISE 15.6 ORDERING: ELISA TEST FOR A VIRAL PROTEIN OR ANTIGEN

Instructions: Match the steps of performing an ELISA antigen test in the proper order by placing the appropriate number (1 through 5) in the space provided.

A. _____ Add an enzyme-labeled secondary antibody to the well or membrane, and incubate as directed.

B. _____ Read the color change.

C. _____ Wash the well or membrane as directed.

D. _____ Place a patient sample in the well or on the membrane, and incubate for the recommended time.

E. _____ Wash the well or membrane, and add the substrate for the enzyme.

EXERCISE 15.7 TRUE OR FALSE: COMPREHENSIVE

Instructions: Read the following statements and write "T" for true or "F" for false in the blanks provided. If a statement is false, correct the statement to make it true.

1. _____ When a patient has an infection, it is best to start the patient on antibiotics right away to treat the infection, and then to collect a sample for culture and sensitivity.

2. _____ When collecting microbiologic samples from an abscess, the purulent material in the abscess (pus) is the best source of material for bacterial culture.

3. _____ Urine samples collected by free-catch typically have bacteria in them from the external genitalia and skin.

4. _____ The stain used specifically to identify *Mycobacterium* spp. is the acid-fast stain.

5. _____ Acid-fast organisms stain dark blue, whereas non-acid-fast organisms and the background should stain pink.

6. _____ Broth is typically used for initial isolation of organisms as opposed to solid agar.

7. _____ Plate media should be incubated overnight, right-side up, at 35° C to 37.5° C.

8. _____ When culturing a sample from a site like the GI tract, you should attempt to identify every organism.

9. _____ The catalase test is most commonly used to differentiate staphylococci from streptococci and enterococci.

10. _____ Gram-negative bacteria in the family Enterobacteriaceae are generally oxidase-positive.

11. _____ The organism *Listeria monocytogenes* is the causative agent of strangles in horses.

12. _____ *Mycobacterium* spp. organisms are often challenging to culture because they sometimes take weeks to grow.

13. _____ The causative agent of Lyme disease is the spirochete *Borrelia burgdorferi*.

14. _____ The yeast *Cryptococcus neoformans* is often present in samples from the respiratory and gastrointestinal tract of birds.

15. _____ The pathogen in question (bacteria or virus) must be cultured and isolated before performing PCR testing.

16. _____ DNA sequencing is a way to definitively identify most organisms.

17. _____ A fomite is an animal that is capable of transmitting a nosocomial agent.

18. _____ A person can get a zoonotic infection from a patient, but a patient cannot get one from a person.

19. _____ Bacteria are the most common cause, and viruses are the second most common cause, of nosocomial infections.

20. _____ *Streptococcus equi* subsp. *equi (S. equi)* is frequently implicated as a nosocomial infection in veterinary patients.

EXERCISE 15.8 MULTIPLE CHOICE: COMPREHENSIVE

Instructions: Circle the one correct answer to each of the following questions.

1. Which fungal agent is designated as a "fungal select agent"?
   a. *Malassezia pachydermatis*
   b. *Blastomyces dermatitidis*
   c. *Candida albicans*
   d. *Sporothrix schenckii*

2. Most anticoagulants will interfere with bacterial culture and so cannot be used when collecting samples for culture. When collecting samples that are at risk for clotting, which of the following anticoagulants may be used because it will not interfere with bacterial culture?
   a. EDTA
   b. Sodium citrate
   c. Polyanethol sulfonate
   d. Lithium heparin

3. Which of the following organisms is a common cause of diarrhea?
   a. *Campylobacter jejuni*
   b. *Pasteurella multocida*
   c. *Bordetella bronchiseptica*
   d. *Brucella abortus*

4. Which of the following samples may be frozen prior to bacterial culture?
   a. Urine
   b. Milk
   c. Joint fluid
   d. Transtracheal wash samples

5. The stain used to identify *Nocardia* spp. is
   a. Gram stain
   b. Hematoxylin-eosin stain
   c. Kinyoun modified Ziehl-Nielsen acid-fast stain
   d. Acid-fast stain

6. MacConkey agar is an example of a
   a. Selective media
   b. Differential media
   c. Enrichment media
   d. Selective and differential media

7. The two media most commonly used for initial inoculation and isolation of bacteria are
   a. Mueller-Hinton and TSA
   b. TSA and MacConkey
   c. MacConkey and blood agar
   d. Blood agar and Mueller-Hinton

8. Gram-negative and Gram-positive organisms are _____ and _____ in color, respectively.
   a. Pink and green
   b. Green and pink
   c. Pink and purple
   d. Purple and pink

9. Coagulase-positive, Gram-positive cocci are generally
   a. Pathogenic *Streptococcus* spp.
   b. *Streptococcus* spp. that are indigenous flora
   c. Pathogenic *Staphylococcus* spp.
   d. *Staphylococcus* spp. that are indigenous flora

10. In addition to *Salmonella, Campylobacter,* and *Clostridium,* another causative agent of diarrhea isolated from fecal culture is
    a. *Mycobacterium avium* subsp. *paratuberculosis*
    b. *Streptococcus agalactia*
    c. *Staphylococcus aureus*
    d. *Pseudomonas aeruginosa*

11. When culturing urine, the colonies must be counted by performing a quantified culture. What other sample must be handled in this manner?
    a. Joint fluid
    b. Cerebral spinal fluid
    c. Blood
    d. Milk

12. Which of the following organisms is an agent of contagious mastitis in cattle?
    a. *Clostridium perfringens*
    b. *Listeria monocytogenes*
    c. *Streptococcus agalactiae*
    d. *Mycoplasma* spp.

13. Which of the following organisms are catalase-negative, Gram-positive cocci that in rare but serious cases cause necrotizing fasciitis?
    a. *Erysipelothrix* spp.
    b. *Streptococcus* spp.
    c. *Bordetella* spp.
    d. *Brucella* spp.

14. The Gram-positive, pleomorphic rod *Corynebacterium pseudotuberculosis* is the cause of

    _____ in sheep and goats.
    a. Diamond skin disease
    b. Pigeon fever
    c. Contagious foot rot
    d. Caseous lymphadenitis

15. Pneumonia in foals is caused by the aerobic, CAMP-positive, Gram-positive rod
    a. *Erysipelothrix rhusiopathiae*
    b. *Rhodococcus equi*
    c. *Actinomyces* spp.
    d. *Clostridium perfringens*

16. The partially acid-fast organisms *Nocardia* spp. appear on microscopic examination as
    a. Seagull-shaped spiral organisms
    b. Short, fat coccobacilli
    c. Rods with a "beaded" appearance
    d. Club-shaped rods

17. An organism that is frequently isolated from fish and amphibians with infections is
    a. *Actinobacillus* spp.
    b. *Rhodococcus equi*
    c. *Campylobacter* spp.
    d. *Aeromonas* spp.

18. The colonies of which organism are often hemolytic on blood agar, secrete a green pigment into the surrounding media, and have a metallic appearance?
    a. *Pseudomonas* spp.
    b. *Escherichia coli*
    c. *Staphylococcus* spp.
    d. *Malassezia* spp.

19. The reproductive pathogens *Brucella* spp. are a group of small, oxidase-positive
    a. Gram-positive rods
    b. Gram-negative coccobacilli
    c. Gram-positive cocci
    d. Gram-positive, spore-forming rods

20. Some important pathogens and GI-indigenous flora are Gram-negative anaerobic rods. Which of the following organisms is not a Gram-negative anaerobic rod?
    a. *Bacteroides* spp.
    b. *Fusobacterium* spp.
    c. *Prevotella* spp.
    d. *Clostridium* spp.

21. Which of the following organisms is a cause of renal disease, abortion, and infertility?
    a. *Leptospira* spp.
    b. *Borrelia burgdorferi*
    c. *Brachyspira hyodysenteriae*
    d. *Campylobacter* spp.

22. The organism *Mycoplasma* spp. is
    a. Gram-positive
    b. Gram-negative
    c. Acid-fast-positive
    d. Not visible on Gram stain

23. Which of the following organisms is *not* an obligate intracellular organism?
    a. *Mycoplasma*
    b. *Neorickettsia*
    c. *Chlamydia*
    d. *Ehrlichia*

24. The McFarland standard is used to
    a. Set hospital policy regarding exposure to infectious agents
    b. Determine which antibiotic to use
    c. Estimate bacterial numbers
    d. Evaluate hemolytic reactions

25. The media used to culture dermatophytes are
    a. Sabouraud dextrose agar and salt mannitol agar
    b. Salt mannitol agar and blood agar
    c. Blood agar and DTM
    d. DTM and Sabouraud dextrose agar

26. The pathogenic yeast that is a common cause of otitis externa is
    a. *Coccidioides immitis*
    b. *Malassezia pachydermatis*
    c. *Blastomyces dermatitidis*
    d. *Cryptococcus neoformans*

27. In the polymerase chain reaction (PCR) test, a series of three steps is repeated approximately 40 times to amplify DNA. Which of the following represents the correct order of these steps?
    a. Annealing, denaturing, extension
    b. Extension, denaturing, annealing
    c. Denaturing, annealing, extension
    d. Annealing, extension, denaturing

Instructions: Fill in each of the spaces provided with the missing word or words that complete the sentence.

1. Bacterial agents that are highly infectious and dangerous to the degree that they have potential use as biologic weapons

   are classified by the government as _____ agents and must be reported to the _____ if identified
   in the lab.

2. When submitting urine for bacterial culture, a minimum of _____ mL should be collected by

   _____ and submitted in a blood tube with a top that is _____ in color.

3. A _____ infection is a local infection that spreads to multiple organs.

4. The part of the bacterium that is different in structure between Gram-negative and Gram-positive organisms, which

   therefore takes up stain differently, is the _____ _____.

5. Partially acid-fast organisms stain the color _____, whereas non–acid-fast organisms and the background

   stain _____.

6. When attempting to identify a bacterium isolated on a culture plate, the first step is to determine its _____

   and _____ as observed on a Gram stain.

7. The catalase test determines the presence or absence of this enzyme based on the ability of a bacterial organism to
   convert _____ to _____ and _____.

8. Hemolytic patterns are used to determine the pathogenicity of *Streptococcus* organisms. *Streptococcus* isolates that

   are indigenous flora are generally _____-hemolytic, whereas pathogenic *Streptococcus* isolates are gen-

   erally _____-hemolytic.

9. Diarrhea caused by *Clostridium perfringens* and *Clostridium difficile* correlates with the presence of toxins rather

   than the presence of the organisms themselves. The toxins are typically detected with a(n) _____ test.

10. Each species of animal has characteristic and unique indigenous flora. Whereas the Gram-positive organism *Staph-*

    ylococcus _____ is a member of the indigenous skin flora of dogs, *Staphylococcus* _____ is
    a normal skin inhabitant in cats and large animals.

11. The Gram-positive, spore-forming rod *Bacillus anthracis* is the causative agent of the dangerous zoonotic disease

    _____ and is classified as a _____ agent by the U.S. government.

12. Members of the family Enterobacteriaceae, such as *Escherichia coli, Klebsiella,* and *Salmonella,* are typically

    oxidase-_____.

13. An organism often associated with progressive infections in people with cat bites is _____ _____.

14. The small, Gram-negative coccobacillus _____ _____ is the causative agent of kennel cough,

    a disease also known as _____ _____.

15. A _____ agar plate is used to perform a disc diffusion susceptibility test.

16. The only fungal cultures that are routinely performed in-house are _____ cultures.

17. A _____ lamp is sometimes used to examine suspect dermatophyte lesions because some of these organisms (<50%) will _____ when exposed to long-wavelength ultraviolet light.

18. Oligonucleotides are short segments of _____ that are used as _____ in the PCR test.

19. An infection that a hospitalized patient acquires from the hospital environment or another patient is called a(n) _____ infection. An infection that a patient is incubating at the time of admission but that becomes apparent while the patient is in the hospital is called a _____-_____ infection.

EXERCISE 15.10 CASE STUDY: PERFORMING A QUANTIFIED URINE CULTURE

Tanya, a 3-year-old female Collie, was presented for urinating in the house. The owner reported that during the previous few days, Tanya urinated in the house several times, and when she was outside to "potty," she would often go four or five times in a row. Physical examination revealed no significant findings. The bladder was empty at the time of the examination. Acute cystitis with a possible bacterial infection was suspected, and urine was collected by cystocentesis for urinalysis, a quantified urine culture, and sensitivity testing. The urine was blood tinged, and the urinalysis indicated the presence of leukocytes, red blood cells, and bacteria. Antibiotics were prescribed for 7 days while waiting for culture results.

1. Explain the procedure used to inoculate a plate for a quantified urine culture using both 1 μL and 10 μL loops.

_____

_____

_____

_____

_____

_____

_____

_____

_____

2. The plates were incubated at 37° C overnight, and the colonies were counted the next day. *Staphylococcus pseudointermedius* was isolated. The 1:1000 plate had approximately 90 colonies, and the 1:100 plate was covered with growth. Calculate the number of colony-forming units found on the 1:1000 plate, and explain the significance of these results.

_____

_____

_____

_____

_____

16 Diagnostic Imaging

LEARNING OBJECTIVES

When you have completed this chapter, you will be able to:

1. Pronounce, define, and spell all the key terms in this chapter.
2. Do the following regarding the production of x-rays:
   - Describe the properties of x-radiation.
   - Describe the parts of the x-ray tube and machine, and discuss the role each part plays in generation of x-radiation.
   - Explain the production of the useful x-ray beam and scatter radiation, and discuss the negative consequences of scatter radiation.
3. Do the following regarding x-ray equipment:
   - Describe the features of and uses for portable, mobile, and stationary x-ray equipment.
4. Do the following regarding image production and exposure factors:
   - Explain how *milliamperage*, *exposure time*, *kilovoltage*, and *focal-film distance* are set to produce a quality diagnostic radiograph.
   - Explain the purpose for a technique chart, and describe the procedure used to formulate a technique chart.
5. Do the following regarding digital radiography:
   - Describe the features, advantages and disadvantages of, and uses for computed radiography and digital radiography equipment.
   - Describe common digital radiography artifacts, including how to identify and prevent each one.
   - Explain the roles of *DICOM*, *PACS*, *RIS*, and *teleradiography* in the production and management of digital radiographs.
6. Do the following regarding image formation with film-screen systems:
   - Explain the principles of image formation using nonscreen x-ray film and film-screen cassette-based systems.
7. Do the following regarding film processing:
   - Discuss the design, features, and organization of an x-ray darkroom.
   - Describe the use and maintenance of the equipment used to process x-ray film, including operation of the automatic processor.
8. Do the following regarding radiographic image quality:
   - Explain how *radiographic density, contrast,* and *detail* are controlled by changing milliamperage and kilovoltage to optimize image quality.
   - Describe types of geometric distortion, like magnification and elongation.
   - List the common technical errors and artifacts and the steps that can be taken to minimize them.
9. List and describe methods for labeling and filing radiographic films.
10. Do the following regarding radiation safety:
    - Describe the hazards of x-radiation, and explain the role of beam filtration in minimizing its damaging effects.
    - Discuss the methods used to monitor x-radiation exposure and the units for measuring radiation.
    - Explain the principles and practices used to minimize exposure to x-radiation, including the use of personal protective equipment (PPE).
11. Explain the principles of patient positioning for radiographic studies, including the importance of appropriate restraint.
12. Do the following regarding radiographic contrast agents:
    - List commonly used positive and negative radiographic contrast agents, and explain how they are used in the production of a diagnostic contrast study.
    - Describe the contrast procedures used to image the gastrointestinal (GI) system, urinary system, and spinal cord.
13. Do the following regarding ultrasonography:
    - Describe the indications for and characteristics of ultrasonography in diagnostic imaging.
    - Describe the basic principles of production of an ultrasound image, including the appearance of various tissues and organs on a finished image.
    - Describe how a patient is prepared for ultrasound imaging and the procedure used to conduct an ultrasound examination.
    - Discuss the equipment used to produce a B-mode, M-mode, or Doppler ultrasound image.
    - Describe the appearance of an ultrasound image, as well as the appearance and cause of common artifacts.
14. Describe indications for and characteristics of therapeutic and diagnostic nuclear medicine, fluoroscopy, computed tomography, and magnetic resonance imaging.

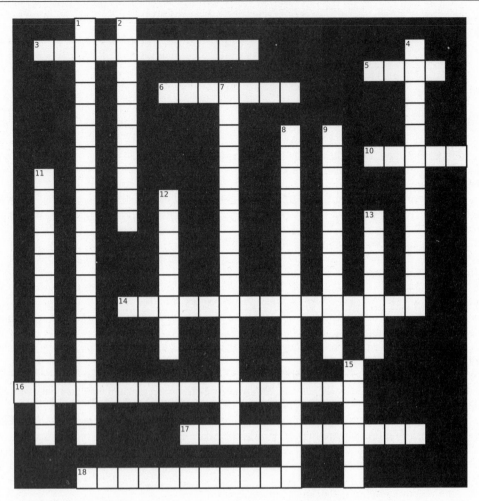

Across

3 The source of the x-ray beam in an x-ray tube. (2 words)
5 A device used to decrease scatter radiation.
6 The general amount of blackness in a radiographic image.
10 Electromagnetic radiation of shorter wavelength than light.
14 The specific type of the part that serves as the source of the x-rays in a dental or portable x-ray machine. (2 words)
16 The distance between the source of the x-rays and the image receptor. (2 words)
17 The range of gray shades, allowing both bone and soft tissues to be seen at the same exposure setting.
18 Weakening of sound waves as they travel through the body.

Down

1 A device used to make grid lines invisible. (2 words)
2 Decrease in the strength of the x-ray beam near the anode. (2 words)
4 The current applied to the cathode filament.
7 The ability to distinguish two adjacent structures on an x-ray image. (2 words)
8 Energy that breaks chemical bonds and damages DNA. (2 words)
9 Controls the speed of travel of the electrons in an x-ray tube.
11 The specific type of the part that serves as the source of the x-rays in a stationary x-ray machine. (2 words)
12 The difference between blacks and whites in a radiographic image.
13 The source of electrons in an x-ray tube.
15 The sharpness of a radiographic image.

EXERCISE 16.2 MATCHING #1: TERMS AND DEFINITIONS

Instructions: Match each term in column A with its corresponding definition in column B by writing the appropriate letter in the space provided.

Column A

1. _____ Anechoic
2. _____ Linear array transducer
3. _____ B-mode
4. _____ Computed radiography
5. _____ DICOM
6. _____ Digital radiography
7. _____ Fluoroscopy
8. _____ Hyperechoic
9. _____ Hz
10. _____ Isoechoic
11. _____ M-mode
12. _____ PACS
13. _____ Rad
14. _____ Rem
15. _____ Teleradiology

Column B

A. A diagnostic technique used to image moving structures.

B. The computer system used to permanently store and transmit digital images to different computer workstations within a single location or between locations.

C. The method of imaging that uses x-rays to view images of anatomy in cross sections.

D. A dark structure on an ultrasound image is said to be _____.

E. A structure that has the same brightness as adjacent structures on an ultrasound image is said to be _____.

F. Used primarily for transrectal reproductive examinations in cattle and horses.

G. A measurement of absorbed radiation that takes into account biologic effectiveness of radiation.

H. A universal digital image format that has allowed for digital images to be shared between different vendors' software.

I. Allows transmission of electronic images across the Internet to referral facilities.

J. Also known as "brightness mode."

K. A structure that produces more echoes than adjacent structures is said to be _____.

L. The unit of absorbed dose of ionizing radiation.

M. A measurement of sound frequency.

N. An imaging technique that doesn't require use of film.

O. An ultrasound display used primarily for echocardiography.

EXERCISE 16.3 MATCHING #2: SCREEN SPEED AND CHARACTERISTICS

Instructions: Match each characteristic in column A with its corresponding screen speed in column B by writing the appropriate letter in the space provided. Note that responses may be used more than once.

Column A

1. _____ Require less radiation.
2. _____ Produce poorer detail.
3. _____ Have larger crystals.
4. _____ Have increased resolution.
5. _____ Also called "detail screens."
6. _____ Best for imaging small exotic animals.
7. _____ Regular screens.

Column B

A. Fast screens

B. Slow screens

C. Intermediate screens

EXERCISE 16.4 MATCHING #3: FACTORS THAT AFFECT RADIOGRAPHIC DENSITY

Instructions: Match each action in column A (assuming no other changes are made) with the way it will affect radiographic density in column B by writing the appropriate letter in the space provided. Note that responses may be used more than once.

Column A

1. _____ Changing the kVp from 50 to 60
2. _____ Changing the object-film distance from 6 inches to 12 inches
3. _____ Changing mA from 300 to 200
4. _____ Changing the exposure time from ½ second to ¼ second
5. _____ Changing from detail screens to fast screens
6. _____ Changing the focal-film distance from 40 inches to 30 inches
7. _____ Removing the grid

Column B

A. Increases radiographic density.

B. Decreases radiographic density.

C. Does not change radiographic density.

EXERCISE 16.5 MATCHING #4: ULTRASOUND ARTIFACTS AND INTERPRETATIONS

Instructions: Match each artifact listed in column A with its corresponding description in column B by writing the appropriate letter in the space provided.

Column A

1. _____ Reverberation artifact
2. _____ Shadowing
3. _____ Acoustic enhancement
4. _____ Edge artifact
5. _____ Mirror-image artifact
6. _____ Slice-thickness artifact

Column B

A. Dark bands at the margins of an early pregnancy vesicle.

B. Caused when the beam encounters intestinal gas.

C. Commonly seen as the duplication of the gallbladder on the far side of the diaphragm.

D. Caused when the beam encounters a bladder stone.

E. The erroneous appearance of debris in the urinary bladder.

F. The tissue deep to the gallbladder appears brighter than adjacent tissue.

EXERCISE 16.6 MATCHING #5: X-RAY RADIOGRAPHIC ARTIFACTS AND TECHNICAL ERRORS

Instructions: Match each of the radiographic technical errors listed in column A with its resulting artifact in column B by writing the appropriate letter in the space provided. Note that each response may be used more than once and that more than one answer may be correct.

Column A

1. _____ mAs or kV setting too high
2. _____ Dirt or debris between the film and screen
3. _____ Focal-film distance too short
4. _____ Contrast medium on tabletop, skin, or cassette
5. _____ mAs or kV setting too low
6. _____ Failure to use a grid
7. _____ Focal-film distance too long
8. _____ Defective cassette that does not close properly, exposing margins of film to light
9. _____ Anatomic part undermeasured
10. _____ Outdated film
11. _____ Crescent mark from rough handling
12. _____ Static electricity
13. _____ Anatomic part overmeasured
14. _____ Grid out of focal range or upside-down
15. _____ Defect or crack in screen
16. _____ Speed of intensifying screen too slow
17. _____ Film exposed to scatter radiation
18. _____ Film stored in hot or humid environment
19. _____ Speed of intensifying screen too fast
20. _____ Gridlines

Column B

A. Increased film density

B. Decreased film density

C. Black marks

D. White marks

E. Gray film (film fog)

F. Parallel lines

EXERCISE 16.7 PHOTO QUIZ: PARTS OF THE X-RAY TUBE

Instructions: Identify each part of an x-ray tube with the appropriate description from the list below by writing the appropriate letter in the space to the left; then name the part by writing the name in the space to the right.

Letter corresponding with the part

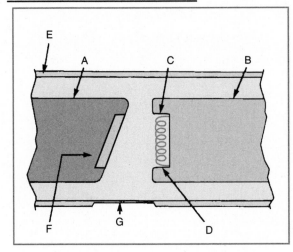

Description: Name of the part

1. _____ The part through which the x-rays exit the tube: _____.

2. _____ This part produces an electron cloud when current is applied: _____.

3. _____ The high-voltage circuit controls the electrical potential between the cathode and this part: _____.

4. _____ The part that encases the other parts of the tube: _____ _____.

5. _____ The x-rays do not emanate from this negatively charged pole: _____.

6. _____ This part directs the electrons toward the anode: _____ _____.

7. _____ The electrons directly impact this part to produce x-rays: _____ _____.

EXERCISE 16.8 TRUE OR FALSE: COMPREHENSIVE

Instructions: Read the following statements and write "T" for true or "F" for false in the blanks provided. If a statement is false, correct the statement to make it true.

1. _____ Radiographs are considered to be a part of a patient's legal medical record.

2. _____ X-rays are a type of electromagnetic radiation with a lower frequency than visible light, radio signals, and TV signals.

3. _____ Rotating anodes are generally used in dental machines and small portable machines.

4. _____ Scatter radiation reduces density.

5. _____ Fluoroscopy is used to study moving structures such as beating of the heart and motility of the esophagus.

6. _____ Computed radiography (CR) and digital radiography (DR) are two names for the same thing.

7. _____ One advantage of digital radiography systems is that they require less radiation to produce a diagnostic image than film/screen systems.

8. _____ CR and DR systems are not as sensitive to under- and overexposures as conventional film/screen systems.

9. _____ A radiology information system (RIS) is a digital imaging device that is used to evaluate blood flow.

10. _____ The exposure time is related to the number of x-ray photons produced—as one goes up, the other does also.

11. _____ Kilovoltage affects radiographic density but not radiographic contrast.

12. _____ The focal-film distance influences radiographic density.

13. _____ A technique chart is used to provide appropriate machine settings and must be custom-made for each machine.

14. _____ If you get new cassettes or get a new processor, your technique chart will not have to be updated as long as the cassettes are exactly the same type and the processor is the same brand.

15. _____ Intensifying screens are very durable and don't need to be replaced as long as they are not damaged.

16. _____ X-ray film and intensifying screens must be matched for proper function.

17. _____ Barium sulfate has a low atomic number and absorbs a small amount of radiation, resulting in increased radiographic opacity.

18. _____ Automatic processors standardize, speed up, and simplify film processing and decrease the required maintenance.

19. _____ X-ray film is more sensitive after exposure and before development than at any other time.

20. _____ Rem is an abbreviation used for the equivalent dose.

21. _____ Film badges should be stored outside of the x-ray room.

22. _____ Technicians should always remember that x-ray effects are cumulative.

23. _____ Myelograms may be performed with the patient awake or anesthetized.

24. _____ Most radiographic studies require only one view.

25. _____ When x-raying large dogs, it may be necessary to use two films per view to image the entire abdomen.

26. _____ Manual restraint of patients for radiographic studies is routine and not a safety concern as long as protective equipment is used.

27. _____ The ultrasound machine transducer both emits the sound and receives reflected waves.

28. _____ When adjacent tissues are very dissimilar in density, little of the ultrasound wave bounces off the tissue interface.

29. _____ Like radiographic artifacts, ultrasound artifacts do not contribute useful information.

30. _____ The most common use for computed tomography (CT) scans in veterinary patients is examination of the central nervous system.

31. _____ Any animal receiving a CT scan should have cotton placed in its ears to protect its hearing from the high decibel noise generated by the CT machine.

Instructions: Circle the one correct answer to each of the following questions.

1. The shorter the wavelength of x-rays,
   a. The greater the energy and the penetration
   b. The greater the energy but the lower the penetration
   c. The lower the energy but the greater the penetration
   d. The lower the energy and the penetration

2. The kilovoltage electrical circuit controls the
   a. Electrical potential across the filament
   b. Number of electrons created
   c. Electrical potential between the cathode and the anode
   d. Number of the x-rays created

3. The "target" in an x-ray tube is the area where the
   a. X-rays impact the anode
   b. Electrons impact the cathode
   c. Electrons impact the anode
   d. X-rays impact the cathode

4. Information regarding the maximum safe exposure time that can be used without damaging the machine may be found on the
   a. Technique chart
   b. Tube rating chart
   c. X-ray log
   d. Safe-operating procedures

5. Which of the following factors does *not* increase scatter radiation?
   a. Thickness of the body part
   b. Size of the x-ray field
   c. Type of cassette
   d. Kilovoltage

6. The three primary machine controls that influence x-ray production are
   a. Focal-film distance, kilovoltage, and milliamperage
   b. Kilovoltage, exposure time, and focal-film distance
   c. Milliamperage, exposure time, and kilovoltage
   d. Milliamperage, focal-film distance, and exposure time

7. Which of the following x-ray machines usually has a maximum mA output of 300 to 2000 and a maximum kVp output of 100 to 150?
   a. Dental machine-ray unit
   b. Portable machine-ray unit
   c. Mobile machine-ray unit
   d. Stationary machine-ray unit

8. Which type of unit is used to image the changing diameter of the trachea during inspiration and expiration?
   a. Mobile
   b. Portable
   c. Fluoroscope
   d. Stationary

9. Dynamic range refers to which of the following image characteristics?
   a. Range of sharpness
   b. Size
   c. General amount of blackness
   d. Number of shades of gray

10. A photostimulable phosphor plate is used to capture the image in the following type of x-ray system:
    a. Computed radiography
    b. Digital radiography
    c. Film/screen
    d. Nonscreen film

11. A digital artifact called Uberschwinger artifact appears as
    a. A grainy appearance to the image
    b. Black spots or dots on the image
    c. Loss of part of the image
    d. A lucent halo around metal implants

12. A universal format or standard for digital image storage, display, manipulation, and retrieval is
    a. DICOM
    b. PACS
    c. RIS
    d. ALARA

13. A computerized system used to move, transmit, and store digital images is
    a. LAN
    b. PACS
    c. RIS
    d. ALARA

14. The images from which of the following digital modalities must be viewed on a high-resolution monitor because the images are inherently high resolution and so require this type of monitor?
    a. Computed tomography
    b. Magnetic resonance imaging
    c. Ultrasound
    d. Digital radiography

15. If the kilovoltage setting is increased,
    a. The radiographic density and contrast will increase
    b. The radiographic density will increase but the contrast will decrease
    c. The radiographic density will decrease but the contrast will increase
    d. The radiographic density and contrast will decrease

16. As compared with screen film, nonscreen film
    a. Produces images with less detail
    b. Cannot be used for intraoral dental studies
    c. Requires a much longer exposure time to get a diagnostic image
    d. Requires the use of expensive cassettes

17. When compared with calcium tungstate, rare earth screens
    a. Require less radiation and emit green light
    b. Require less radiation and emit blue light
    c. Require more radiation and emit green light
    d. Require more radiation and emit blue light

18. The light- and x-ray-sensitive granules in the emulsion of x-ray film are usually made of
    a. Calcium tungstate
    b. Molybdenum
    c. Silver bromide
    d. Carbon fiber

19. The primary purpose of a grid is to
    a. Decrease the settings needed
    b. Minimize distortion
    c. Decrease radiation exposure
    d. Control scatter radiation

20. Grids are placed
    a. Above the patient
    b. Between the tube and the table
    c. Between the patient and the cassette
    d. Under the cassette

21. A grid should be used when x-raying body parts that are
    a. More than 5 cm thick
    b. Less than 10 cm thick
    c. More than 10 cm thick
    d. More than 20 cm thick

22. Silver can be recovered from
    a. X-ray film and fixer solution
    b. Fixer solution and developer solution
    c. Developer solution and rinse water
    d. Rinse water and x-ray film

23. Radiographic detail is improved by
    a. Using a larger focal spot
    b. Increasing the exposure time
    c. Decreasing the focal-film distance
    d. Minimizing the object-film distance

24. Low-contrast radiographs have many shades of gray. Low contrast is preferred for
    a. Spinal radiographs
    b. Thoracic radiographs
    c. Tibial radiographs
    d. Carpal radiographs

25. The machine setting that has the greatest influence on radiographic contrast is
    a. Milliamperage
    b. Exposure time
    c. Focal-film distance
    d. Kilovoltage

26. A "rad" is a measure of the
    a. Biologic effect of the radiation
    b. Absorbed dose of x-ray energy/unit mass of tissue
    c. Machine output
    d. Maximum permissible dose

27. The small animal abdominal organ which is the least echogenic is which of the following?
    a. Prostate
    b. Liver
    c. Renal medulla
    d. Spleen

28. The maximum permissible dose (MPD) is the dose of radiation a person is allowed to receive from occupational exposure over a certain time. The annual MPD for occupational personnel is
    a. 0.03 Sv/year
    b. 0.05 Sv/year
    c. 0.10 Sv/year
    d. 0.15 Sv/year

29. Protective equipment including aprons, thyroid shields, and gloves should have _____ mm lead equivalent minimum.
    a. 0.25
    b. 0.5
    c. 1
    d. 2

30. Barium sulfate is contraindicated
    a. If bowel perforation is suspected
    b. For esophageal studies
    c. For upper GI exams
    d. For lower GI exams

31. Soluble, radiopaque ionic contrast media should not be used for
    a. Esophageal studies
    b. Upper GI studies
    c. Cystography
    d. Myelography

169

32. Which of the following contrast studies requires that images be taken right after barium sulfate contrast is given and also 15, 30, and 60 minutes after contrast administration?
    a. Positive-contrast cystogram
    b. Upper gastrointestinal series
    c. Barium enema
    d. Myelogram

33. An intravenous pyelogram (IVP) or excretory urogram is used to evaluate the urinary system. This study involves
    a. Administration of barium sulfate intravenously
    b. Administration of air in the bladder
    c. Intravenous administration of an ionic organic iodide
    d. Infusion of an ionic organic iodide into the bladder

34. An ultrasound echo is produced whenever the ultrasound beam crosses a boundary between two tissues of differing acoustic impedance (opposition to flow of the beam). The main factor that influences acoustic impedance is the
    a. Speed of the sound
    b. Density of the tissue
    c. Intensity of the sound
    d. Frequency of the sound

35. Which ultrasound display mode has little value in performing abdominal or cardiac exams and therefore is not used?
    a. A mode
    b. B mode
    c. M mode
    d. Doppler mode

36. M mode ultrasound is used primarily for
    a. Abdominal ultrasonography
    b. Pregnancy exams
    c. Large animal tendon exams
    d. Echocardiography

37. Linear array ultrasound transducers are not particularly useful for examination of the
    a. Bladder from a transabdominal approach
    b. Heart from an intercostal approach
    c. Small animal uterus from a transabdominal approach
    d. Large animal reproductive tract from a transrectal approach

38. The most appropriate transducer frequency for an ultrasound exam on a cat is
    a. 7.5 MHz
    b. 5 MHz
    c. 3 MHz
    d. 1 MHz

39. A structure on an ultrasound image that is brighter than an adjacent structure is said to be _____ in relation to the adjacent structure.
    a. Anechoic
    b. Echogenic
    c. Isoechoic
    d. Hyperechoic

40. Ultrasound cannot be used to image which of the following tissues?
    a. Liver
    b. Heart
    c. Brain
    d. Blood vessels

41. What alternative modality is used to treat thyroid tumors?
    a. Magnetic resonance imaging
    b. Nuclear medicine
    c. Computed tomography
    d. Ultrasonography

42. The substance technetium-99m is an agent used to perform which of the following examinations?
    a. Magnetic resonance imaging
    b. Nuclear medicine imaging
    c. Computed tomography
    d. Ultrasonography

43. Which alternative imaging technique produces an image by using a thin x-ray beam to measure x-ray attenuation?
    a. Magnetic resonance imaging
    b. Nuclear medicine imaging
    c. Computed tomography
    d. Ultrasonography

44. Some computed tomography scanners have a "helical scan mode." What is the chief advantage of this capability?
    a. It requires less radiation.
    b. It produces a better image.
    c. It does not require the patient to be still.
    d. It is faster.

45. Both magnetic resonance imaging (MRI) and computed tomography (CT) create cross-sectional views of the patient's anatomy. What is the primary difference between MRI and CT scanning in terms of the way they work?
    a. MRI does not use ionizing radiation.
    b. CT does not use x-rays.
    c. CT uses radio waves.
    d. MRI uses radionuclides.

46. Which of the following alternate imaging modalities involves use of a strong magnetic field?
    a. Magnetic resonance imaging
    b. Nuclear medicine imaging
    c. Computed tomography
    d. Ultrasonography

47. Which of the following scans are usually performed once without contrast and again with contrast?
    a. Magnetic resonance imaging (MRI) and nuclear medicine
    b. Nuclear medicine and ultrasound
    c. Ultrasound and computed tomography (CT)
    d. CT and MRI

EXERCISE 16.10 FILL-IN-THE-BLANK: COMPREHENSIVE

Instructions: Fill in each of the spaces provided with the missing word or words that complete the sentence.

1. Information that must be on a diagnostic radiograph, in addition to the name of the facility where the study was taken, includes the name of the _____, the name of the _____ (or the patient ID #), and the _____.

2. There are two electrical circuits in an x-ray machine. The high voltage circuit (also known as the _____ circuit) controls the penetration of the x-ray beam. The low voltage circuit (also known as the _____ circuit) controls the number of the x-rays created.

3. A cathode with a larger filament produces a larger electron beam and thus decreases the _____ of the image.

4. Rotating anodes have a "two-step" exposure switch. When the first step is activated, the anode starts _____, and when the second step is activated, _____ are produced.

5. Most of the energy generated by the electrons impacting the anode target is converted into heat. In fact, _____% of the energy is lost as heat, and _____% of the energy is converted to x-ray energy.

6. Scatter radiation is undesirable because it _____ film quality and _____ exposure of personnel.

7. Severe underexposure of a digital image receptor will result in a finished image with a grainy appearance, an effect known as _____ _____ or "noise."

8. When a digital image is overexposed, thin parts of the body may appear _____ in color and will never be visible, not even after the image density and contrast are adjusted.

9. If dust, hair, or other particles are trapped in a CR cassette, spots will be visible on the finished image that are _____ in color.

10. The exposure factors that must be set on any x-ray machine regardless of age or type are _____, _____, and _____ _____.

11. When milliamperage (mA) is increased, radiographic density increases or, in other words, the image gets _____. Conversely, when mA is decreased, radiographic density decreases, or the image gets _____.

12. When kilovoltage (kV) is increased, radiographic density _____. This is because the x-rays produced are more penetrating.

13. The effect of focal-film distance on the number of x-rays reaching the image receptor is governed by the "inverse square law." This law predicts that if the focal-film distance is doubled, the number of x-rays reaching the receptor will be reduced by a factor of _____.

14. Grids should be used for tissues that are greater than _____ cm in thickness.

15. The term *screen speed* refers to the ability of an intensifying screen to convert absorbed _____ energy into _____.

16. The artifact produced by using old intensifying screens, which appears as a white speckled pattern, is known as _____ _____.

17. Screen x-ray film is sensitive primarily to _____, whereas nonscreen film is more sensitive to _____.

18. Grids absorb part of the primary x-ray beam and thus require the use of _____ machine settings to produce a given film density.

19. A Potter-Bucky diaphragm moves the grid across the film during the exposure so that the _____ _____ are not visible.

20. When a grid is used, the exposure settings must be increased to compensate for the radiation absorbed by the grid. Either exposure time should be increased by a factor of _____, or the kilovoltage must be increased _____%.

21. The primary machine setting that affects radiographic density is _____.

22. In recent years, the old units of measurement of radiation have been replaced by international units. The "rad" has been replaced by the _____, and the "rem" has been replaced by the _____.

23. Positive-contrast agents _____ radiographic opacity, whereas negative-contrast agents _____ radiographic opacity.

24. Carbon dioxide is preferred over room air as a contrast agent because it is less likely to cause _____ _____, a serious, sometimes fatal, complication.

25. When a GI perforation is suspected, ionic or nonionic organic _____ should be used.

26. A lower gastrointestinal positive contrast study is also known as a _____ enema.

27. The frequency of the ultrasound waves emitted by a transducer is used to rate the output. Most transducers have an output of 2.5 to 12 megahertz (MHz). 1 Hertz (Hz) = 1 _____ per _____. Because the prefix "mega" means "million," a 5 MHz transducer emits sound at a frequency of _____ cycles/second.

28. The ultrasound transducer emits sound waves approximately _____% of the time and receives reflected waves approximately _____% of the time.

29. An ultrasound beam is weakened or _____ by absorption, reflection, scattering, refraction, and diffraction.

30. Ultrasound cannot be used to image through bone or gas because _____% of the beam is reflected off of a fat–bone interface, and 100% of the beam is reflected off of a _____-_____ interface.

31. A patient receiving an ultrasound examination of the abdomen should be placed in lateral or _____ recumbency, and a patient receiving a cardiac examination should be placed in lateral or _____ recumbency.

32. The ultrasound transducer should be oriented in relationship to the animal's body such that when acquiring a sagittal view, the patient's head should appear on the _____ side of the screen, and when acquiring a transverse view, the patient's left side should appear on the _____ side of the screen.

33. Electromagnetic radiation that originates from radionuclides is referred to as _____ radiation.

EXERCISE 16.11 CASE STUDY #1: DEVELOPING A TECHNIQUE CHART

The practice you work for has purchased a new x-ray machine. The decision was made to delay changing to a digital image-receptor system for a few years, so for now, you are going to be using a rare earth film/screen image-receptor system that the practice bought a few years ago until the upgrade to digital occurs. The doctor has asked you to develop a technique chart for this new x-ray machine.

1. Answer the following questions regarding the steps you will take to develop a variable kVp technique chart for the canine abdomen by following the principles outlined in this chapter.

   a. What machine setting must be checked prior to developing the chart?

   _____

   _____

   b. What would you do to prepare the automatic processor prior to starting?

   _____

   _____

   c. What characteristics would you look for in the animal that would be used for the trial exposures?

   _____

   _____

   d. What kVp setting would you select for the trial exposure?

   _____ kVp

   e. It is suggested that you use a setting of 7.5 mAs. The machine you are using has mA stations of 100, 200, and 300. What mA and exposure time settings would you choose to arrive at the desired mAs? Express the exposure time in seconds, in milliseconds, and as a fraction.

   Milliamperage: _____ mA

   Exposure time: _____ seconds

_____ milliseconds

_____ (expressed as a fraction)

f. You have chosen an animal with a ventrodorsal measurement of 15 cm and a lateral measurement of 15 cm for the trial exposures. The first trial exposure of the ventrodorsal view is overexposed. What kVp setting should you choose for the second trial exposure?

_____ kVp

g. The second trial exposure is slightly overexposed. What kVp setting should you choose for the third trial exposure?

_____ kVp

h. The third trial exposure is optimum in density. Fill out the chart (on the next page) with the settings for this view and thickness.

i. The first trial exposure of the lateral view is also overexposed. What kVp setting should you choose for the second trial exposure?

_____ kVp

j. The second trial exposure is slightly underexposed. What kVp setting should you choose for the third trial exposure?

_____ kVp

k. The third trial exposure is optimum in density. Fill out the chart (on the next page) with the settings for this view and thickness.

l. Continue to fill in the chart (on the next page) according to the principles indicated in the chapter.

CANINE or FELINE Kodak Lanex Medium Rare Earth Screens and T MAT L Film	ABDOMEN _____ mA _____ ms _____ mAs GRID: YES	
	kVp	
CM Thickness	**VD**	**LAT**
8		
9		
10		
11		
12		
13		
14		
15		
16		
17		
18		
19		
20		
21		
22		
23		
24		
25		
26		
27		
28		
29		
30		

EXERCISE 16.12 CASE STUDY #2: MINIMIZING RADIATION EXPOSURE

Your first job following graduation is as a veterinary technician in a small animal practice. This is a busy multiple doctor practice, and you are responsible for acquiring approximately 10 to 15 sets of x-rays a day. As any good technician, you are concerned about your safety and are eager to follow protection practices to minimize your exposure to ALARA (as low as reasonably achievable). While in school you had committed them to memory and thus want to recall these practices in anticipation of minimizing your risk. Review the practices as they relate to each of the following areas.

a. Collimation

_____

b. Filter

_____

c. Prevent retakes

_____

d. Exposure to the primary beam

_____

e. Use of protective equipment

_____

f. Use of accessory equipment to position the patient

_____

g. Use of chemical restraint

_____

h. Restrictions on personnel involved in the procedure

_____

i. Positioning your body while restraining the patient to limit exposure

_____

Other Important Principles:

j. Avoid dose creep

_____

k. Use fast screens

_____

l. Calibrate regularly

_____

m. Follow state radiation safety codes

_____

17 Basic Necropsy Procedures

When you have completed this chapter, you will be able to:
1. Pronounce, define, and spell all of the key terms in this chapter.
2. List and discuss the indications for a necropsy.
3. Explain how to write a necropsy report, including how to describe lesions.
4. Discuss sample collection for laboratory testing, including the uses for the following collections: fixed tissue, fresh tissue, swabs, and whole blood, serum, fluids, and feces. In addition, perform rabies procedure.
5. Discuss the importance of correctly shipping diagnostic specimens.
6. Describe the facilities, instruments, and supplies needed to perform a necropsy, including protective clothing.
7. Do the following regarding the necropsy procedure for a small mammal:
   - Describe how to open the carcass.
   - Explain the principles of preliminary and external examination of the carcass.
   - Describe the initial steps of a necropsy dissection, including reflection of the skin and limbs, and examination of superficial organs and body cavities.
   - Describe the steps for dissection and examination of the skull and brain, neck and thoracic viscera, abdominal cavity, female and male urogenital tracts, abdominal aorta, rectum, and anal glands, vertebral column, and spinal cord.
   - Outline all of the steps for an entire necropsy procedure.
8. Do the following with regard to necropsy variations:
   - Describe variations in necropsy procedure specific to ruminants, horses, and pigs, as well as to fetuses, birds, and laboratory animals.
   - Explain the differences between a complete necropsy and a cosmetic necropsy.

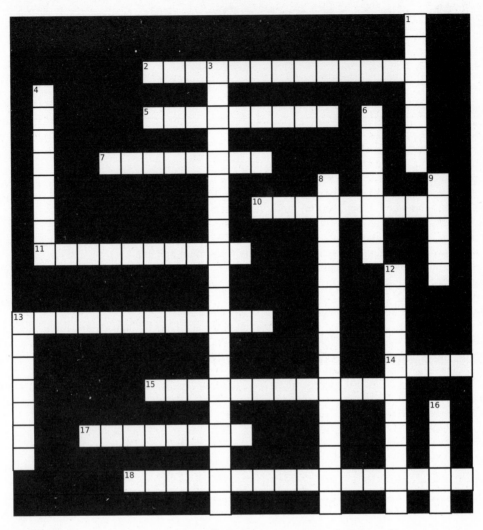

Across

2 The spinal cord exits the skull here. (2 words)
5 Contraction of the _____ causes air to be drawn into the lungs.
7 This structure is located between the stomach and the jejunum.
10 The master gland.
11 The _____ becomes diseased in cardiomyopathy.
13 You must be careful to avoid this structure when giving an IM injection in the rear limb. (2 words)
14 The second cervical vertebra.
15 All parts of the ruminant stomach except for the abomasum.
17 Membranes between the brain and calvarium.
18 The tricuspid valve is an _____ valve.

Down

1 Attachment sites within the hoof.
3 Collective term for the bones of the appendages. (2 words)
4 A cow's true stomach.
6 Part of the mesentery.
8 Takes deoxygenated blood to the lungs. (2 words)
9 The _____ bones have to be cut to remove the tongue and larynx.
12 Contains the trachea, esophagus, and heart inside the chest.
13 Attaches to the ventral aspect of the ribs.
16 A neck bone that is one half of the atlantooccipital joint.

EXERCISE 17.2 DEFINITIONS: KEY TERMS

Instructions: Define each term in your own words.

1. Necropsy: _____

_____

2. Prosector: _____

_____

3. Pathology: _____

_____

4. Gross pathology: _____

_____

5. Histopathology: _____

_____

6. Pathogenesis: _____

_____

7. Lesions: _____

_____

8. Autolysis: _____

_____

9. In situ: _____

_____

10. Hydronephrosis: _____

_____

EXERCISE 17.3 MATCHING: INSTRUMENTS AND SUPPLIES USED FOR A NECROPSY

Instructions: Match each instrument or supply in column A with its corresponding use in column B by writing the appropriate letter in the space provided.

Column A

1. _____ Stryker saw
2. _____ Pruning shears
3. _____ String
4. _____ Tissue cassettes
5. _____ Clip-on laundry tags
6. _____ Screw-top plastic containers containing formalin
7. _____ Sealable, plastic bags and plastic vials
8. _____ Meat cutter's band saw

Column B

A. To hold small tissues

B. To hold refrigerated and frozen samples

C. To cut ribs

D. To hold tissues for histopathology

E. To close off bowel ends

F. To remove the brain

G. To remove the spinal cord in a horse

H. To identify tissues

EXERCISE 17.4 ORDERING: PERFORMING A NECROPSY

Instructions: To perform a complete necropsy, 36 steps must be followed that can be grouped in the following categories:

1. *Examination of external and superficial structures*
2. *Examination of the body cavities*
3. *Examination of the head and CNS*
4. *Examination of the thoracic viscera*
5. *Examination of the abdominal viscera*
6. *Final steps*

Within each category, place the steps of performing a complete necropsy in the proper order from first to last by placing the appropriate number (1, 2, 3, etc.) in the space provided.

1. **Examination of external and superficial structures** *(steps 1 through 7)*

   A. _____ Dissect and examine, section, and collect skin, lymph nodes, salivary glands, and testes or mammary glands.

   B. _____ Remove the eyes.

   C. _____ Dissect and examine, section, and collect the synovium, skeletal muscle, sciatic nerve, and bone marrow.

   D. _____ Make a midline skin incision, reflect the limbs, and extend the incision rostrally to the mandibular symphysis and caudally to the perineum.

   E. _____ Weigh the animal.

   F. _____ Open the coxofemoral, stifle, and scapulohumeral joints.

   G. _____ Perform an external examination.

2. **Examination of the body cavities** *(steps 8 through 13)*

   A. _____ Dissect and examine, section, and collect thyroid, parathyroid, and adrenal glands.

   B. _____ Examine organs and vascular structures.

   C. _____ Remove the tongue from the oral cavity, and reflect the tongue, tonsils, larynx, and esophagus caudally.

   D. _____ Open the chest by cutting the ribs.

   E. _____ Open the abdomen on the midline and puncture the diaphragm.

   F. _____ Open the pericardium.

3. **Examination of the head and CNS** *(steps 14 through 19)*

A. _____ Transect the cranial nerves, and remove the brain and the pituitary gland.

B. _____ Cut the spinal cord and vertebral column at atlantooccipital joint.

C. _____ Section the head longitudinally and examine nasal and oral cavities.

D. _____ Cut the calvaria and remove the caudal-dorsal portion of the calvaria and dorsal meninges.

E. _____ Open the tympanic bullae.

F. _____ Remove skin and muscle from calvaria.

4. **Examination of the thoracic viscera** *(steps 20 through 24)*

A. _____ Section the lungs, saving one section from each lobe.

B. _____ Remove the tongue, tonsils, esophagus, trachea, lungs, heart, and thoracic aorta as a unit.

C. _____ Serially section the tongue.

D. _____ Examine, weigh, and collect sections of the heart.

E. _____ Open the esophagus and trachea.

5. **Examination of the abdominal viscera** *(steps 25 through 31)*

A. _____ Serial section the spleen.

B. _____ Weigh, section, and collect samples from the liver.

C. _____ Remove the distal duodenum, jejunum, ileum, colon, and mesenteric lymph nodes as a unit.

D. _____ Open the gallbladder and collect samples from the stomach, duodenum, and pancreas.

E. _____ Open the stomach and duodenum.

F. _____ Express the gallbladder.

G. _____ Remove the liver, duodenum, pancreas, stomach, and spleen as a unit.

6. **Final steps** *(steps 32 through 36)*

A. _____ Remove the spinal cord if necessary.

B. _____ Remove the floor of pelvis.

C. _____ Dissect and examine, section, and collect the small intestine, colon, and mesenteric lymph nodes.

D. _____ Dissect and examine, section, and collect tissues from all parts of the urogenital system.

E. _____ Dissect and examine, section, and collect tissues from the rectum, anal glands, and abdominal aorta.

EXERCISE 17.5 TRUE OR FALSE: COMPREHENSIVE

Instructions: Read the following statements and write "T" for true or "F" for false in the blanks provided. If a statement is false, correct the statement to make it true.

1. _____ A body may either be frozen or refrigerated between death and the necropsy to prevent degeneration of tissues.

2. _____ Ten percent buffered formalin is a carcinogen and so should not contact skin.

3. _____ Tissues, fluids, and stomach contents that are being tested for toxins may be frozen.

4. _____ When sending in tissues for histopathologic examination, the excess formalin in the bottle should never be removed until the tissues arrive at the lab, or tissue artifacts will result.

5. _____ Formalin-fixed material should be refrigerated and then kept on ice until arrival at the lab.

6. _____ When performing a necropsy on a dog, cat, horse, or cow, the patient should be placed in right lateral recumbency.

7. _____ Unlike other soft tissues, the brain should not be sectioned until it is thoroughly fixed.

8. _____ The heart is removed from the thoracic cavity separately from the lungs and other viscera.

9. _____ Fluid content of the lungs can be assessed by gently squeezing them.

10. _____ After removing but before slicing each kidney, the capsule should be peeled off.

11. _____ As with other animals, a fetus should be placed in left lateral recumbency.

12. _____ Birds have only a left ovary.

13. _____ The lungs should be inflated with formalin before the lungs and heart are removed from the thorax in small rodents (mice, hamsters, and gerbils).

14. _____ Sample collection for prion diseases is sometimes necessary in any large animal.

15. _____ Transmissible spongiform encephalopathies (TSE) are caused by abnormal prions.

EXERCISE 17.6 MULTIPLE CHOICE: COMPREHENSIVE

Instructions: Circle the one correct answer to each of the following questions.

1. When preserving most tissues for histopathology, which of the following fixatives should be used?
   a. 10% buffered formalin, with a fixative to tissue ratio of 10:1 by volume
   b. 50% buffered formalin with a fixative to tissue ratio of 10:1 by volume
   c. 10% buffered formalin with a fixative to tissue ratio of 1:10 by volume
   d. 50% buffered formalin with a fixative to tissue ratio of 1:10 by volume

2. Ten percent buffered formalin is made by mixing dibasic anhydrous sodium phosphate and monobasic sodium phosphate with
   a. Three parts water and one part 37% to 40% formaldehyde solution
   b. Nine parts 50% formalin and one part 37% to 40% formaldehyde solution
   c. Nine parts water and one part 37% to 40% formaldehyde solution
   d. One part 50% formalin and nine parts 37% to 40% formaldehyde solution

3. Fifty percent formalin is made by mixing
   a. One part water and one part 37% to 40% formaldehyde solution
   b. One part 10% formalin and one part 37% to 40% formaldehyde solution
   c. One part water and one part 10% formalin
   d. One part 10% formalin and five parts 37% to 40% formaldehyde solution

4. Some tissues should be preserved in Bouin fixative, because it produces less tissue shrinkage and better preservation of cellular detail. Which of the following tissues should be preserved in Bouin fixative?
   a. Brain
   b. Liver
   c. Eyes
   d. Lung

5. To avoid decomposition, a complete necropsy should begin with dissection of the
   a. Lungs
   b. Liver
   c. Brain
   d. Eyes

6. Once removed, the interior of the eye can be examined by immersion in
   a. Alcohol
   b. Bouin fixative
   c. Cool water
   d. 10% formalin

7. When performing a complete necropsy on a dog or cat, some joints should be routinely opened and examined. Which of the following joints should be examined in this way?
   a. Stifle joint
   b. Elbow joint
   c. Carpal joints
   d. Metacarpal–phalangeal joints

8. A "Stryker saw" is typically used to
   a. Cut the ribs
   b. Open the joints
   c. Open the calvaria
   d. Cut the hyoid bones

9. When examining the spinal cord, a dorsal laminectomy must be performed by cutting the laminae of each vertebra with bone shears or a Stryker saw. Which cervical vertebrae are more difficult to cut than the others?
   a. The sixth and seventh
   b. The first and last
   c. The fourth and fifth
   d. The first and second

10. When performing a necropsy on very small birds such as hummingbirds and finches
    a. The same technique should be used as with other birds
    b. The entire body should be put in a formalin jar undissected
    c. The body cavities should be opened before placing the body in the formalin jar
    d. The body should be sectioned into two halves before fixing it

11. In very small mammals, such as mice, hamsters, and gerbils,
    a. The entire vertebral canal with the spinal cord inside should be removed
    b. The spinal cord should be removed as for a dog or cat
    c. The spinal cord should be removed from the vertebral canal after the vertebral column is separated from the rest of the body
    d. The spinal cord should be removed by performing a dorsal laminectomy

12. A cosmetic necropsy is appropriate
    a. As an alternative to a complete necropsy
    b. When the disease is limited to the abdomen and chest
    c. When the cause of death is known before beginning
    d. When tissues do not need to be collected

13. Samples for prion disease surveillance should be
    a. Fixed in Bouin fixative
    b. Frozen
    c. Refrigerated
    d. Fixed in formalin

14. Prions are classified as
    a. Viruses
    b. Bacteria
    c. Proteins
    d. Parasites

15. A transmissible spongiform encephalopathy of sheep is
    a. Chronic wasting disease
    b. Scrapie
    c. BSE
    d. Creutzfeldt–Jakob disease

EXERCISE 17.7 FILL-IN-THE-BLANK: COMPREHENSIVE

Instructions: Fill in each of the spaces provided with the missing word or words that complete the sentence.

1. It is important to perform a necropsy as soon as possible after death to avoid _____.

2. The fixative 50% formalin is specifically used for the following tissues: (a) _____, (b) _____, _____, and (c) _____.

3. Tissues for virus isolation must be collected aseptically to prevent contamination and either refrigerated in a sterile container or immersed in sterile _____ buffered _____ and preserved by freezing, although fresh, refrigerated tissue immersed in _____ _____ medium is the preferred method of tissue submission.

4. Paired organs can be cut on different planes to distinguish them. When harvesting tissue from the kidneys, to differentiate one from the other, the left kidney should be cut _____ and the right one should be cut _____.

5. Organs removed during a necropsy should be measured and/or weighed if they have an abnormal _____ or _____.

6. To free the tongue, larynx, pharynx, trachea, and esophagus, the _____ bones must be cut.

7. Patency of the bile duct can be determined by squeezing the _____.

8. The ureters should be opened and examined if they or the renal pelvis are _____.

9. Ruminoreticular contents should be examined for _____ objects and undesirable _____ material.

10. When performing a necropsy in a horse and dissecting the head and neck, special attention should be given to the _____, _____, and the _____ veins.

11. Because enteric diseases occur frequently in pigs, attention should be focused on the _____ system.

12. The gestational age of a large animal fetus can be estimated by _____ or _____ it.

EXERCISE 17.8 CASE STUDY: PERFORMING A NECROPSY ON A RABIES SUSPECT

Signalment: 8-year-old, castrated, male Labrador Retriever mix

History: The patient exhibits acute onset of progressive neurologic disease (seizures, ataxia, cranial nerve abnormalities, and a change in behavior) and an elevated body temperature. The patient had not seen a veterinarian in the 2 years prior to admission, and routine vaccinations, including the rabies vaccination, are 6 months overdue.

A basic diagnostic workup (blood work, parasite screen, urinalysis, and x-rays) did not reveal a cause of the neurologic illness. Over the next few days, despite supportive treatment, the neurologic signs continued to progress. Three days after presentation, in view of the severity of the condition and the significant expense that would be necessary to continue with the workup and treatment, the owners elected euthanasia and requested a necropsy. Although this patient had no known exposure to a potentially rabid animal, and a number of other differentials were being considered, infection with rabies virus could not be ruled out.

When performing a necropsy on a rabies suspect such as this patient, precautions must be taken by the prosector. Answer the following questions about the precautions you would take if involved in the necropsy of this patient.

1. Should restrictions be placed on which hospital personnel are permitted to handle this patient antemortem, handle the body postmortem, and participate in the necropsy? If so, what are they?

   _____

   _____

   _____

   _____

   _____

   _____

2. It is decided that you meet the criteria to assist the doctor with the necropsy. What protective equipment should you use to minimize the risk of transmission?

   _____

   _____

   _____

   _____

   _____

   _____

3. What tissue or other sample is needed to test this patient for rabies, and how is it harvested?

   _____

   _____

   _____

   _____

   _____

   _____

4. How should the tissue sample be prepared and stored between harvesting and transport to the lab?

_____

_____

_____

5. How should the carcass be handled after completion of the necropsy?

_____

_____

_____

6. How should the table, instruments, and other equipment be cleaned?

_____

_____

_____

18 Diagnostic Sampling and Therapeutic Techniques

LEARNING OBJECTIVES

When you have completed this chapter, you will be able to:

1. Pronounce, define, and spell all the key terms in this chapter.
2. List and describe general guidelines for the collection of samples for laboratory testing, exhibit proficiency in the administration of medication in the small animal:
   - Describe indications and methods for administration of medication to cats and dogs using each of the following approaches: oral, orogastric, transdermal, ophthalmic, aural, intrarectal, intranasal, intradermal, subcutaneous, intramuscular, intravenous, intratracheal, intraosseous, and intraperitoneal.
   - Compare and contrast placement of IV catheters in the peripheral and jugular veins in cats and dogs. Describe the specific steps to carry out placement of through-the-needle (TTN), over-the-needle (OTN), and multilumen catheters.
3. Compare and contrast patient preparation, positioning, and procedures for blood collection using venipuncture and arterial blood sampling techniques.
4. List and describe procedures for collection of urine samples in cats and dogs, including advantages and limitations of each method.
5. Describe the indications, materials needed, and procedures for performing fecal sample collection, thoracocentesis, and abdominocentesis.
6. Describe diagnostic peritoneal lavage (DPL), and list its indications and contraindications. Compare and contrast percutaneous and endotracheal lavage techniques.
7. Define arthrocentesis, and list indications for performing it in the cat or the dog. List materials needed, and explain the procedure.
8. Explain the procedure of collecting bone marrow aspirate samples, including indications, contraindications, and potential complications. Compare and contrast the procedure if the sample is obtained from the ilium, humerus, or femur, and explain how the procedure of fine-needle aspiration differs.
9. Describe the methods of orally administering medication to large animal species.
10. Compare and contrast the procedures for administering large volumes of medication via nasogastric tubes in the horse and orogastric tubes in ruminants and swine.
11. Do the following regarding intravenous administration of medication in the large animal:
    - Describe the procedure for intravenous administration of medications in the horse using the jugular vein, intravenous catheterization utilizing the cephalic vein, and lateral thoracic vein.
    - List indications for use of specific veins for intravenous administration of medication in ruminants and swine.
    - Compare and contrast the materials needed and procedures for placing IV catheters in camelids and food animal species.
12. List possible sites of intramuscular administration for each large animal species, and describe limitations and contraindications.
13. Compare and contrast the methods used for administration of medication to horses and food animal species using each of the following approaches: subcutaneous, intradermal, intraperitoneal, intranasal, intramammary (cows only), ophthalmic, epidural, transdermal, intrasynovial, rectal, and intramuscular, including limitations and contraindications in food animals.
14. Compare and contrast venous and arterial blood collection techniques in equine, camelid, and food animal species.
15. List and describe procedures for collection of urine and fecal samples in equine, camelid, and food animal species. List advantages and limitations of each method.
16. Describe procedures for collection and evaluation of milk samples from dairy animals.
17. Describe procedures for collection of rumen fluid in large animals.
18. Describe the indications, materials needed, and procedures for performing a thoracocentesis, transtracheal wash, bronchoalveolar lavage (BAL), abdominocentesis, and cerebrospinal fluid collection in equine, camelid, and food animal species.

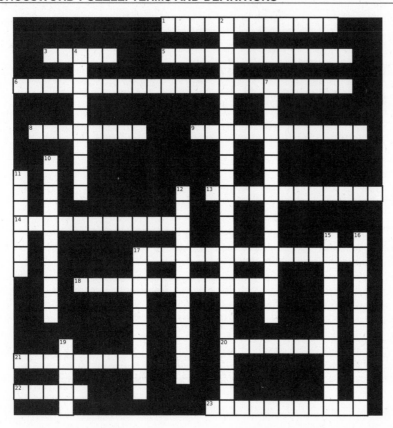

Across

1   Application of 70% isopropyl alcohol to a venipuncture site results in improved visualization of the vein because it causes this.
3   Low-profile gastrostomy tubes are made of silicone and cause less irritation of the _____ when compared with traditional latex gastrostomy tubes.
5   When this occurs with certain intravenous chemotherapeutic drugs, as much of the drug should be removed from the site as possible by aspirating 5 mL of blood back through the catheter.
6   An in vitro technique used to rapidly synthesize large quantities of a given DNA segment. (3 words)
8   Improper compression of the vein following venipuncture may cause this complication.
9   This type of catheter can be placed in the femur.
13 An increased number of white blood cells.
14 Passing through the skin.
17 A decrease in circulating platelets.
18 A common site for this procedure to be performed is the carpal joint.
20 Prolonged loss of appetite.
21 Forcibly ejecting collected blood through the syringe needle into the collection tube can cause this sample artifact.
22 Passage of an orogastric tube into this organ allows for sample collection of fluid that is then analyzed for diagnosis of diseases of the forestomachs.
23 In a patient with this white blood count abnormality, a bone marrow aspirate is indicated.

Down

2   Infusion of isotonic fluids into the abdomen for the express purpose of retrieval of the fluid for diagnostic fluid analysis. (3 words)
4   The concentration of osmotically active particles in a solution.
7   A potential complication of this procedure is abdominal pain and distention.
10 The act of surgically making an opening in the abdominal wall and into the stomach, usually for the placement of a feeding tube.
11 Performing this action during a transtracheal wash will help loosen mucus and encourage the animal cough, thereby enhancing sample collection.
12 Although a common procedure in small animals, this urine collection technique is not performed in most large animals.
15 Often a cause of leukocytosis.
16 An overall decrease in red blood cells, white blood cells, and platelets.
17 Potential complication of an indwelling intravenous catheter involving a blood clot obstructing flow, which is characterized by a vein that "stands up" without being held off.
19 This self-retaining catheter is an ideal choice for urinary catheterization of mares.

EXERCISE 18.2 MATCHING #1: INDICATIONS FOR CLINICAL PROCEDURES

Instructions: Match each clinical procedure in column A with its corresponding indication in column B by writing the appropriate letter in the space provided.

Column A

1. _____ Cystocentesis
2. _____ Thoracentesis
3. _____ Milk sample collection
4. _____ Abdominocentesis
5. _____ Epidural
6. _____ Bone marrow aspirate
7. _____ Arthrocentesis
8. _____ Fine-needle aspiration
9. _____ Bronchoalveolar lavage
10. _____ Cerebrospinal fluid tap

Column B

A. Analgesia

B. Chronic productive cough

C. Skin mass

D. Seizure

E. Mastitis

F. Lameness

G. Pleural effusion

H. Hematuria

I. Ascites

J. Pancytopenia

EXERCISE 18.3 MATCHING #2: SUPPLIES FOR CLINICAL PROCEDURES

Instructions: Match each clinical procedure in column A with the corresponding list of supplies in column B by writing the appropriate letter in the space provided.

Column A

1. _____ Fine-needle aspiration
2. _____ Transtracheal wash
3. _____ Abdominocentesis
4. _____ Sterile milk collection

Column B

A. 16-gauge catheter, 3.5-French polypropylene urinary catheter, 20-mL syringe filled with sterile saline

B. Teat cannula, scalpel blade

C. Clean hands, culture collection tubes

D. 3-mL syringe with a 22-gauge needle, microscope slides

EXERCISE 18.4 MATCHING #3: URINE COLLECTION IN LARGE ANIMALS

Instructions: Match each large animal species in column A with the corresponding technique used to collect urine by free-catch in column B by writing the appropriate letter in the space provided.

Column A

1. _____ Horse
2. _____ Male pig
3. _____ Cow
4. _____ Alpaca
5. _____ Female goat

Column B

A. Wait for the animal to rise after a period of recumbency.

B. Take the animal to the dung pile.

C. Stroke prepuce with soft brush.

D. Stroke the skin beneath the vulva.

E. Place fresh bedding in the stall.

Chapter **18** Diagnostic Sampling and Therapeutic Techniques

EXERCISE 18.5 MATCHING #4: SITES FOR SUBCUTANEOUS INJECTION

Instructions: Match each species in column A with its corresponding site for subcutaneous injection of medication in column B by writing the appropriate letter in the space provided.

Column A

1. _____ Dog
2. _____ Pig
3. _____ Goat
4. _____ Horse
5. _____ Cow

Column B

A. Base of ear

B. Behind the elbow

C. Base of neck

D. Axillary region

E. Lateral hip

EXERCISE 18.6 TABLE #1: ROUTES OF MEDICATION ADMINISTRATION IN SMALL ANIMALS

Instructions: For each route of medication administration in the left column, indicate an associated important potential complication and the action you should take to prevent it.

Route of Medication Administration in the Small Animal Patient	Important Potential Complication	Actions Taken to *Prevent* the Complication
Oral administration of liquid suspension		
Oral administration of a capsule		
Intramuscular injection		
Administration of topical ophthalmic ointment		
Intravenous administration of a chemotherapeutic agent		

EXERCISE 18.7 TABLE #2: OROGASTRIC TUBE PLACEMENT

Instructions: Regarding orogastric tube placement in either dogs or cattle, give a rationale or reason for each of the following procedural steps.

Procedural Step	Rationale
Measure the selected tube against the patient from the tip of the nose to the 13th rib or end of the rib cage. Mark this measurement on the tube.	
Coat the tip of the tube with a water-soluble gel.	
Place a mouth gag or speculum in the patient's mouth.	
Advance the tube into the esophagus. If coughing is heard, stop and withdraw the tube.	
Palpate for "two separate tubes" in the ventral cervical neck area.	
After the fluid has been administered, kink the tube to occlude it and withdraw the tube in a downward direction.	

Instructions: Read the following instructions for peripheral vein catheterization in the small animal patient. Circle all incorrect steps, and write in the corrected procedural step in the space provided. Then, in the space provided, enter the number of each incorrect step you circled, and describe the complications that could arise if the procedural step was performed as written.

1. Generously clip the fur from the area.	
2. Spray alcohol once over the area.	
3. Have assistant apply digital pressure proximal to the insertion site.	
4. Extend the leg to visualize the vein.	
5. Use your thumb to stabilize the vein.	
6. With the bevel up, insert the stylet and catheter through the skin at a 45-degree angle.	
7. Advance the catheter into the vessel.	
8. When a flash of blood is seen, advance the stylet and catheter fully into the vessel lumen.	
9. Advance the catheter off the stylet and into the vessel lumen.	
10. Cap the catheter with a T-set or injection cap, and flush with heparinized saline.	
11. Secure the catheter to the leg with white tape.	
12. Wrap roll gauze around the leg proximally and distally to the insertion site, and affix to the leg with white tape.	
13. Make sure the entire bandage is very tight around the leg.	

Step #	Complication

EXERCISE 18.9 TABLE #4: ARTERIAL BLOOD SAMPLE COLLECTION

Instructions: Read the following protocol for arterial blood sample collection in the small or large animal patient using a regular needle and syringe. Circle all incorrect steps and write in the corrected procedural step in the space provided. Then, in the space provided below the table, enter the number of each incorrect step you circled and describe the patient complication or erroneous blood gas analysis result(s) that could arise if the procedural step was performed as written.

1. Choose a site, and locate the artery by palpating the pulse.	
2. Clean the site using the appropriate aseptic technique.	
3. Attach an appropriate-sized needle to a syringe, and draw a small amount of heparin into the syringe. Expel this small amount of heparin from the syringe into the needle.	
4. Occlude the artery.	
5. Insert the needle into the artery, and firmly pull back on the syringe plunger multiple times to aspirate blood into the syringe.	
6. Withdraw the needle, and have the assistant hold off on the puncture site for 20 to 30 seconds.	
7. Expel any air bubbles from the syringe, and replace the needle cap onto the needle.	
8. Roll the syringe between your hands to distribute the anticoagulant throughout the sample.	
9. Immediately perform blood gas analysis.	

Step #	Complication

EXERCISE 18.10 PHOTO QUIZ #1: DIAGNOSTIC SAMPLING AND THERAPEUTIC TECHNIQUES

Instructions: Name the procedure being performed in each photo.

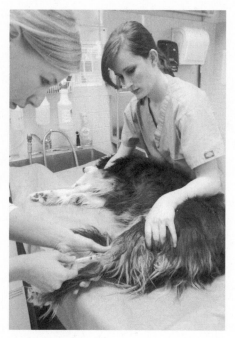

1. _____

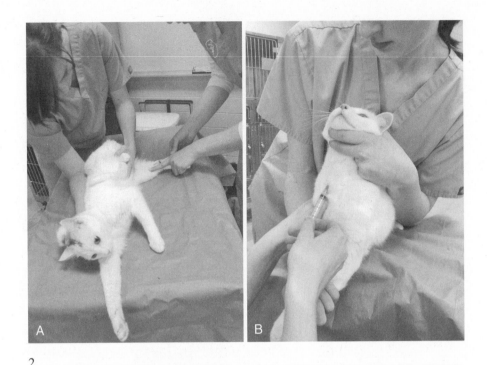

2. _____

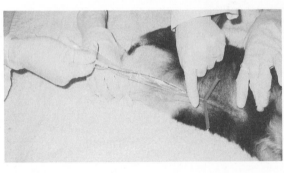

3. _____

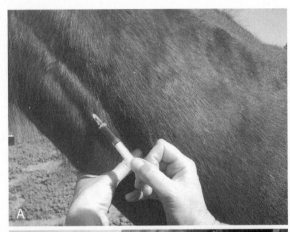

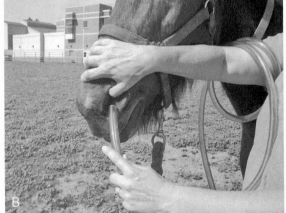

4. _____

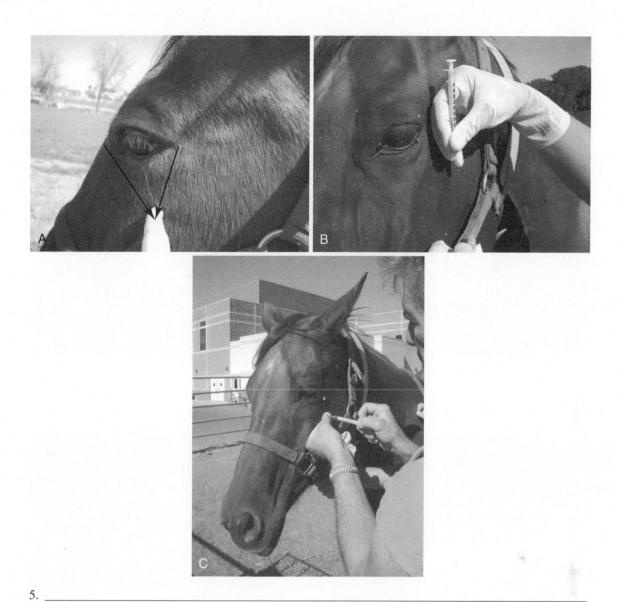

5. _____

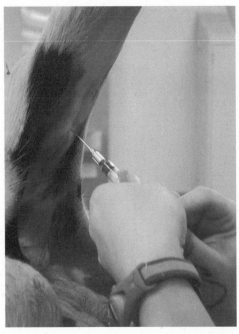

6. _____

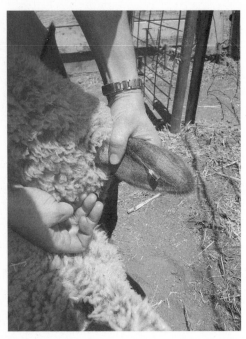

7. _____

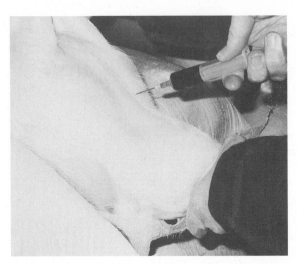

8. _____

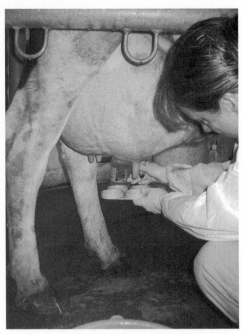

9. _____

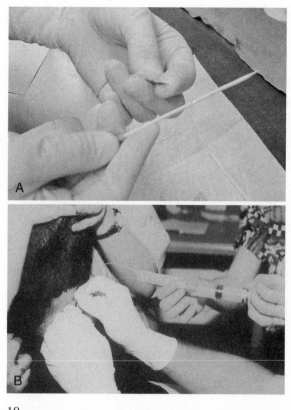

A

B

10. _____

EXERCISE 18.11 PHOTO QUIZ #2: INTRAVENOUS CATHETERS

Instructions: Answer the following questions by writing the appropriate letter in the space provided. (Note that each letter will be used only once.)

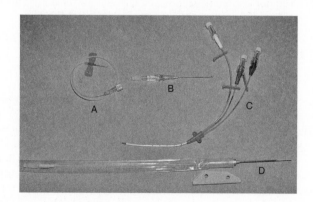

1. _____ Which IV catheter can be used to administer multiple yet separate infusions?

2. _____ Which IV catheter is commonly used for a quick, one-time administration of medication?

3. _____ Which IV catheter is commonly placed as an indwelling catheter in the cephalic vein?

4. _____ Which IV catheter is commonly placed as an indwelling catheter in the jugular vein?

Instructions: Read the following statements and write "T" for true or "F" for false in the blanks provided. If a statement is false, correct the statement to make it true.

1. _____ If antiseizure medication cannot be administered to a convulsing dog by the intravenous route, it may be given intranasally or intrarectally.

2. _____ To prevent the needle from going through-and-through the skin while giving a subcutaneous injection, it is important to insert the needle perpendicular to the long axis of the skin fold.

3. _____ In a severely dehydrated patient, intravenous administration of medications or isotonic fluids is preferred over subcutaneous administration.

4. _____ When placing a jugular catheter in a dog, the catheter is always placed with the tip of the catheter directed toward the heart.

5. _____ Marginal ear venipuncture is an appropriate blood collection technique for a coagulation profile.

6. _____ Male dogs may not require sedation for the placement of a urinary catheter, whereas male cats are usually sedated for this procedure.

7. _____ When using a Vacutainer blood collection system, it is important to not connect the needle to the blood collection tube prior to venipuncture because doing so will break the vacuum in the collection tube and the blood will not flow into the tube.

8. _____ When performing a cranial vena cava venipuncture on a pig, it is preferred to use the left side because it reduces the risk of damaging the phrenic nerve.

9. _____ When instilling both an ophthalmic ointment and a solution into a patient's eye, the correct order of administration is to apply the ointment first followed by the solution because the ointment will help the solution "stick" to the eye.

10. _____ When performing an equine abdominocentesis, at least 0.5 mL of fluid must be collected and placed into a 2-mL EDTA tube to ensure accurate analysis of the abdominal fluid.

EXERCISE 18.13 MULTIPLE CHOICE: COMPREHENSIVE

Instructions: Circle the one correct answer to each of the following questions.

1. A common indication for placing an orogastric tube in a small animal patient is to
   a. Obtain a sample of stomach contents for analysis
   b. Administer activated charcoal to absorb an ingested toxin
   c. Administer water to correct severe dehydration
   d. Obtain a sample of tracheal secretions for analysis

2. Trauma to the sciatic nerve is a potential complication when administering an intramuscular injection into which of following muscles?
   a. Triceps muscle
   b. Lumbosacral muscle
   c. Cranial thigh muscle
   d. Semimembranosus muscle

3. Jugular vein catheterization is preferred over peripheral vein catheterization in the small animal patient for which of the following treatment scenarios?
   a. Single administration of an IV medication
   b. Administration of fluids that have an osmolality of less than 600 mosm/L
   c. Administration of total parenteral nutrition
   d. Administration of blood products for a transfusion

4. The Seldinger guidewire technique refers to the placement of
   a. A spinal needle during a cerebrospinal tap
   b. A Foley catheter during a urinary catheter placement
   c. A multilumen catheter during a jugular catheter placement
   d. An over-the-needle catheter during a transtracheal wash

5. Which of the following small animal procedures requires strict adherence to aseptic technique, including the placement of a surgical drape over the exposed area of the patient?
   a. Cystocentesis
   b. Bone marrow aspiration
   c. Nasoesophageal feeding tube placement
   d. Dorsal metatarsal artery puncture

6. Your patient is a 2-week-old female DSH brown tabby who is severely dehydrated as the result of an *Isospora* (coccidia) infection causing profuse diarrhea. Administration of fluids is ordered. You are unable to place an intravenous catheter. Which of the following routes of administration would be the next best choice?
   a. Oral
   b. Intrarectal
   c. Intraosseous
   d. Subcutaneous

7. The doctor has ordered a urine culture and sensitivity to be collected and submitted on your next patient, a neutered male Boston Terrier named "Kyle." Which of the following collection methods is preferred for this test?
   a. Free-catch
   b. Bladder expression
   c. Cystocentesis
   d. Urinary catheterization

8. When premeasuring a urinary catheter for placement in a male dog, the measurement is taken from
   a. The base of the prepuce to the caudal portion of the bladder
   b. The base of the prepuce to the cranial portion of the bladder
   c. The tip of the prepuce to the caudal portion of the bladder
   d. The tip of the prepuce to the cranial portion of the bladder

9. It is often necessary to monitor urine production in a small animal patient with an indwelling urinary catheter. For a normovolemic dog weighing 27 pounds, 8 ounces, how much urine should be produced in 24 hours?
   a. 25 mL
   b. 55 mL
   c. 600 mL
   d. 1300 mL

10. Bone marrow aspirates are very painful. Which part of the procedure is responsible for causing the most amount of pain to the patient?
    a. Infiltrating the skin with 2% lidocaine
    b. Making the stab incision into the skin with a scalpel blade
    c. Inserting the stylet into the bone
    d. Aspirating the bone marrow fluid

11. Which of the following size needles is most appropriate for performing a jugular venipuncture in a cow?
    a. 18 gauge
    b. 20 gauge
    c. 22 gauge
    d. 25 gauge

12. At certain venipuncture sites, it is not possible to directly visualize or palpate the vessel prior to inserting the needle. Instead, anatomic landmarks are used to direct the positioning of the needle. This is called a "blind stick." Which of the following is a "blind stick"?
    a. Cephalic venipuncture in a cat
    b. Lateral saphenous venipuncture in a dog
    c. Jugular venipuncture in a horse
    d. Coccygeal venipuncture in the cow

13. In the llama, which cervical vertebra is used as the landmark for low neck jugular venipuncture?
    a. Fourth
    b. Fifth
    c. Sixth
    d. Seventh

14. Placement of an intravenous catheter in the auricular vein is common practice in which species?
    a. Cat
    b. Horse
    c. Cow
    d. Pig

15. Which of the following muscles is appropriate to use for medication administration in the cow and pig?
    a. Gluteal muscle
    b. Cervical (neck) muscle
    c. Semimembranosus muscle
    d. Shoulder muscle

16. Tuberculosis testing is conducted via a(n)
    a. Intramuscular injection
    b. Intradermal injection
    c. Subcutaneous injection
    d. Intraperitoneal injection

17. Meningitis is a potential complication associated with
    a. Cerebrospinal fluid tap
    b. Pleural tap
    c. Diagnostic peritoneal lavage
    d. Arthrocentesis

18. In which of the following patients is it correct to use a balling gun to administer oral tablets?
    a. A foal
    b. A pig
    c. A horse
    d. A steer

19. The most appropriate method for administering mineral oil to a horse is
    a. Through a nasogastric tube
    b. Through an orogastric tube
    c. Via drenching
    d. Mixing it in with feed

20. What is the purpose of a subpalpebral lavage system?
    a. To facilitate gastric lavage
    b. To administer ophthalmic medications
    c. To facilitate joint lavage
    d. To administer rectal medications

EXERCISE 18.14 CASE STUDY: RESPIRATORY DISTRESS IN A CAT

Patient name: "Louie" Hansen
Signalment: 2-year-old, neutered male DSH brown Tabby; indoor-outdoor cat
Presenting complaint: Trouble breathing; seems painful
Relevant triage physical examination findings: Patient is in respiratory distress as evidenced by tachypnea and open-mouthed breathing with abdominal effort. Patient is cyanotic.

1. After completing the triage examination, what should you do next? *(Choose the correct response.)*
   a. Complete a full examination to discover what is causing the respiratory distress.
   b. Bring the patient to the radiology suite for radiographs.
   c. Place an IV catheter and administer shock doses of an isotonic fluid.
   d. Bring the patient into the treatment area, and administer oxygen.

As you are completing this, the doctor comes in to listen to Louie's chest. As she is putting her stethoscope into her ears, she discusses with you her concern that Louie may have pleural effusion or a pneumothorax.

2. Define pleural effusion.

   _____

   _____

3. Define pneumothorax.

   _____

Based on the chest auscultation, the doctor believes that Louie has pleural effusion and wants to proceed with a thoracocentesis.

4. Define thoracocentesis.

   _____

   _____

5. Describe the purpose of each of the following supplies that are needed for this procedure:

   a. Butterfly catheter: _____

   _____

   b. Three-way stopcock: _____

   _____

   c. 20-mL syringe: _____

   _____

The thoracocentesis site has been aseptically prepared.

6. Based on the doctor's assessment, describe where you insert the needle to perform the thoracocentesis.

   _____

   _____

The thoracocentesis was successful, with 70 mL of fluid drained from the left side and 130 mL drained from the right side. The fluid sample is packaged and awaiting courier pickup from the lab.

   Louie's breathing has returned to normal, and his mucous membranes are returning to a healthy pink color. He appears to be comfortable in his oxygen cage. However, even though he appears stable at the moment, you know his status can change quickly if he develops any complications following the procedure or if the fluid builds back up in the pleural space.

7. What should you monitor in your patient to assess his respiratory function?

   _____

   _____

   _____

Now that Louie is stable, the doctor orders a complete blood count, chemistry panel, serum thyroid level, and urinalysis. You know that minimizing stress during restraint is important for Louie since he has respiratory compromise.

8. With this in mind, describe which venipuncture approach you will choose and why you made this choice.

   _____

   _____

   _____

The pleural fluid analysis reveals that Louie's pleural effusion is pus. He has a pyothorax (pus in the thoracic cavity). Louie is being admitted to the hospital to have bilateral chest tubes placed to drain the pus from his chest. He will be given intravenous analgesics, antibiotics, and fluids.

   It is the next morning, and you are giving Louie his morning treatments. You notice the bandage around his IV catheter is soaking wet.

9. What problems may have occurred with his IV catheter to cause his bandage to become wet?

_____

_____

_____

As you are changing Louie's bandage to inspect the catheter and catheter site, you also assess the area for phlebitis.

10. Define phlebitis.

_____

11. What are the signs of phlebitis?

_____

_____

_____

You discover and fix the cause of Louie's catheter malfunction, confirm he does not have phlebitis, and rebandage his catheter.

    After 7 days of intensive nursing care, Louie is finally ready to go home! Louie has been prescribed two oral antibiotic pills he will need to take for the next 2 weeks.

12. Explain to Mrs. Hansen how to administer an oral tablet to Louie using common language.

_____

_____

_____

_____

_____

Mrs. Hansen looks horrified as she listens to you and watches you demonstrate administering a tablet to Louie. When you are finished, she asks, "Wouldn't it be easier to just put the pill in some food and feed it to him? That is the way we gave antibiotic pills to our dog, Chester, last year when he had that skin infection, remember? That was so easy!"

13. What is your reply to Mrs. Hansen's question?

_____

_____

_____

_____

19 Small Animal Medical Nursing

LEARNING OBJECTIVES

When you have completed this chapter, you will be able to:

1. Pronounce, define, and spell all key terms in this chapter.
2. Explain the relationship between the "Five Freedoms of Animal Welfare" and the responsibilities of the veterinary technician.
3. List in order the four steps that constitute the veterinary technician practice model and describe what is involved in carrying out each step of the nursing process.
4. Explain the relationship between etiology, pathogenesis, lesions, and clinical signs.
5. Do the following regarding respiratory disease and cardiovascular disease in the small animal:
   - Compare and contrast the clinical relevance of upper versus lower respiratory disease in dogs and cats, and describe how inflammation might be related to nasal discharge, coughing, dyspnea, and hypoxia.
   - Discuss the etiology and pathogenesis of cardiovascular disease in dogs and cats and list and describe the most common cardiovascular diseases.
6. Discuss the etiology and pathogenesis of digestive and hepatobiliary diseases in dogs and cats and list and describe the most common digestive and hepatobiliary diseases.
7. Do the following regarding urinary, endocrine, and immune-mediated disease in dogs and cats:
   - Discuss the etiology and pathogenesis of urinary disease and list and describe the most common urinary diseases.
   - Discuss the etiology and pathogenesis of endocrine disease and list and describe the most common endocrine diseases.
   - Discuss the etiology and pathogenesis of immune-mediated disease and list and describe the most common immune-mediated diseases.
8. Do the following regarding infectious disease in dogs and cats:
   - Discuss the etiology and pathogenesis of infectious disease.
   - List and describe special protocols needed to provide nursing care for dogs and cats with infectious diseases.
   - Explain how to educate clients about stopping the spread of infectious disease.

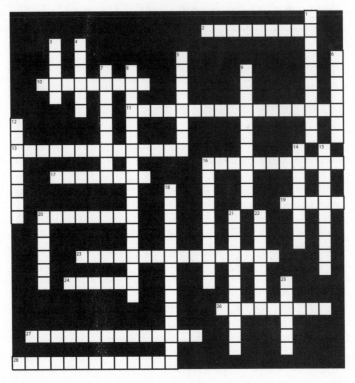

Across

2   The term for the acute disease involving inflammation of the intestinal mucosa.

10   Classification of tumors capable of invasion and destruction of local tissue and of metastasis.

11   The treatment of MG includes administration of anticholinesterase inhibitors and _____ drugs.

13   To diagnose MG, we test for the presence of _____ against AChRs.

16   Tumors of the membranes that surround the brain and spinal cord.

17   Cancer _____ is a syndrome characterized by weight loss and muscle wasting and is caused by the physical presence of a tumor.

19   The type of therapy used to prevent or treat dehydration, ensure hydration in patients with chronic constipation, and treat electrolyte imbalances.

20   The category of tumors that arise from mesenchymal tissues.

23   The type of obstruction involving the stomach, small bowel, or large bowel.

24   GI _____ occur as a result of mucosal layer defects caused by the administration of NSAIDs, neoplasia, and disease of the liver.

26   The acute inflammatory disease of the stomach mucosa often caused by ingestion of toxic plants, spoiled food, foreign objects, or irritating drugs.

27   The syndrome caused by hormones or other substances that are synthesized by the tumor and that circulate systemically, affecting multiple organ systems.

28   The term for a large dilated esophagus.

Down

1   An important risk associated with megaesophagus and regurgitation.

3   The type of hematoma characterized by blood-filled swelling on the inner surface of the pinna.

4   Classification of tumors that do not invade or destroy surrounding normal tissues or metastasize.

5   Generalized _____ that is worse with exercise and resolves with rest is the primary clinical sign of MG.

6   The treatment of choice for localized cancer in dogs and cats.

7   Tumors of _____ glands cause an abnormal hormone secretion and subsequent disruption of body function.

8   The type of inhibitor medication that improves muscle strength by prolonging the action of acetylcholine at the synapses.

9   The term for inflammation of the esophagus.

12   The name of the condition caused by reduced drainage of the aqueous humor through the ciliary body and anterior chamber of the eye.

14   A patient with osteoarthritis often exhibits orthopedic pain and reduced _____.

15   The category of tumors that arise from epithelial tissues.

16   The process by which cancer cells spread from the primary tumor to distant locations such as lymph nodes and the lungs.

18   The term for the disease of the eye involving inflammation of the conjunctiva.

20   The _____ of the tumor's name generally indicates whether the tumor is benign or malignant.

21   The diagnostic tool most commonly used to determine if megaesophagus is present.

22   The term for pathologic lens opacity.

25   The prefix of a tumor's name indicates the specific tissue of _____.

EXERCISE 19.2 DEFINITIONS: KEY TERMS

Instructions: Define each term in your own words.

1. Pathogenesis: _____

   _____

2. Nasal and sinus congestion: _____

   _____

3. Stertor: _____

   _____

4. Stridor: _____

   _____

5. Cough: _____

   _____

6. Hemoptysis: _____

   _____

7. Pleural effusion: _____

   _____

8. Dyspnea: _____

   _____

9. Orthopnea: _____

   _____

10. Hypoxemia: _____

    _____

11. Cardiomyopathy: _____

    _____

12. Systemic hypertension: _____

    _____

13. Regurgitation: _____

    _____

14. Vomiting: _____

_____

15. Hematemesis: _____

_____

16. Hematochezia: _____

_____

17. Melena: _____

_____

18. Tenesmus: _____

_____

19. Hyperthermia: _____

_____

20. Pain: _____

_____

21. Urethral obstruction: _____

_____

22. Diarrhea: _____

_____

23. Constipation: _____

_____

24. Colitis: _____

_____

EXERCISE 19.3 MATCHING #1: TERMS AND DEFINITIONS

Instructions: Match each term in column A with the corresponding definition in column B by writing the appropriate letter in the space provided.

Column A

1. _____ Diarrhea
2. _____ Hepatitis
3. _____ Nausea
4. _____ Secondary immune-mediated hemolytic anemia (IMHA)
5. _____ Serous
6. _____ *Escherichia coli*
7. _____ Hepatic encephalopathy
8. _____ Constipation
9. _____ Mucopurulent
10. _____ Mucoid
11. _____ Hemorrhagic
12. _____ Portosystemic shunts
13. _____ Feline lower urinary tract disease
14. _____ Primary immune-mediated hemolytic anemia

Column B

A. Clear liquid discharge.

B. Opaque and sticky discharge.

C. Green-yellow and mucoid discharge.

D. Bloody discharge.

E. A sign that often precedes vomiting. Characterized by anxiety, hypersalivation, vocalization, and lip smacking.

F. A symptom characterized by frequent passage of loose, unformed, and often watery stool.

G. A condition characterized by infrequent and often difficult passage of hard stool.

H. The result of exposure of the brain to GI toxins.

I. Inflammation of the liver parenchyma.

J. Extrahepatic or intrahepatic vascular abnormalities that connect the systemic and portal circulations.

K. The most common cause of bacterial cystitis in small animals.

L. The term used to describe the constellation of signs indicating bladder and urethra irritation in the cat.

M. A type of IMHA in which the immune system develops autoantibodies against components of the red blood cell membrane.

N. A type of IMHA in which the immune system attacks RBC pathogens adhered to the membrane, but then also indiscriminately destroys normal RBCs.

Instructions: Match each disease or condition in column A with its corresponding description in column B by writing the appropriate letter in the space provided.

Column A

1. _____ Heartworm disease
2. _____ Hypoadrenocorticism
3. _____ Hyperthyroidism
4. _____ Hepatic lipidosis
5. _____ Myasthenia gravis
6. _____ Hemolytic anemia
7. _____ Infectious disease
8. _____ Hyperadrenocorticism
9. _____ Kidney disease
10. _____ Diabetes mellitus
11. _____ Immune-mediated disease
12. _____ Acute cholangitis

Column B

A. Mosquito-borne infectious disease affecting dogs and cats.

B. The disease of cats caused by a derangement of lipid metabolism associated with anorexia of approximately 7 days.

C. The acute disease of the bile ducts caused by an ascending bacterial infection from the small intestines and characterized by neutrophilic inflammation.

D. A disease characterized by irreversible, progressive loss of renal function.

E. A disease that affects cats in which the thyroid gland is overactive, producing abnormally large amounts of thyroid hormones.

F. A disease caused by either insufficient production of insulin by the pancreatic beta cells or by insulin resistance characterized by the body's inability to respond properly to endogenous insulin.

G. A disease that primarily affects dogs and is characterized by elevated circulating levels of cortisol produced by the adrenal cortex.

H. A disease caused by adrenal gland atrophy or destruction resulting in inadequate secretion of glucocorticoids and mineralocorticoids.

I. A disease in which the immune system has lost tolerance of self and damages organs.

J. A disease characterized by RBC destruction.

K. A disorder of neuromuscular transmission that causes muscle weakness.

L. A disease in which pathogenic microorganisms invade and colonize the fluids and tissues of a host.

Instructions: Read the following statements and write "T" for true or "F" for false in the blanks provided. If a statement is false, correct the statement to make it true.

1. _____ Etiology is defined as the cause of a disease.

2. _____ Anorexia is a complete or partial loss of appetite.

3. _____ Hypovolemia is an increase of intravascular fluid.

4. _____ Regurgitation is the forceful expulsion of contents from the stomach and/or intestines.

5. _____ The use of anti-inflammatory drugs in the treatment of lower respiratory disease specifically targets the airways.

6. _____ In dogs, sneezing is most commonly associated with upper respiratory viral infections, whereas sneezing in cats is usually the result of inhalation of foreign material.

7. _____ Cats do not normally pant, so the presence of open-mouth breathing with noticeable chest movements indicates dyspnea.

8. _____ Coughing is a common sign of CHF in cats.

9. _____ Treatment of feline heartworm disease is unrewarding because a safe and effective adulticide protocol has yet to be found.

10. _____ In dogs, exocrine pancreatic insufficiency is commonly caused by chronic pancreatitis.

11. _____ A urolith is a pathologic stone formed from mineral salts in the urinary tract.

12. _____ In resistant or recurrent UTI cases, a 2-week course of antibiotics is needed.

13. _____ Hypothyroidism primarily affects dogs, although a rare congenital form can be seen in kittens.

14. _____ Dogs tend to develop type-2 diabetes mellitus, whereas cats are more prone to type-1 diabetes mellitus.

15. _____ Diabetes mellitus will often progress to a condition called diabetic ketoacidosis despite diagnosis and treatment.

16. _____ Immune-mediated diseases are those in which the immune system has failed to protect the patient from invasion by microorganisms.

17. _____ Acquired myasthenia gravis is more common in cats than it is in dogs.

18. _____ Vaccination, maintenance of proper health, and proper nutrition strengthen host defense systems.

19. _____ Benign tumors do not invade or destroy surrounding normal tissues or spread to a new site.

20. _____ Carcinomas arise from mesenchymal tissue.

21. _____ A disadvantage of cryosurgery is that the completeness of tumor removal cannot be determined because there is no tissue to submit for margin evaluation.

Instructions: Circle the one correct answer to each of the following questions.

1. The veterinary technician may be responsible for everything except
   a. Gathering a patient's data
   b. Identifying and prioritizing technician evaluations
   c. Developing a nursing care plan
   d. Interpreting lab tests

2. A disease of the heart muscle seen in cats that is characterized by an increase in the thickness of the left ventricle wall and a small ventricular lumen is classified as
   a. Dilated
   b. Hypertrophic
   c. Arrhythmogenic
   d. Restrictive

3. Diagnosing heart disease relies partly on diagnostic procedures, including all of the following except
   a. Diagnostic ultrasonography
   b. Radiographs
   c. Endoscopy
   d. Electrocardiography

4. Dilated cardiomyopathy is the most common canine cardiomyopathy. It is characterized primarily by
   a. Enlarged atrial and ventricular lumina with decreased contractility
   b. Thromboembolism with increased contractility
   c. Increased contractility and ventricular arrhythmias
   d. Atrial enlargement with normal ventricular function

5. Treatment of canine heartworm disease may include any of the following except
   a. Adulticide therapy
   b. Microfilaracide therapy 3 to 4 weeks later
   c. Surgical removal of worms
   d. A gradual increase in activity over 3 to 4 weeks

6. Nursing care for patients suffering from regurgitation includes
   a. Elevating food and water bowls
   b. Keeping the patient's head and forelimbs elevated for 10 minutes postmeal
   c. Changing the form of food and monitoring for signs of aspiration
   d. All of the above

7. The premature activation of trypsin in the pancreas is associated with what condition?
   a. Tenesmus
   b. Exocrine pancreatic insufficiency
   c. Pancreatitis
   d. Hepatic lipidosis

8. Clinical signs associated with feline pancreatitis typically include
   a. Vomiting, weight gain, hyperthermia, lethargy, and hypotension
   b. Hypothermia, diarrhea, anorexia, vomiting, and hypotension
   c. Vomiting, diarrhea, regurgitation, and hypothermia
   d. Vomiting, lethargy, weight loss, anorexia, and hypothermia

9. Management of acute hepatic encephalopathy includes all of the following except
   a. Fluid therapy
   b. Correcting electrolyte imbalances
   c. Analgesia
   d. Treatment of seizures

10. Chronic hepatitis indicates a history of liver disease for a prolonged period of time, usually greater than
    a. 2 to 3 weeks
    b. 6 to 8 weeks
    c. 2 to 3 months
    d. 4 to 6 months

11. Cholangitis refers to
    a. Inflammation of the bile ducts
    b. Inflammation of the liver
    c. Inflammation of the pancreas
    d. Inflammation of the gallbladder

12. Medical management of chronic kidney disease focuses on
    a. Slowing the progression
    b. Treating concurrent diseases
    c. Correcting electrolyte imbalances
    d. All of the above

13. UTI is a common secondary complication in all of the following except
    a. Diabetes mellitus
    b. Chronic kidney disease
    c. Hyperadrenocorticism
    d. Hypothyroidism

14. Feline lower urinary tract disease is typically classified as
    a. Nonhemorrhagic or hemorrhagic
    b. Nonobstructive or obstructive
    c. Noninvasive or invasive
    d. Nonpainful or painful

15. Clinical signs of hyperthyroidism include
    a. Increased activity
    b. Weight gain
    c. Decreased appetite
    d. Decreased urine output

16. Treatment of feline hyperthyroidism falls into two categories:
    a. Curative and palliative
    b. Symptomatic and supportive
    c. Acute and chronic
    d. Primary and secondary

17. The treatment of diabetes mellitus is different for dogs and cats. Dogs require lifelong treatment that includes the administration of insulin, glucose monitoring, and a high-fiber diet. In contrast, a high-protein/lower-fat diet is recommended for cats. In addition, which of the following is true of cats?
    a. Aggressive treatment with insulin is often associated with spontaneous remission within 3 to 4 months.
    b. Cats require lifelong treatment with insulin and lifelong daily glucose monitoring.
    c. Blood glucose is monitored and insulin therapy is incorporated as needed.
    d. Most cats respond well long term to the administration of oral hypoglycemics.

18. Hyperadrenocorticism or Cushing syndrome can be caused by
    a. A functional adrenal gland tumor
    b. A functional anterior pituitary tumor
    c. Immune damage of the adrenal gland
    d. Either A or B
    e. Either B or C

19. Feline Cushing syndrome is rare and, when diagnosed, is often seen concurrently with
    a. Mastitis
    b. Osteosarcoma
    c. Pancreatitis
    d. Diabetes mellitus

20. Which of the following is not typically a sign of hypoadrenocorticism (Addison disease)?
    a. Diarrhea
    b. Vomiting
    c. Polydipsia
    d. Hyperactivity

21. Secondary immune-mediated disease can result from
    a. Infection
    b. Cancer
    c. Vaccine administration
    d. All of the above

22. If a patient with myasthenia gravis has megaesophagus, common presenting signs are
    a. Dry mouth and vomiting
    b. Vomiting and diarrhea
    c. Diarrhea and hypersalivation
    d. Hypersalivation and regurgitation

23. Which of the following is contagious directly between animals or indirectly through fomites?
    a. Canine heartworm disease
    b. *Borrelia burgdorferi*
    c. Feline calicivirus
    d. Rocky Mountain spotted fever

24. Neoplasia is
    a. The process of healing through the controlled growth of new cells
    b. The natural process by which dead and dying cells are replaced
    c. The formation of a tissue mass because of uncontrolled cell growth
    d. Changing the appearance of a body part surgically

25. Hyperbilirubinemia will cause the mucous membranes to be
    a. Pale
    b. Cyanotic
    c. Icteric
    d. Brick red

26. In lung auscultation, "crackles" are associated with
    a. Bronchial and pleural disease
    b. Pleural and pulmonary disease
    c. Pulmonary disease and effusion
    d. Effusion and bronchial disease

27. An increased PCV and TP indicates
    a. Dehydration
    b. Hypovolemia caused by blood loss
    c. Hypothermia
    d. Cardiac insufficiency

28. Which of the following is *not* associated with restoration of normovolemia?
    a. Pink/dry mucous membranes
    b. CRT less than 2 seconds
    c. Normal cardiac function
    d. Normal blood pressure

29. A temperature less than 99° F, shivering, prolonged CRT, bradycardia, cyanosis, and decreased respirations are symptoms of
    a. Pain
    b. Hypothermia
    c. Electrolyte imbalance
    d. Cardiac insufficiency

30. Symptoms of cardiac insufficiency include
    a. Tachypnea
    b. Tachycardia
    c. Prolonged CRT
    d. All of the above

31. A body condition score of 4 or higher out of 5 indicates
    a. Obesity
    b. Overhydration
    c. Neurologic depression
    d. Decreased muscle mass

32. Malnutrition leads to all of the following except
    a. Multisystemic organ dysfunction
    b. Electrolyte imbalance
    c. Dehydration
    d. Pancreatitis

33. Loss of gag and swallow reflexes commonly occur in all of the following except
    a. Sedation or anesthesia
    b. Megaesophagus
    c. Damage to cranial nerves
    d. Hyperadrenocorticism

34. Clinical signs of feline bronchitis include all of the following except
    a. Cough
    b. Stridor
    c. Wheezing
    d. Dyspnea

EXERCISE 19.7 FILL-IN-THE-BLANK: COMPREHENSIVE

Instructions: Fill in each of the spaces provided with the missing word or words that complete the sentence.

1. Nasal discharge results from irritation or inflammation of the nasal mucosa and can be described as _____ (green-yellow and mucoid), _____ (bloody), _____ (clear liquid), or _____ (opaque and sticky).

2. A patient with nasal discharge, sneezing, and/or congestion should be closely examined for facial _____ that can accompany some causative diseases such as fungal infections, tooth root abscess, and neoplasms.

3. A cough may be _____, meaning fluid, mucus, or blood is brought up from the airway.

4. A _____ cough is sometimes referred to as a "dry cough."

5. The presence of pleural effusion can be confirmed via _____, ultrasonography, or radiography.

6. In an extreme situation, stressing a dyspneic patient can result in _____.

7. Heart disease can be caused by a pathologic abnormality affecting the _____, _____, rhythm conduction, or the overall structure of the heart.

8. The first respiratory sign that heart disease has progressed to heart failure is often _____.

9. Degenerative atrioventricular valve disease affects the cardiac valve _____ or _____ and is characterized by thickening of the tissue.

10. Patients with high heartworm burdens and severe cardiopulmonary disease are at high risk for pulmonary _____ and must be stabilized prior to the administration of adulticide for heartworm treatment.

11. For both dogs and cats the key to avoiding heartworm disease is to _____ infection. This is achieved through the use of approved _____ class preventatives.

12. Once high blood pressure is diagnosed, treatment with _____ medication is begun immediately.

13. Systemic hypertension is often secondary to another disease such as chronic _____ disease, _____, _____, or diabetes mellitus.

14. Difficulty eating is also referred to as _____.

15. _____ material typically consists of undigested or partially digested food.

16. Vomiting patients are prone to _____ and _____ imbalances, so monitoring for and treating these secondary problems is of importance when providing complete patient care.

17. Hematochezia usually indicates a problem with the _____ or _____.

18. Tenesmus of GI origin is usually the result of _____ disease and often accompanies diarrhea or constipation.

19. Pancreatitis occurs when the digestive enzyme _____ is prematurely activated within the _____ tissue instead of within the duodenum.

20. Pancreatitis may be chronic or acute in nature. The frequency of each type varies among species. Chronic cases are seen more commonly in _____, whereas acute cases are seen more commonly in _____.

21. Chronic pancreatitis can lead to the endocrine disease _____ _____.

22. _____ _____ _____ is caused by insufficient production and secretion of digestive enzymes by the pancreas.

23. In dogs, EPI is most commonly the result of pancreatic acinar _____.

24. The loss of digestive enzymes leads to maldigestion and malabsorption of ingested nutrients causing clinical signs of polyphagia; _____ _____; and chronic pale, fatty, and voluminous diarrhea.

25. Patients with severe hepatobiliary disease may develop _____ _____ as a result of exposure of the brain to GI toxins.

26. Symptomatic treatment of HE focuses on decreasing the amount of _____ in the systemic circulation, which can be achieved by decreasing production within the _____.

27. Feline hepatic lipidosis is caused by a derangement of lipid _____ associated with _____ of approximately 7 days.

28. _____ portosystemic shunts are congenital and typically involve one or two vessels that connect the portal vein to the vena cava.

29. _____ portosystemic shunts can be congenital or acquired secondary to portal hypertension and are multiple shunts within the hepatic parenchyma.

30. Chronic feline cholangitis is characterized by _____-_____ inflammation. The cause of this condition is _____.

EXERCISE 19.8 CASE STUDY #1: DISEASES AFFECTING THE THYROID GLAND

Signalment: Petunia, a 10-year-old, spayed female domestic long hair cat.
Chief Complaint: The owner reports that Petunia has been losing weight gradually over the past several months.
Minimum Database: Petunia's appetite is good, but she is acting more lethargic lately. The physical examination confirms weight loss (body weight of 5.7 pounds and a body condition score of 2/5), an elevated heart rate, an unkempt hair coat, and a palpable thyroid nodule. Blood testing revealed an elevated serum T_4 level, along with a number of other changes in chemistry values. The attending veterinarian diagnosed hyperthyroidism.

1. Briefly describe hyperthyroidism. Specifically explain the causes of this condition, how it is diagnosed, common clinical signs, and treatment options.

   a. Brief description of hyperthyroidism: _____

   _____

   _____

   b. Causes: _____

   _____

   c. Diagnosis: _____

   _____

   _____

   d. Clinical signs: _____

   _____

   e. Treatment options: _____

   _____

   _____

   _____

2. Unlike cats, which much more frequently develop hyperthyroidism, dogs much more frequently develop hypothyroidism. These diseases differ greatly and are in many ways opposites. Explain the causes of hypothyroidism, how it is diagnosed, common clinical signs, and treatment options.

   a. Brief description of hypothyroidism: _____

   _____

   _____

b. Causes: _____

_____

c. Diagnosis: _____

_____

_____

d. Clinical signs: _____

_____

e. Treatment options: _____

_____

_____

_____

3. Finally, explain the key differences between these diseases of the thyroid gland.

_____

_____

_____

_____

_____

_____

_____

_____

EXERCISE 19.9 CASE STUDY #2: THE VETERINARY TECHNICIAN PRACTICE MODEL

Signalment: Molly, a 10-year-old, spayed female Terrier mix-breed dog.

Chief Complaint: The owner reports that Molly has been coughing lately, doesn't have much energy, and tires quickly after going on walks.

Database: After gathering a complete history and performing a physical examination, the doctor orders a complete workup to evaluate Molly's heart, including blood work and thoracic radiographs. He is concerned about valvular heart disease but wants more data before a treatment plan is developed. Consider the following facts gleaned from Molly's patient database.

Physical findings:

- Tachycardia and tachypnea
- Open-mouth breathing, increased respiratory effort, and slight cyanosis
- Grade V/VI systolic heart murmur
- Increased lung sounds (crackles)

Diagnostic workup:

- Radiographs reveal left-sided heart enlargement and evidence of fluid in the lungs (pulmonary edema).
- Blood work results are unremarkable.

The doctor believes Molly may have degenerative A-V valve disease and secondary congestive heart failure. In animals with this condition, the heart valves degenerate and thicken, allowing blood to flow backwards from the ventricles, into the atria. This causes a backup of blood in the heart and subsequent development of fluid in the lungs, as well as a decrease in forward flow. The cause of this disease is unknown, although there may be a genetic predisposition, as dogs of certain breeds are especially prone to this condition.

1. Any disease, including this one, can be defined by its etiology, pathogenesis, associated lesions, and clinical signs.

   a. Define each of these terms.

   i. Etiology: _____

   _____

   ii. Pathogenesis: _____

   _____

   iii. Lesion: _____

   _____

   iv. Clinical signs: _____

   _____

   b. What is the relationship between each of these elements?

   _____

   _____

   _____

   c. What are Molly's main clinical signs?

   _____

   _____

   _____

2. Use of the technician practice model in this case will ensure that Molly is provided with consistently excellent care. The first step is to help gather patient data, which you have already done.

    a. What would be the next steps?

        _____

        _____

    b. List two technician evaluations shown in Table 19-4 that would apply to Molly. What evidence do you have that each of these evaluations applies?

        i. _____

          _____

          _____

        ii. _____

          _____

          _____

          _____

    c. What technician interventions would be indicated to help Molly?

        _____

        _____

        _____

        _____

        _____

    d. How will you know that Molly is responding to your interventions?

        _____

        _____

        _____

        _____

        _____

Large Animal Medical Nursing

LEARNING OBJECTIVES

When you have completed this chapter, you will be able to:

1. Pronounce, define, and spell all key terms in the chapter.
2. Explain the importance of a thorough physical examination and medical record for large animal patients; in addition, list normal values for temperature, pulse, and respiration in the horse.
3. List and describe the most common diseases and conditions of the horse for the respiratory, cardiovascular, hemolymphatic, gastrointestinal, liver, neurologic, urinary tract, dermatologic, and ophthalmologic systems, including the causes and pathogenesis of each.
4. Discuss the care of the hospitalized equine patient, including patient monitoring, therapeutics, and laboratory studies.
5. List and describe the most common diseases and conditions of ruminants for the digestive, respiratory, reproductive/mammary gland, metabolic, hemolymphatic, cardiovascular, nervous, ophthalmologic, musculoskeletal, dermatologic, and urinary systems, including special care and conditions of the neonate.
6. Do the following regarding common diseases and conditions of swine:
   - Discuss common diseases and conditions of swine, including neonatal care, multisystemic diseases, gastrointestinal disease, and diseases of the respiratory, reproductive, nervous, and musculoskeletal systems.
   - Discuss normal and abnormal behaviors of swine.
7. Do the following regarding common diseases and conditions of camelids:
   - Discuss common diseases and conditions of camelids, including special care and conditions of the neonate.
   - List and describe the most common diseases of camelids for the digestive, metabolic, and nervous systems.
   - List preventive health measures in the management of camelids.

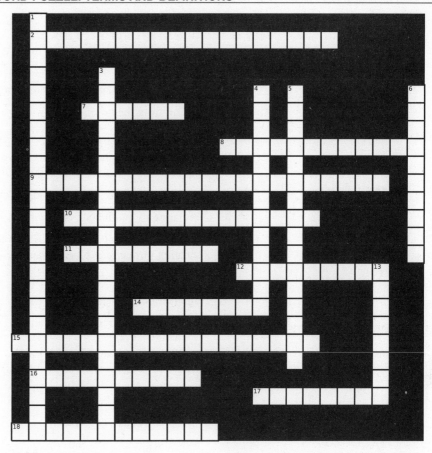

Across

2 Adjective describing a pathologic condition in which the body forms few or no antibodies.
7 A bacterial toxin that has been weakened by heat or chemical treatment.
8 Lower-than-normal levels of blood glucose.
9 Condition characterized by altered function of the central nervous system in which brain swelling and inflammation lead to necrosis of brain tissue.
10 A common reproductive condition in goats that may develop in does with or without exposure to a buck.
11 An antibody that neutralizes a specific biologic toxin. The antibody is produced in response to a particular toxin such as tetanus.
12 First milk containing antibodies.
14 Slow or difficult labor or delivery of a newborn.
15 Necrosis of a large area of a mammary gland or glands secondary to infection. (2 words)
16 Invasion of the bloodstream by microorganism (usually bacteria) from a focus of infection.
17 Inflammation of muscle.
18 A condition that is characterized by the formation or presence of calculi in the urinary tract.

Down

1 Deficient levels of antibodies absorbed by the gut in animals dependent upon colostrum for immunologic protection. (4 words)
3 A neurologic deficit in which the animal loses awareness of body position and movement in space. (2 words)
4 A cancer of lymphocytes and lymphoid tissues that is the third most common cancer diagnosed in dogs.
5 Condition that occurs in ewes during the last few weeks of pregnancy when there is a sudden demand for energy by fast-growing fetuses. (2 words)
6 Abnormal position of the eyes.
13 Inflammation of the mammary gland.

EXERCISE 20.2 MATCHING #1: TERMS AND DEFINITIONS

Instructions: Match each term in column A with its corresponding definition in column B by writing the appropriate letter in the space provided.

Column A

1. _____ Endotoxemia
2. _____ Epistaxis
3. _____ Keratoconjunctivitis
4. _____ Ketosis
5. _____ Pericarditis
6. _____ Persistent infection
7. _____ Serosanguineous
8. _____ Serous
9. _____ Stranguria

Column B

A. Inflammation of the pericardial membrane surrounding the heart.

B. Bleeding from the nose.

C. Straining to urinate.

D. Condition in high-producing dairy cows caused by the buildup in the blood of products of fat breakdown.

E. Chronic infection that does not resolve despite use of antimicrobials.

F. Of, relating to, producing, or resembling serum.

G. A group of clinical signs caused by bacteria-associated toxins circulating through the bloodstream.

H. Containing or consisting of both blood and serous fluid.

I. Combined inflammation of the cornea and conjunctiva.

EXERCISE 20.3 MATCHING #2: DISEASES OF RUMINANTS

Instructions: Match each disease or causative organism of disease in column A with the primary body system that it affects in column B by writing the appropriate letter in the space provided. (Note that responses may be used more than once.)

Column A

1. _____ Grain overload
2. _____ Nervous ketosis
3. _____ BVD
4. _____ Listeriosis
5. _____ Infectious bovine rhinotracheitis
6. _____ Traumatic reticuloperitonitis
7. _____ *Pasteurella multocida*
8. _____ Caprine arthritis encephalitis
9. _____ *Mycoplasma bovis*
10. _____ Salmonellosis
11. _____ Rabies
12. _____ Coronavirus

Column B

A. Central nervous system

B. Respiratory system

C. Gastrointestinal system

EXERCISE 20.4 MATCHING #3: DISEASES OF PIGS

Instructions: Match each description in column A with its corresponding disease of pigs in column B by writing the appropriate letter in the space provided. (Note that responses may be used more than once, and some responses may not be used.)

Column A

1. _____ Infection causes a high fever and may produce characteristic diamond skin lesions.

2. _____ Infection in baby pigs results in development of neurologic signs and, in some cases, vomiting and diarrhea.

3. _____ Infection results in pneumonia.

4. _____ Weaning and growing pigs exhibit fever; pneumonia; a dry, nonproductive cough; and flu-like signs.

5. _____ Respiratory signs include labored breathing, increased secondary respiratory infections, increased postweaning mortality, and decreased rate of gain and feed efficiency.

6. _____ Infection in adults may cause reproductive problems, including early embryonic death, abortion, or stillbirths, in pregnant sows or gilts.

7. _____ Reproductive signs include abortion, stillbirths, fetal mummies, and the birth of weak piglets.

Column B

A. Rhinotracheitis

B. Pseudorabies

C. Erysipelas

D. Rabies

E. Porcine reproductive and respiratory syndrome

EXERCISE 20.5 MATCHING #4: BODY CONDITION SCORE (BCS) FOR SHEEP

Instructions: Match each description in column A with its corresponding body condition score for sheep in column B by writing the appropriate number in the space provided.

Column A

A. _____ Slight bulging (convexity) between the dorsal and transverse spinous processes.

B. _____ Mild concavity between the dorsal and transverse spinous processes.

C. _____ Absence of lumbar musculature and subcutaneous fat, leaving a profound depression between the tips of the dorsal and transverse spinous processes.

D. _____ No depression (straight line) between the dorsal and transverse spinous processes.

E. _____ Moderate concavity between the dorsal and transverse spinous processes.

F. _____ Profound convexity between the dorsal and transverse spinous processes (cannot palpate spinous processes).

Column B

0

1

2

3

4

5

Instructions: Read the following statements and write "T" for true or "F" for false in the blanks provided. If a statement is false, correct the statement to make it true.

1. _____ Horses with upper respiratory tract problems have obvious abnormalities when the lungs are auscultated.

2. _____ Bastard strangles is characterized by development of an abscess in an abnormal location in the equine patient.

3. _____ A life-threatening side effect of guttural pouch infections can be the growth of plaque over the internal carotid artery.

4. _____ Heaves can be cured in the equine patient.

5. _____ Second-degree atrioventricular (AV) block is an arrhythmia in horses that is a medical emergency.

6. _____ Horses are predisposed to atrial fibrillation because of the small atria and high vagal tone.

7. _____ Equine contagious arteritis is a bacterial disease that produces limb swelling, conjunctivitis, abortion, and respiratory disease in horses.

8. _____ Choke is an indication of a tracheal obstruction.

9. _____ Eastern, Western, and West Nile equine encephalitis vaccines are highly effective, and vaccinated horses rarely get sick.

10. _____ Equine patients with Wobbler syndrome are more likely to be female than male.

11. _____ Horses with equine herpes virus must be isolated to stop the spread of the disease.

12. _____ Addison disease in the horse is a common cause of polyuria and polydipsia.

13. _____ Changing the diet of a hospitalized equine patient is OK as long as you ask the owner.

14. _____ Bovine respiratory disease syndrome (BRDS) is caused by a single organism, *Pasteurella multocida*.

15. _____ BRDS in feedlot cattle is often referred to as shipping fever.

16. _____ Milk fever predominantly occurs in first-calf heifers.

17. _____ Pregnancy toxemia in ewes occurs in late gestation.

18. _____ Goats are more prone to copper toxicity than sheep.

19. _____ Small ruminants are susceptible to tetanus and should receive toxoid/antitoxin prior to surgery.

20. _____ Most cases of lameness in ruminants occur in the foot as opposed to the upper limb.

21. _____ Orf is treated with antibiotics, as it is caused by a bacterium.

22. _____ Neonatal pigs easily become hyperthermic, and care must taken to keep them cool and comfortable.

Instructions: Circle the one correct answer to each of the following questions.

1. Normal temperature for the adult horse is
   a. 89° F to 91.5° F
   b. 96° F to 101.5° F
   c. 99° F to 101.5° F
   d. 100° F to 103.5° F

2. A normal pulse in the adult horse is
   a. 18 to 34 bpm
   b. 28 to 44 bpm
   c. 38 to 54 bpm
   d. 48 to 64 bpm

3. Normal respiration for the adult horse is
   a. 4 to 8 breaths/min
   b. 6 to 16 breaths/min
   c. 16 to 26 breaths/min
   d. 34 to 48 breaths/min

4. Strangles is caused by the bacterial pathogen
   a. *Neorickettsia risticii*
   b. *Clostridium perfringens*
   c. *Salmonellosis equi*
   d. *Streptococcus equi*

5. The most common cause of a fungal infection of the guttural pouches is
   a. *Aspergillus* spp.
   b. *Salmonellosis* spp.
   c. *Streptococcus* spp.
   d. *Neorickettsia* spp.

6. Abortion secondary to equine herpesvirus occurs in which month of gestation?
   a. 1 to 3
   b. 3 to 5
   c. 6 to 8
   d. 7 to 11

7. Heaves most commonly occurs in horses that are
   a. Older than 2 years of age
   b. Older than 5 years of age
   c. Older than 10 years of age
   d. Older than 15 years of age

8. Potomac horse fever is caused by
   a. *Salmonella* spp.
   b. *Neorickettsia risticii*
   c. *Clostridium perfringens*
   d. Larval cyathostomiasis

9. The secondary hosts of the causative agent of equine protozoal myelitis (EPM) are
   a. Raccoons
   b. Opossums
   c. Birds
   d. Mice

10. Which ophthalmic disease is most common in horses?
    a. Corneal ulceration
    b. Recurrent uveitis
    c. Entropion
    d. Glaucoma

11. Monitoring of the equine patient with an infectious disease should occur
    a. Every 1 to 2 hours
    b. Every 3 to 4 hours
    c. Every 4 to 6 hours
    d. Every 8 to 12 hours

12. Equine patients unable to defecate because of recumbency should have the feces manually removed
    a. Once per day
    b. Twice per day
    c. Three times per day
    d. Only when the patient is uncomfortable

13. The recumbent equine patient should be repositioned every
    a. 2 hours
    b. 4 hours
    c. 6 hours
    d. 8 hours

14. The following agents are used in the equine patient. Which one has no analgesic properties?
    a. Xylazine
    b. Acepromazine
    c. Detomidine
    d. Butorphanol

15. The normal range for the PCV in the equine patient is
    a. 12% to 17%
    b. 19% to 32%
    c. 32% to 45%
    d. 45% to 57%

16. Endotoxins can cause margination and sequestration of the
    a. White blood cells
    b. Red blood cells
    c. Platelets
    d. Plasma

17. The equine patient has a yellow tint to the blood serum because
    a. It doesn't have a gallbladder
    b. Of the large cecum
    c. Of the large muscle mass
    d. The liver is small in comparison to the patient's size

18. What chemistry test is an indicator of muscle damage?
    a. Phosphate
    b. Blood urea nitrogen
    c. Albumin
    d. Creatine phosphokinase

19. Normal equine urine pH is
    a. 2 to 4
    b. 5 to 7
    c. 7 to 9
    d. 9 to 10

20. Small ruminants should be vaccinated for enterotoxemia
    a. Every 2 months
    b. Every 4 months
    c. Every 6 months
    d. Once a year

21. The normal pH of the rumen is
    a. 6.0 to 6.4
    b. 6.5 to 6.8
    c. 7.2 to 7.8
    d. 7.5 to 8.8

22. Which disease affects both cattle and small ruminants?
    a. Johne
    b. BVD
    c. Nervous ketosis
    d. BRDS

23. In the ruminant foot, which claws bear the most weight?
    a. Front lateral and hind lateral claws
    b. Front medial and hind lateral claws
    c. Front medial and hind medial claws
    d. Front lateral and hind medial claws

24. PPV causes death and mummification of the fetus
    a. At less than 30 days of gestation
    b. Between 30 and 70 days of gestation
    c. After 70 days of gestation
    d. At any stage of gestation

25. PPV causes death and resorption of the fetus
    a. At less than 30 days of gestation
    b. Between 30 and 70 days of gestation
    c. After 70 days of gestation
    d. At any stage of gestation

26. Which animals listed below are classified as old world camelids? *(Choose all that apply.)*
    a. Guanaco
    b. Bactrian camels
    c. Vicuña
    d. Dromedary camels
    e. Llama
    f. Alpaca

27. Which animals listed below are classified as new world camelids? *(Choose all that apply.)*
    a. Guanaco
    b. Bactrian camels
    c. Vicuña
    d. Dromedary camels
    e. Llama
    f. Alpaca

28. Which animal is the normal host of *Parelaphostrongylus tenuis*?
    a. Llama
    b. White-tailed deer
    c. Mule deer
    d. Alpaca

EXERCISE 20.8 CASE STUDY #1: EQUINE INFECTIOUS ANEMIA

Your client, Mrs. Ratcliff, has called the clinic and asked why it is important to test her horses for equine infectious anemia (EIA) and why everyone thinks it is such a serious issue.

1. What do you tell her?

_____

_____

_____

_____

_____

_____

_____

_____

EXERCISE 20.9 CASE STUDY #2: EQUINE GASTRIC ULCERS

Mr. Fredrickson received a call from his farm manager. Many of the young horses on his farm are developing gastric problems, and they think it is ulcers. Mr. Fredrickson calls you to discuss the predisposing factors in horses that may contribute to the formation of gastric ulcers and what signs to be aware of so that he can address this issue with the farm manager.

1. What do you tell him?

_____

_____

_____

_____

_____

_____

EXERCISE 20.10 CASE STUDY #3: DERMATOPHILOSIS AND *CULICOIDES* HYPERSENSITIVITY

Dr. Rainy has been to see the horses at Mr. Robinson's barn. Several of them have dermatophilosis, and a couple of his older mares have *Culicoides* hypersensitivity.

Dr. Rainy prescribed medication for the affected horses and directed Mr. Robinson to call you so you could talk to him about what he could do with regard to the environment to help these horses recover and not become affected each year.

1. What do you tell Mr. Robinson when he calls?

_____

_____

_____

_____

_____

_____

_____

_____

_____

_____

_____

_____

EXERCISE 20.11 CASE STUDY #4: REARING LAMBS

Mrs. Rogers has just started a small sheep operation, and she is interested in raising lambs. She has contacted your clinic to ask questions about how best to make sure her lambs are born healthy, how to prevent lamb rejection, and how to prevent lamb stealing by ewes. Your DVM has indicated that you can share the standard protocol the clinic recommends with Mrs. Rogers, and that she should also schedule a herd wellness check prior to breeding season.

1. What do you tell her?

_____

_____

_____

_____

_____

_____

_____

_____

_____

_____

_____

_____

_____

_____

_____

_____

_____

_____

EXERCISE 20.12 CASE STUDY #5: CARE OF NEONATAL CRIAS

Mrs. Jones has just purchased a pair of llamas, and the female is pregnant. Mrs. Jones is concerned about the birth of the cria and what she needs to do to make sure that everything goes well after the birth. She also asks what to look for that would warn her that the cria is in trouble.

1. What information will you share with Mrs. Jones?

_____

_____

_____

_____

_____

_____

_____

_____

21 Veterinary Oncology

LEARNING OBJECTIVES

When you have completed this chapter, you will be able to:
1. Pronounce, define, and spell all key terms in this chapter.
2. Discuss the pathogenesis of cancer, including:
   - Define oncology and explain mechanisms by which tumors cause clinical signs.
   - Differentiate between malignant and benign tumors.
   - List the classifications of tumors by tissue origin and provide examples of each.
   - Describe the difference between staging and grading and explain how each can be used to make treatment decisions.
3. Discuss the epidemiology of cancer, including:
   - List and describe common tumor types.
4. List clinical warning signs that can be associated with cancer.
5. Describe general staging diagnostics for patients with cancer, including:
   - Describe what is involved in an initial data base for a patient.
   - Discuss how imaging can be used to evaluate a patient.
   - Describe the difference between cytology and histology and list the advantages and limitations of each.
6. Discuss the process of staging cancer.
7. Describe therapeutic options in veterinary oncology, including surgery, radiation, chemotherapy, and palliative and comfort care, as well as discuss safety concerns and side effects related to administration and use of both oral and IV chemotherapy, along with ways to address such concerns and ways to reduce risks of side effects.
8. Discuss complementary, alternative, and integrative therapy. Explain why oncologists usually reject alternative medicine but embrace complementary and integrative therapies.
9. List and discuss common tumors of horses and cattle.

EXERCISE 21.1 MATCHING #1: IDENTIFYING TYPES OF TUMORS

Instructions: Match each term in column A with its corresponding definition in column B by writing the appropriate letter in the space provided.

Column A

1. _____ Neoplasm
2. _____ Lymphoma
3. _____ Mast cell tumor
4. _____ Osteosarcoma
5. _____ Carcinomas
6. _____ Oral tumors
7. _____ Hemangiosarcoma

Column B

A. Primarily affects bones of the appendicular skeleton.

B. Characterized by unrestrained proliferation of abnormal cells.

C. Common in larger, middle-age to older aged dogs; commonly found on the skin, heart, liver, and spleen.

D. The most common malignant skin tumors in dogs.

E. Affects primarily older animals.

F. Cancer of immune system cells.

G. Tumors of epithelial tissues.

EXERCISE 21.2 MATCHING #2: TYPES OF MEDICINE

Instructions: Match each description in column A with its corresponding type of medicine practice in column B by writing the appropriate letter in the space provided.

Column A

1. _____ Emphasizes the relationship between the veterinarian, patient, and pet owner.

2. _____ Used with conventional medicine to bring about health.

3. _____ Shiatsu massage.

4. _____ Makes use of all appropriate therapies to bring about optimal health and healing.

5. _____ Emphasizes wellness within a supportive relationship.

6. _____ Acupressure treatments.

Column B

A. Complementary medicine

B. Integrative medicine

EXERCISE 21.3 FUNDAMENTAL CHARACTERISTICS OF CANCER CELLS

Instructions: Identify 5 of the 8 characteristics of cancer cells.

1. _____

2. _____

3. _____

4. _____

5. _____

EXERCISE 21.4 MATCHING #3: TUMOR CLASSIFICATION

Instructions: Match each item in column A with the appropriate tissue of origin in column B.

Column A

1. _____ Osteosarcoma

2. _____ Lymphosarcoma

3. _____ Adenoma

4. _____ Leiomyosarcoma

5. _____ Sarcoma

6. _____ Liposarcoma

Column B

A. Glandular tissue

B. Mesenchymal tissue

C. Lymph cells

D. Smooth muscle tissue

E. Bone

F. Fat cells

Instructions: Fill in each of the spaces provided with the missing word or words listed below and complete the sentence. Terms may be used more than once.

Lymphoma

Mast cell tumor

Osteosarcoma

Melanoma

Hemangiosarcoma

Carcinomas

Squamous cell

1. _____ are tumors of epithelial tissue that arise from many sites.

2. _____ often present as an emergency with pale gums, poor or snappy pulses, distended abdomens, and extreme lethargy.

3. _____ is the most common oral tumor in dogs.

4. When lameness is presented, radiographs are recommended to rule out the presence of _____.

5. _____ is typically found under the tongue in cats.

6. Cells of a _____ tumor are filled with vesicles containing histamine.

7. A dog with a _____ most commonly presents with acute history of collapse and abdominal swelling.

8. The most common presentation of _____ in dogs is multiple, nonpainful, enlarged lymph nodes.

9. The most common presentation of _____ in cats is a subacute to chronic history of weight loss, possible vomiting, decreased appetite, and diarrhea.

EXERCISE 21.6 TRUE OR FALSE: COMPREHENSIVE

Instructions: Read the following statements and write "T" for true or "F" for false in the blanks provided. If a statement is false, correct the statement to make it true.

1. _____ Neoplasm is another term for new blood.

2. _____ Not all cells can become cancerous.

3. _____ The term neoplasia describes only malignant tissue.

4. _____ Radiation, certain chemicals such as radon gas, and pesticides are examples of mutagenic substances.

5. _____ When a mutagen gives rise to a formation of cancer, the process is called angiogenesis.

6. _____ A tumor that grows large and causes discomfort is likely malignant.

7. _____ The grade of a tumor can only be determined by a pathologist.

8. _____ Tumor size and how far it has spread are part of the grade of the tumor.

9. _____ One of the leading causes of disease-related deaths in the small animal species is coronary artery disease.

10. _____ Flat-Coated Retrievers are at higher risk of cancer than other dog breeds.

11. _____ An elevated score in a TK1 test can be an indication of a higher risk of cancer.

12. _____ The most common feline presentation of lymphoma is in the kitten.

13. _____ The most common malignant skin tumor in dogs is melanoma.

14. _____ Degranulation is the result of exostosis of the cells in a mast cell tumor.

15. _____ Tissue biopsy is the only definitive proof of hemangiosarcoma.

16. _____ Pain medication is of little use in the dog.

17. _____ "Watch and wait" is the best approach during early diagnosis procedures.

18. _____ The CT scan is considered the standard of care for assessment of thoracic lesions.

19. _____ Fine needle aspiration is a good choice when immediate diagnosis is desired.

20. _____ Results of the needle biopsy are considered the "gold standard."

21. _____ Staging a tumor is essential for planning appropriate and effective treatment.

22. _____ The primary goal of treatment in veterinary oncology is to prolong the life of the animal.

23. _____ Rarely is surgery recommended for a patient with metastasis.

24. _____ A form of radiation therapy that is effective in veterinary medicine is the placement of radioactive "seeds" in the body.

25. _____ Radiation does not specifically target cancer cells.

26. _____ Severe reactions to radiation are common.

27. _____ Leukotrachia is common following radiation therapy.

28. _____ Chemotherapeutic drugs all work to target cell replication.

29. _____ Chemotherapy is not useful in treating every type of cancer, and not all chemotherapy has negative side effects.

30. _____ Chronic exposure to chemotherapeutic agents is of particular concern for pregnant veterinary staff.

31. _____ ATLS is usually fatal unless treatment is immediate.

32. _____ The nadir of neutrophil count is approximately 5 to 7 days following the administration of chemotherapy.

33. _____ Home-cooked meals containing high-quality protein and fat sources provide the best balance to meet the long-term feeding needs of pets.

34. _____ Canned pumpkin is a good addition to the diet to help with loose stools.

35. _____ Veterinary technicians are responsible for identifying potential nutritional problems in their patients.

EXERCISE 21.7 FILL-IN-THE-BLANK: COMPREHENSIVE

Fill in each blank with the missing information to form a correct statement.

1. _____ is the most common type of skin tumor in horses; it is locally invasive but rarely metastatic.

2. _____ _____ _____ tumors are associated with prolonged exposure to the sun and are therefore more commonly seen in open-ranged cattle.

3. _____ tumors are cutaneous tumors derived from melanocytes.

4. _____ is one of the most common tumors in the frog of a horse's foot.

5. Cutaneous tumors are common in horses and are often found on _____, _____, _____, _____, _____-_____, and _____ _____.

6. The diet recommended over the use of generic brands is a(n) _____-approved diet.

7. An all-natural herbal supplement known to stop bleeding, used by herbalists and acupuncturists, is _____ _____.

8. Nonmainstream therapies used instead of standard medical treatments are known as _____ treatments.

9. Therapy that includes adjuvant treatments used in combination with conventional medical treatments is called _____ therapy.

10. Comfort care is often used synonymously with _____ _____.

11. Disciplined use of the _____ _____ _____ _____ ensures oncology patients will receive consistently excellent medical care and will reduce or eliminate chemotherapy-related errors.

12. The nadir of the neutrophil count occurs at approximately _____ to _____ days following the administration of chemotherapy.

13. The most abundant type of WBC with a short half-life and rapid turnover is the _____.

14. A serious and potentially life-threatening allergic reaction is known as _____.

15. A dog with four white feet may carry the _____ mutation, making them more likely to have a toxicity reaction to chemotherapeutic agents.

16. In the scale produced by the VCOG that standardizes the reporting of adverse drug events, a grade 1 and 2 toxicity is considered to be _____.

17. The most common side effects of chemotherapy are _____, _____ _____, _____, and _____.

18. PPEs that should be worn when working with chemotherapeutic drugs include _____, _____, _____, and _____ _____.

19. Chemotherapy acts on the molecular level with the intent of obstructing the _____, _____, and _____ requirements of cancer cells.

20. The chemotherapeutic agent that directly damages DMS, preventing mitosis, is a(n) _____ _____.

21. _____ prevent nausea caused by other chemotherapeutic drugs.

22. _____ inhibitors cause DNA strands to separate, blocking DNA replication.

23. Radiation causes damage to DNA _____ and _____ through the formation of highly charged particles (called free radicals) that damage DNA.

24. The histologic appearance of the tumor and how closely (or not) it resembles normal tissue is known as the tumor _____.

25. Histologic examination of the primary tumor requires either a _____ or a _____ of the mass.

26. For abdominal imaging, _____ is usually the diagnostic choice in veterinary medicine.

27. To assess cell morphology and to confirm that proper technique was used during blood collection and handling, a _____ _____ should be performed.

28. The standard of care for cancer patients that may undergo treatment includes _____, _____, _____, _____, and _____.

29. Two of the most important factors for long-term treatment success are _____ and _____.

30. It is estimated that _____ million dogs and cats are annually diagnosed with cancer.

EXERCISE 21.9 CASE STUDY: BLADDER CANCER IN BUFFY, A MIXED-BREED DOG

Buffy, a Cocker Spaniel mix, age 14, has been brought to the clinic. The owner reports that Buffy has been urinating frequently, and he has seen blood in Buffy's urine on and off for about 2 weeks. Buffy appears to strain a bit upon urination and has been urinating more frequently than in the past but otherwise seems "normal, but maybe not quite himself, ya know, a bit tired." The HHHHHMM Score is 40. The initial examination involved palpation and a rectal examination, and an initial suspicion of bladder cancer was suggested.

1. The veterinarian asks you to prepare the tests for an initial cancer evaluation. What tests need to be provided for Buffy?

_____

_____

_____

_____

2. As you prepare to take a blood draw from the jugular vein and capture a thoracic radiograph, an assistant in the practice pulls you aside and asks, "Why are we taking a thoracic radiograph if we think this is a bladder tumor?" You respond:

_____

_____

_____

_____

3. The assistant further inquires, "Why are we taking blood from the jugular vein rather than a peripheral vein like we usually do?" You respond:

_____

_____

_____

_____

4. The vet asks that you not use cystocentesis when collecting urine from Buffy. Why would such a request be made?

_____

_____

_____

_____

5. You know that the thoracic CT scan is more sensitive than radiographs and more likely to detect smaller and more subtle lesions. Why do you think radiographs are always recommended prior to taking a CT scan?

_____

_____

_____

_____

6. The vet assistant asks you if there is a noninvasive method that could be used to see the bladder structure. You respond:

_____

_____

7. The presence of a transitional cell carcinoma (TCC) has been suggested, with no evidence of metastasis, and Buffy is prepared for a needle biopsy. The veterinarian wants an immediate read on the malignant or benign status of the tumor as well as definitive diagnosis. Explain the process necessary to provide this information.

_____

_____

_____

_____

_____

_____

_____

_____

8. A fine needle biopsy is completed on Buffy, during which no cancer cells are noted. The cells have been sent to a pathologist for verification. Is it appropriate to tell the owner, "Good news! The tumor is benign"?

_____

_____

_____

_____

9. What four aspects should be considered during the process of staging a cancer?

_____

_____

_____

_____

10. The pathology report confirms TCC. Due to the grade of the tumor, the course of chemotherapy that has been elected by the veterinarian, and agreed to by Buffy's owner, will include several weeks of therapy during which a drug of low-vesicant potential and effective in the treatment of TCC will be used. If mitoxantrone is the drug selected, what side effects can be expected, and what is the nadir?

_____

_____

_____

_____

11. The vet has asked you to explain to Buffy's owner what type of side effects should be expected when Buffy returns home following treatments and any needed *human* safety precautions regarding contact with the chemotherapeutic agent. You indicate the following to Buffy's owner:

_____

_____

_____

_____

_____

_____

_____

_____

12. Buffy's owner asks about nutrition and wants to begin an organic, all-natural diet for him. The owner says, "He is such a member of our family; he deserves home-cooked meals, like the rest of us." How would you respond?

_____

_____

_____

_____

_____

_____

_____

_____

_____

_____

13. The veterinary assistant wonders if the drugs are safe for staff to handle. You respond by detailing that several safety protocols are in place in your clinic, including the following:
- PPE
- Chemotherapy drug preparation
- Administration

a. You say the following about PPE:

_____

_____

_____

_____

b. You explain the following about chemotherapy drug preparation:

_____

_____

_____

_____

_____

_____

_____

_____

c. Finally, you indicate the following about administration:

_____

_____

_____

_____

_____

_____

_____

_____

14. The veterinarian is considering a metronomic approach to dosing and asks if you know what this means. You respond:

_____

_____

_____

_____

22 Neonatal Care of Puppies, Kittens, and Foals

When you have completed this chapter, you will be able to:

1. Pronounce, define, and spell all the key terms in this chapter.
2. Define the neonatal period for puppies and kittens, obtain an accurate and thorough clinical history for all littermates and parents, and describe the procedure for physical examination of a neonate, including equipment needed and potential abnormalities.
3. Explain the timeline of normal development in neonatal puppies and kittens.
4. Do the following regarding performance of diagnostic procedures and routine maintenance in neonatal puppies and kittens:
   - Discuss how to perform diagnostic procedures on a neonatal puppy or kitten.
   - Discuss appropriate times to administer medical treatments to neonatal puppies and kittens; explain proper nutrition, preventive medicine, and normal behavior to the owner.
5. Do the following regarding common concerns and disorders in the puppy and kitten:
   - Explain common concerns of neonatal puppies and kittens, such as hypothermia, dehydration, hypoglycemia, malnutrition, fading puppy or kitten syndrome, and neonatal isoerythrolysis in kittens.
   - Discuss proper care of an orphaned neonatal puppy or kitten and common complications involved with orphaned neonates.
6. Do the following regarding the perinatal period and the high-risk mare:
   - Differentiate between normal and abnormal perinatal periods in the mare, and explain how to care for a high-risk mare.
   - Identify the stages of labor in a mare, and describe how to treat any complications that may arise at each stage.
7. Describe the normal development of a neonatal foal that occurs during the first 24 hours after birth, and identify normal vital signs and behavior.
8. Do the following regarding care of the sick foal:
   - List the signs of a critically ill foal, including symptoms of prematurity and dysmaturity and classic early clinical signs of disease.
   - Identify common sites and procedures for venous and arterial blood collection, as well as appropriate needles, syringes, and restraint techniques to be used in the neonatal foal.
   - Identify parameters that should be monitored in the hospitalized foal, and describe complications that may arise during hospitalization.
   - Describe proper nursing care for the foal to prevent contamination, including washing of hands and injection sites, changing of IV fluid lines, and maintenance of IV and jugular catheters.
   - Explain appropriate physical therapy for the recumbent foal, the necessity for being kept in sternal position and frequent changes in recumbency, and proper restraint techniques that can be used for the ambulatory foal.
9. Explain alternative methods that can be used to ensure that nutritional needs are met if a foal is unable to nurse from the mare.

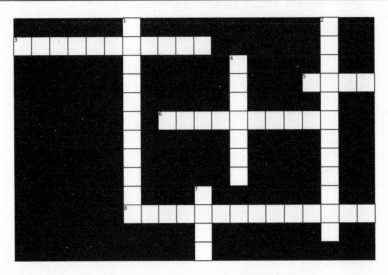

Across

3 Abnormally low body temperature. The measured body temperature must be compared with what is normal for the age group because neonates have lower body temperatures than adults.
5 A juvenile horse nursing from its mother.
6 Born with a specific condition. Can be genetic or environmentally induced.
8 In puppies and kittens, the first 2 to 4 weeks of life are characterized by complete dependence on the mother because of incomplete neurologic functions, such as audio and visual abilities and proper spinal reflexes.

Down

1 Abnormal depletion of body fluids.
2 Lower than normal levels of blood glucose resulting in lack of fuel to the brain and other organ systems.
4 When one parent or both parents transmit disease-causing genes to the offspring, that disease is described as_____.
7 Adult female horse.

EXERCISE 22.2 DEFINITIONS: COMMON DISEASES AND CONDITIONS OF NEONATAL FOALS

Instructions: Define each disease or condition of neonatal foals in your own words.

1. Sepsis or septic shock: _____

   _____

2. Neonatal encephalopathy: _____

   _____

3. Failure of passive transfer (FPT): _____

   _____

4. Neonatal nephropathy: _____

   _____

5. Neonatal isoerythrolysis: _____

   _____

6. Dysmaturity: _____

   _____

7. Neonatal gastroenteropathy: _____

   _____

8. Colitis: _____

   _____

9. Musculoskeletal abnormalities: _____

   _____

10. Patent urachus: _____

    _____

11. Ruptured bladder: _____

    _____

12. Entropion: _____

    _____

13. Septic arthritis or septic physitis: _____

    _____

14. Meconium retention: _____

_____

15. Prematurity: _____

_____

EXERCISE 22.3 MATCHING: THE NEONATAL FOAL

Instructions: Match each word in column A with its corresponding definition in column B by writing the appropriate letter in the space provided.

Column A

1. _____ Urachus
2. _____ Nosocomial
3. _____ Omphalitis
4. _____ Bacteremia
5. _____ Petechiae
6. _____ Pinna
7. _____ Insufflation
8. _____ Colostrum
9. _____ Hypovolemia
10. _____ Foaling
11. _____ Icterus
12. _____ Water breaking
13. _____ Fibrinogen
14. _____ Dysmaturity
15. _____ Hypoxemia
16. _____ Waxing
17. _____ Entropion
18. _____ Glucosuria
19. _____ Bucket baby
20. _____ Primiparous
21. _____ Injected
22. _____ Miotic

Column B

A. Parturition in a mare.

B. Beads of milk on the tip of a mare's teats prior to delivery.

C. Another name for a maiden mare.

D. Mare's first milk.

E. Rupture of a mare's placenta releasing allantoic fluid.

F. Low oxygen blood levels.

G. A foal raised as an orphan.

H. Small-molecular-weight polymers that result from plasmin cleavage of fibrinogen and fibrin.

I. Infection in the bloodstream.

J. The state resulting in a foal with a longer-than-expected gestation.

K. The word used to describe dark purple mucous membranes with prominent vessels.

L. Yellow sclerae and mucous membranes.

M. Small areas of hemorrhaging.

N. Foal's outer ear.

O. A condition in which the lower eyelids roll inward.

P. Decreased blood volume.

Q. A term used to describe constricted pupils.

R. Administration of intranasal oxygen.

S. Sugar present in the urine.

T. A canal in the umbilicus that connects to the urinary bladder.

U. Inflammation of the umbilicus.

V. Resistant infections acquired in the hospital.

Instructions: Read the following statements and write "T" for true or "F" for false in the blanks provided. If a statement is false, correct the statement to make it true.

1. _____ When obtaining a comprehensive history on puppies and kittens, the history of the number of ill animals, the method by which they were raised, and the queen or bitch's vaccination history should be included.

2. _____ Painting the toenails of neonates is an acceptable method of identification.

3. _____ A mercury thermometer is more practical to use than a digital thermometer when obtaining the body temperature of a neonate.

4. _____ When assessing the hydration status of a neonate, checking the skin turgor is the preferred method.

5. _____ Normal neonatal puppies and kittens often have sparse hair coats.

6. _____ Bluish or dark red skin may be normal in a neonatal puppy or kitten.

7. _____ A bloated abdomen in a neonatal puppy or kitten should not be ignored.

8. _____ Neonates lack neuromuscular reflexes.

9. _____ Normal neonates may have irregular heart and respiratory rates.

10. _____ When neonates are born, they are capable of maintaining their own body temperature.

11. _____ The abdominal component to breathing is absent in neonatal puppies and kittens.

12. _____ Dog testicles do not descend until 6 to 8 weeks of age.

13. _____ Cystocentesis is a safe method of urine collection in neonates.

14. _____ Undesirable behavior is one of the most common reasons for abandonment of dogs and cats younger than 1 year of age.

15. _____ Puppies get their energy from protein during the first few weeks of life.

16. _____ The fluid requirement of neonates is much higher than that of adult animals.

17. _____ There is less risk of aspiration associated with tube feeding than with syringe and bottle feeding in neonates.

18. _____ Mares with multiple pregnancies often deliver around the same time each pregnancy.

19. _____ Foals are born without a menace response.

20. _____ The packed-cell volume (PCV) of the normal foal during the first 24 hours of life is less than that of an adult horse.

Instructions: Circle the one correct answer to each of the following questions.

1. The time period of a puppy or kitten's life that is considered to be the neonatal phase is
   a. 1 to 2 weeks
   b. 2 to 4 weeks
   c. 4 to 6 weeks
   d. 6 to 8 weeks

2. Neonatal puppies and kittens are unable to regulate their own body temperature during the first _____ weeks of life.
   a. 2
   b. 3
   c. 4
   d. 6

3. Normal developing puppies and kittens will nurse as frequently as every _____ during their first week of life.
   a. 1 to 2 hours
   b. 2 to 4 hours
   c. 3 to 6 hours
   d. 3 to 5 hours

4. The age at which puppies and kittens should be able to lift their head is
   a. 1 day
   b. 2 days
   c. 3 days
   d. 4 days

5. The age at which puppies and kittens begin to crawl in a coordinated manner is
   a. 1 week
   b. 2 weeks
   c. 3 weeks
   d. 4 weeks

6. At birth, the sex of puppies is
   a. Unambiguous
   b. Easily detected
   c. Determined by descended testicles
   d. Determined by anus to tail position

7. Kittens and puppies begin to open their eyes at the age of
   a. 3 to 7 days
   b. 5 to 10 days
   c. 7 to 12 days
   d. 10 to 14 days

8. The external ear canals of puppies and kittens will open at the age of
   a. 10 to 12 days
   b. 12 to 14 days
   c. 14 to 16 days
   d. 16 to 18 days

9. When obtaining blood from a neonate, the percentage of the circulating blood volume obtained over the course of 1 week should not exceed
   a. 5%
   b. 10%
   c. 15%
   d. 20%

10. At what age do puppies and kittens have a temperature that is similar to an adult's temperature?
    a. 2 weeks
    b. 4 weeks
    c. 6 weeks
    d. 8 weeks

11. Blood can easily be obtained from neonates by using the
    a. Cephalic vein
    b. Jugular vein
    c. Saphenous vein
    d. Femoral artery

12. Puppies and kittens are able to stand with good postural reflexes at the end of week
    a. 2
    b. 3
    c. 4
    d. 5

13. If a neonatal puppy or kitten weighs 300 g, the maximum volume of blood that can be drawn in the course of 1 week would be
    a. 1.5 cc
    b. 2.0 cc
    c. 3.0 cc
    d. 3.5 cc

14. To obtain urine samples in the neonate,
    a. Use an ultrasound
    b. Perform cystocentesis
    c. Stimulate the bladder by gently rubbing the genital area with a moistened cotton ball
    d. Forcefully express the bladder

15. Because neonatal animals have immature kidneys, it is considered normal to find urine with a specific gravity between
    a. 1.010 and 1.015
    b. 1.012 and 1.020
    c. 1.015 and 1.025
    d. 1.020 and 1.030

16. The age puppies and kittens should be taken to the veterinarian for their first official health examination is
    a. 4 to 6 weeks
    b. 6 to 8 weeks
    c. 8 to 10 weeks
    d. 10 to 14 weeks

17. A neonate is considered hypothermic if at birth the body temperature drops below
    a. 90° F
    b. 92° F
    c. 94° F
    d. 97° F

18. When treating hypothermic neonatal puppies, it is important to withhold the administration of oral food until the animal has
    a. Audible gut sounds and is moderately warmed
    b. Audible gut sounds and is fully rewarmed
    c. No gut sounds but is moderately rewarmed
    d. No gut sounds but is fully rewarmed

19. Any disease process or fluid or electrolyte imbalance in neonatal animals will quickly lead to
    a. Hypothermia
    b. Colic
    c. Lethargy
    d. Dehydration

20. Acceptable routes of fluid administration in the neonate include
    a. IV only
    b. IV or IO only
    c. IV, IO, and IP
    d. IV, IO, IP, and SC

21. When administering fluids intraosseously to a neonate, an 18- or 19-gauge needle can be placed in the
    a. Proximal tibia or proximal femur
    b. Proximal tibia or distal femur
    c. Distal tibia or distal femur
    d. Distal tibia or proximal femur

22. Failure of a neonate to suckle will result in _____ after 24 to 36 hours as a consequence of depletion of hepatic storage.
    a. Hypothermia
    b. Hyperthermia
    c. Hypoglycemia
    d. Hyperglycemia

23. Dextrose solutions should never be administered

    _____, as they may cause tissue damage.
    a. Intravenously
    b. Subcutaneously
    c. Intraosseously
    d. Intraperitoneally

24. Occasionally a mare will develop a problem in late-term pregnancy. These mares are referred to as
    a. Primiparous mares
    b. High-risk mares
    c. Late-term mares
    d. Problem mares

25. The average gestational length for the mare is
    a. 200 days
    b. 240 days
    c. 300 days
    d. 340 days

26. The veterinarian will perform a rectal examination and transrectal ultrasound on a pregnant mare at approximately
    a. 15 days and 30 days
    b. 15 days, 30 days, and 90 days
    c. 30 days and 90 days
    d. 30 days, 90 days, and 120 days

27. In late-term pregnancy, the foal's heart rate will fall within the range of
    a. 20 to 80 bpm
    b. 30 to 100 bpm
    c. 40 to 150 bpm
    d. 80 to 180 bpm

28. Mares often foal
    a. First thing in the morning
    b. In the afternoon
    c. In the evening
    d. At night

29. Agitation, pacing, nickering, lifting the tail head, turning and biting at sides, and kicking the abdomen occur during which stage of labor in the mare?
    a. Stage 1
    b. Stage 2
    c. Stage 3
    d. Stage 4

30. Sweating around the shoulders of a mare in labor is indicative of
    a. Dystocia
    b. Foaling within 30 minutes
    c. Colic
    d. Nothing significant

31. The mare will pass her placenta during _____ of labor.
    a. Stage 1
    b. Stage 2
    c. Stage 3
    d. Stage 4

EXERCISE 22.6 FILL-IN-THE-BLANK: NEONATOLOGY OF PUPPIES AND KITTENS

Instructions: Fill in each of the spaces provided with the missing word or words that complete the sentence.

1. When performing a physical examination on a neonate, the use of a _____ stethoscope with a 2-cm bell is helpful.

2. When a neonate is born, hair will be present on most of the body, excluding the _____ abdomen.

3. The only motor skills present in a neonatal puppy or kitten are _____, _____, and distress _____.

4. Urination and defecation of neonates is initiated by the bitch or queen licking the _____ area.

5. The body temperature of puppies and kittens at birth will be lower than in adult animals and will rise to 94.7° F to 100.1° F during their first _____ of life.

6. A neonate's umbilical cord will dry out during its first day of life and is expected to fall off by day _____ to _____.

7. The flexor tone present at birth in puppies and kittens will switch over to the extensor tone after the _____ day of life.

8. Neonates generally tolerate a(n) _____ examination better than a radiography examination when imaging techniques are used.

9. At the beginning of week _____ of life, puppies and kittens should receive their first deworming treatment of pyrantel pamoate.

10. Deworming treatment in puppies and kittens is aimed mainly toward eliminating a common intestinal parasite called _____.

11. As long as neonates remain close to their mother and specifically the mammary glands, they will be able to maintain their _____ balance.

12. A neonate is considered hypothermic if its body temperature drops below _____.

13. When hypothermic neonates are tube fed, milk replacer is either regurgitated and aspirated, resulting in _____, or the ingesta may ferment, leading to _____.

14. Clinical signs in a chilled neonate with a body temperature above 88° F include restlessness, continuous crying, _____ mucous membranes, and skin that feels _____ to the touch.

15. When the body temperature of a small animal neonate falls into the range of _____° F to _____° F, the neonate appears lethargic and uncoordinated.

16. When the body temperature of a small animal neonate is below _____° F, the animal will appear to be dead.

17. _____ also contributes significantly to hypothermia in the neonate, thus proper ventilation or oxygen should be administered when possible.

18. Warm air and _____ in a human neonatal incubator is optimal for rewarming hypothermic animal neonates.

19. _____ rewarming of a neonate will result in heat prostration with increased respiratory rate and effort.

20. Raising the body temperature of a neonate more than _____° F is usually fatal because of delayed organ failure.

21. The hydration status of a neonate is best checked by looking at the oral _____

    _____.

22. All fluids should be warmed to _____ before administration to the neonate.

23. Tacky or dry mucous membranes in a neonate indicate _____% to _____% dehydration.

24. When a neonate has reached _____% dehydration, the oral mucous membranes will be dry, with a noticeable decrease in skin elasticity.

25. Fluid requirements are _____ in neonates; however, total fluid volumes that can be administered are _____.

26. When administering intravenous fluids to a neonate, it is often easiest to place a short 23- or 25-gauge catheter in the _____ vein.

27. The key element to nursing a dehydrated neonate back to health is _____

    _____.

28. _____ and _____ are the first indications that a neonate is not doing well.

29. Hypoglycemic neonates will have serum glucose less than _____ mg/dL.

30. A _____ solution is used to treat a neonate with hypoglycemia.

31. One of the most common causes of seizures in neonatal puppies and kittens is _____.

EXERCISE 22.7 CASE STUDY: POSTPARTUM EXAMINATION OF A LITTER OF PUPPIES

Signalment: Roxanne, a 3-year-old female Rottweiler with her litter of six 4-day-old puppies.

Chief Complaint: Roxanne and her puppies are presented for a routine postpartum examination, including puppy tail docking and dewclaw removal. The owner reports that Roxanne delivered the six puppies uneventfully 4 days prior to presentation. This is Roxanne's second pregnancy, and she is accepting and caring for the puppies. All of the puppies seem to be nursing vigorously and gaining weight. Answer the following questions regarding this case.

a. What are the ways in which examination of neonates differs from examination of adult animals?

_____

_____

_____

_____

b. What special equipment is needed when examining neonates?

_____

_____

_____

_____

c. What are the components of a complete neonatal examination, including specific abnormalities you would look for?

_____

_____

_____

_____

_____

_____

_____

_____

23 Care of Birds, Reptiles, and Small Mammals

LEARNING OBJECTIVES

When you have completed this chapter, you will be able to:

1. Pronounce, define, and spell all key terms in this chapter.
2. Do the following regarding the intake process and examination of birds:
   - Collect an accurate and thorough clinical history for an avian patient and explain proper capture and restraint techniques for an effective and timely examination with minimal stress to the patient.
   - Discuss the physical examination process.
3. Explain sample collections and diagnostic procedures commonly used in birds, as well as proper anesthetic techniques.
4. Describe common routes for administering medication to birds, gavage and hand-feeding, and grooming.
5. Discuss avian nutrition, as well as managing the hospitalized avian patient.
6. List the materials needed to properly treat and handle reptile species in the veterinary hospital and discuss the information needed for an accurate and thorough clinical history of a reptile patient.
7. Discuss reptile nutrition and lighting, obtain sample collections, and perform diagnostic procedures commonly used in reptiles.
8. Understand anesthesia and intubation recommendations for the chelonian, snake, and lizard.
9. Describe husbandry requirements for the reptilian patient, including temperature, humidity, lighting, and substrate requirements and discuss *Salmonella*.
10. Explain the proper care of a ferret, including handling and grooming, phlebotomy, anesthesia, hospital management, and nutritional requirements and list the common presenting complaints in this species.
11. Explain the proper care of a rabbit, including nutritional requirements, anesthetic techniques, and intravenous access and list the common presenting complaints in this species.
12. Explain the proper care of rodents, including antibiotic therapy, anesthetic techniques, antiparasitic agents, and nutritional requirements and specifically discuss guinea pigs, hamsters, gerbils, rats, and chinchillas.
13. Describe the proper care of hedgehogs and sugar gliders, including husbandry requirements, dietary requirements, and common disease conditions.

EXERCISE 23.1 DEFINITIONS: KEY TERMS

Instructions: Define each term in your own words, including the species or general type of animal to which it applies.

1. Cloaca: _____

   _____

2. Ecdysis: _____

   _____

3. Conjunctivitis: _____

   _____

4. Colonic wash: _____

   _____

5. Medial metatarsal vein: _____

   _____

EXERCISE 23.2 FILL-IN-THE-BLANK: TERMS AND DEFINITIONS

Instructions: Fill in each of the spaces provided with the missing term that completes the sentence.

1. The use of penicillin antibiotics in guinea pigs often causes _____ to occur.

2. The _____ is a muscular outpouching of the esophagus located above a bird's sternum

   where food is stored prior to digestion. In birds, the neutrophils are known as _____.

3. A turtle is an example of a _____.

EXERCISE 23.3 MATCHING: TERMS AND DEFINITIONS

Instructions: Match each term in column A with its corresponding definition in column B by writing the appropriate letter in the space provided.

Column A

1. _____ *Giardia*
2. _____ Glottis
3. _____ Palpebral edema
4. _____ Perineum
5. _____ Gram-positive organisms
6. _____ Basilic vein

Column B

A. Located on the wing of birds.

B. Inflammation of the eyelid.

C. Organisms inhabiting the digestive system in most pet bird species.

D. The opening into the trachea.

E. The area around the anus and vulva.

F. A protozoan GI parasite that affects birds.

EXERCISE 23.4 TRUE OR FALSE: COMPREHENSIVE

Instructions: Read the following statements and write "T" for true or "F" for false in the blanks provided. If a statement is false, correct the statement to make it true.

1. _____ Most medical problems in exotic pets are caused by the owner's lack of knowledge about basic nutrition and proper husbandry.

2. _____ A choanal culture is recommended when birds are exhibiting upper respiratory signs.

3. _____ The left jugular vein is much larger than the right jugular vein in birds.

4. _____ Injectable anesthetics are most commonly used to restrain birds for radiography.

5. _____ The primary feathers are often clipped in pet bids to prevent flight.

6. _____ The best method to medicate birds is by putting their drugs in the water.

7. _____ Most pet birds should be weighed on a gram scale.

8. _____ The most common nutritional deficiency in captive turtles is vitamin A deficiency.

9. _____ Seed diets are acceptable for smaller psittacine birds.

10. _____ Birds do not have sweat glands.

11. _____ A significant contributing factor to many disease processes in reptiles is improper feeding.

12. _____ Positive pressure ventilation is recommended with isoflurane anesthesia in chelonians.

13. _____ NSHP is one of the more common bone diseases prevalent in captive reptiles.

14. _____ It is vital that clients purchase full spectrum lights for reptiles.

15. _____ Tortoises are primarily herbivores.

16. _____ Hypovitaminosis in chelonians can be prevented by providing a diet that supplies earthworms, small fish, and orange or yellow vegetables.

17. _____ Lizards are strict carnivores.

18. _____ Ferrets are induced ovulators.

19. _____ There is a distemper vaccine approved for use in ferrets.

20. _____ Ferrets are very susceptible to vaccine reactions.

21. _____ *Otodectes cynotis* is common in ferrets.

22. _____ Guinea pigs should be fed a diet high in calcium.

23. _____ Wire cage bottoms may cause footpad ulcers in guinea pigs.

24. _____ Guinea pigs lack the enzyme L-gulonolactone oxidase.

25. _____ Hamsters should be housed separately.

26. _____ Gerbils have cheek pouches.

27. _____ Nasal discharges in rats may turn red, but this is not usually caused by blood.

28. _____ Hedgehogs in captivity are prone to obesity.

29. _____ Sugar gliders consume large quantities of sugar or fruit.

EXERCISE 23.5 MULTIPLE CHOICE: COMPREHENSIVE

Instructions: Circle the one correct answer to each of the following questions.

1. Which is a protozoan parasite that may be found on a crop wash?
   a. *Candida*
   b. *Capillaria*
   c. *Giardia*
   d. *Trichomonas*

2. Where is the basilic vein found on the bird?
   a. Medial surface of the wing
   b. At the back of the head
   c. On the lower leg
   d. In the roof of the mouth

3. Which muscles are most commonly used for injections in birds?
   a. Pectoral
   b. Epaxial
   c. Gluteal
   d. Biceps

4. Which is the recommended site for placement of intraosseous catheters in birds?
   a. Distal humerus
   b. Proximal tibia
   c. Distal femur
   d. Distal ulna

5. Which pet population is growing steadily, requiring high-quality veterinary care for these pets?
   a. Cat
   b. Rat
   c. Reptile
   d. Rabbit

6. The size of rodent to feed a snake should be which of the following?
   a. Twice the diameter of the snake's body
   b. About the same diameter as the snake's body
   c. No more than 4 inches long
   d. Length and size are not important

7. Which radiographic view is used routinely in turtles but not in snakes, lizards, or birds?
   a. Lateral
   b. Hanging VD
   c. AP (or frontal)
   d. Lateral oblique

8. How often does a snake feed?
   a. Once every 1 to 2 weeks
   b. Every 3 to 6 days
   c. Once a month
   d. Every 48 to 56 hours

9. Metabolic bone disease is least likely to occur in which of the following?
   a. Iguana
   b. Bearded dragon
   c. Burmese python
   d. Box turtle

10. If a ferret-specific commercial diet is not available, then _____ can be substituted.
    a. Canned dog food
    b. Insectivore diet
    c. Kitten food
    d. Rodent chow

11. Which is the best place for IV access in the rabbit?
    a. Ear
    b. Foot
    c. Jugular vein
    d. Saphenous vein

12. Human influenza is seen in which of the following animals?
    a. Hedgehog
    b. Prairie dog
    c. Ferret
    d. Guinea pig

13. Which mite most commonly affects the fur of rabbits?
    a. *Sarcoptes*
    b. *Microsporum*
    c. *Demodex*
    d. *Cheyletiella*

14. Which animal produces precocious young?
    a. Ferret
    b. Rabbit
    c. Guinea pig
    d. Sugar glider

15. Which antibiotic is least likely to cause dysbiosis in rabbits and rodents?
    a. Amoxicillin
    b. Streptomycin
    c. Tetracycline
    d. Ciprofloxacin

16. An adult female ferret with a swollen vulva and hair loss most likely has which disorder?
    a. Hyperadrenocorticism
    b. Hypothyroidism
    c. Ovarian neoplasia
    d. Hyperthyroidism

17. Which animal requires vitamin C in its diet?
    a. Rabbit
    b. Sugar glider
    c. Hedgehog
    d. Guinea pig

18. Which of the following is a social animal and needs special attention if housed singly?
    a. Guinea pig
    b. Sugar glider
    c. Hamster
    d. Rabbit

19. The cranial vena cava is often the preferred site for blood collection in which animal?
    a. Rabbit
    b. Ferret
    c. Parrot
    d. Snake

20. Which animal has the enzyme atropinase, which can interfere with atropine administration?
    a. Ferret
    b. Snake
    c. Sugar glider
    d. Rabbit

21. Ferrets should be vaccinated against which disease?
    a. Feline panleukopenia
    b. Canine distemper
    c. Measles
    d. Leptospirosis

22. Which of the following animals has cheek pouches that it can stuff with food?
    a. Sugar glider
    b. Guinea pig
    c. Ferret
    d. Hamster

23. Seizures are an inherited disorder seen in which of the following?
    a. Gerbils
    b. Hamsters
    c. Rabbits
    d. Ferrets

24. Which animal originally comes from Australia?
    a. Gerbil
    b. Sugar glider
    c. Hedgehog
    d. Hamster

25. Which rodent is used most commonly in research?
    a. Rabbit
    b. Guinea pig
    c. Mouse
    d. Hamster

26. Which of the following should be fed an insectivore diet?
    a. Hedgehog
    b. Prairie dog
    c. Sugar glider
    d. Iguana

27. Which of the following rodents has hypsodontic teeth?
    a. Hamster
    b. Rabbit
    c. Guinea pig
    d. Gerbil

28. Which of the following animals should be examined for dental malocclusion, trichobezoars, and dehydration?
    a. Anorexic rabbit
    b. Obese guinea pig
    c. Bulemic turtle
    d. Stressed bird

29. Which of the following animals should be on heartworm preventive medication if kept outdoors in an area with a high prevalence of heartworm?
    a. Rabbit
    b. Prairie dog
    c. Sugar glider
    d. Ferret

30. Which animal should be housed in a tall wire enclosure with branches and places to hide?
    a. Hedgehog
    b. Sugar glider
    c. Guinea pig
    d. Prairie dog

1. A client calls and states that her daughter received an adult guinea pig for Christmas but does not have any knowledge on what or how to feed it. On further questioning, she mentions that she is feeding it the same diet she feeds her rabbit. What advice should you give her?

_____

_____

_____

_____

_____

_____

_____

_____

_____

_____

_____

_____

24 Physical Therapy, Rehabilitation, and Alternative Medical Nursing

LEARNING OBJECTIVES

When you have completed this chapter, you will be able to:

1. Pronounce, define, and spell all of the key terms in this chapter.
2. List commonly used nutraceuticals and chondroprotectants, and describe their therapeutic uses.
3. Do the following regarding the use of herbal medicine:
   - List commonly used Western herbs, Chinese herbs, and Ayurvedic herbs, and describe their therapeutic uses.
4. Explain the principles and techniques of acupuncture and describe the role of the veterinary technician in acupuncture therapy.
5. Describe how veterinary spinal manipulative therapy can benefit animal patients, and explain the role of the veterinary technician.
6. List common indications for veterinary rehabilitation.
7. Compare and contrast the physical therapeutic modalities used in veterinary rehabilitation, including exercise-based therapies, electrical and magnet-based therapies, light and sound-based therapies, and superficial thermal therapies.
8. List supportive and assistive devices commonly used for animal patients.

Instructions: Define each term in your own words.

1. Glucosamine:_____

_____

2. Chondroprotectants:_____

_____

3. Ayurvedic medicine:_____

_____

4. Goniometry:_____

_____

5. Chondroitin:_____

_____

6. Nutraceutical: _____

_____

7. Rehabilitation: _____

_____

8. Hyaluronic acid: _____

_____

9. Modality: _____

_____

10. Polysulfated glycosaminoglycans: _____

_____

EXERCISE 24.2 MATCHING #1: KEY TERMS AND DEFINITIONS

Instructions: Match each term in column A with its corresponding description in column B by writing the appropriate letter in the space provided.

Column A

1. _____ Thermotherapy
2. _____ Acupressure
3. _____ Passive range of motion (PROM)
4. _____ Hydrotherapy
5. _____ Massage
6. _____ Cryotherapy
7. _____ Low-level laser therapy (LLLT)
8. _____ Myotherapy
9. _____ Neuromuscular electrical stimulation (NMES)
10. _____ Ultrasound (therapeutic)
11. _____ TENS
12. _____ Acupuncture
13. _____ Orthotic

Column B

A. Relief of soft-tissue pain resulting from muscle tension or "knots."

B. Applying firm digital pressure to an acupuncture point for a specific length of time.

C. Device applied to the body to limit motion or provide support.

D. Application of light waves that are monochromic and polarized to stimulate healing.

E. Stimulation of a specific point on the body to produce a physiologic effect.

F. Removes heat from the body and causes rebound vasodilatation when removed.

G. The use of electric impulses to release endogenous opioids; flexion and extension of a joint within its normal ability to move by a practitioner.

H. Manual movement or vibration of soft tissue to relieve pain and increase circulation.

I. Contraction of type II muscle fibers through the application of electric current.

J. Used to treat chronic and acute pain through electro-analgesia.

K. Application of heat to the body to reduce pain.

L. Sound waves that can have a thermal effect on the body.

M. Movements occur in water to enhance range of motion and reduce concussion of joints.

EXERCISE 24.3 MATCHING #2: HERB DOSAGE FORMS

Instructions: Match each herb dosing term in column A with its corresponding description in column B by writing the appropriate letter in the space provided. More than one answer may apply.

Column A

1. _____ Poultice
2. _____ *Materia medica*
3. _____ Bulk
4. _____ Extract
5. _____ Ointment
6. _____ Capsule
7. _____ Compress

Column B

A. Form concentrated in alcohol or glycerin.

B. Most often used in preparation for herbivores.

C. Form applied topically and left in place.

D. A formulary for herbs.

E. Form applied topically for short periods.

F. Made by soaking in hot water and allowed to cool.

G. One of two oral forms preferred for carnivores.

Chapter **24 Physical Therapy, Rehabilitation, and Alternative Medical Nursing**

EXERCISE 24.4 MATCHING #3: ALTERNATIVE THERAPIES

Instructions: For the following alternative therapies, identify whether each condition is an indication or contraindication for that therapy by writing an "I" for indication or "C" for contraindication in the space provided.

1. Alternative Therapy: Neuromuscular electrical stimulation

   a. _____ Infection

   b. _____ Thrombophlebitis

   c. _____ Mast cell tumor

   d. _____ Muscle atrophy following surgery

2. Alternative Therapy: Low-level laser therapy

   a. _____ Degenerative joint disease

   b. _____ Intervertebral disc disease

   c. _____ Soft tissue injury

   d. _____ Treatment of trigger points

3. Alternative Therapy: Massage therapy

   a. _____ Bite wound abscess

   b. _____ Toning atrophied muscle

   c. _____ Tendonitis

   d. _____ Surgical site

EXERCISE 24.5 MATCHING #4: REHABILITATION — PHYSICAL DYSFUNCTIONS

Instructions: Match each physical dysfunction in column A with its corresponding description in column B by writing the appropriate letter in the space provided.

Column A

1. _____ Pain
2. _____ Inflammation
3. _____ Reduced range of motion
4. _____ Hypermobility
5. _____ Muscle atrophy
6. _____ Muscle tightness or spasm
7. _____ Trigger points
8. _____ Scarring
9. _____ Abnormal gait
10. _____ Neurologic dysfunction
11. _____ Ataxia
12. _____ Balance and proprioception
13. _____ Bursitis

Column B

A. A response to tissue injury characterized by pain, swelling, redness, and heat.

B. Treated with a balance board exercise.

C. Treated with ischemic compression.

D. Decreased muscle mass.

E. A decrease in the parameter measured by goniometry.

F. Often treated with myotherapy.

G. An unpleasant feeling caused by real or potential tissue damage.

H. Treated with neuromuscular reeducation exercises.

I. Friction is a massage technique that is used to break up this type of tissue.

J. Treated with a clinical application of ultrasound.

K. Common problem of physical dysfunction; therapy option is an underwater treadmill.

L. Uncoordinated gait.

M. Excessive range of motion of a joint.

Instructions: Match each of the therapeutic exercises in column A with its corresponding benefit in column B by writing the appropriate letter in the space provided.

Column A

1. _____ Proprioceptive exercises
2. _____ Endurance exercises
3. _____ Neuromuscular reeducation exercises
4. _____ Balance exercises
5. _____ Strengthening exercises

Column B

A. To decrease muscle atrophy.

B. For the cardiovascular system.

C. To improve stability.

D. To correct posture and gait.

E. To improve body awareness.

EXERCISE 24.7 TRUE OR FALSE: COMPREHENSIVE

Instructions: Read the following statements and write "T" for true or "F" for false in the blanks provided. If a statement is false, correct the statement to make it true.

1. _____ Complementary and alternative medicine is now mainstream and conventional.

2. _____ Ayurvedic herbs are typically formulated with a single herb.

3. _____ The main advantage of using herbal supplements is that, unlike drugs, they are safe and do not cause side effects.

4. _____ Bulk herbs are most commonly used for herbivores.

5. _____ It is important that herbs are purchased from a reputable source that emphasizes quality control.

6. _____ Capsules and tables are more often used for carnivores.

7. _____ Extracts are made by concentrating the herb in alcohol. A standardized extract is unlike a drug in that a specific amount of active ingredient is measured instead of measuring of the herb itself.

8. _____ Similar to drugs, some herbs have a low margin of safety.

9. _____ A veterinarian can use acupuncture to treat birds, dolphins, and elephants.

10. _____ The least invasive form of acupuncture is dry-needle insertion.

11. _____ A chiropractic vertebral subluxation is most often detected on x-rays.

12. _____ Swimming is the best treatment for strengthening both forelimbs and hindlimbs.

13. _____ In the underwater treadmill, the most resistance with the least buoyancy is achieved when the water is at the level of the shoulder.

14. _____ Benefits of a land treadmill are greatest when going up- or downhill.

15. _____ Extracorporeal shockwave is high energy focused to an entire muscle group or zone.

16. _____ The most common use for LLLT is to enhance wound healing.

17. _____ Cryotherapy and heat therapy can be used over areas without sensation as long as the application time is limited to 5 minutes or less.

18. _____ Bruising is reduced by cryotherapy.

19. _____ Regardless of the size of the dog, carts and wheelchairs are recommended for both indoor and outdoor use under close supervision.

20. _____ Wheelchairs, while helpful, are not typically well accepted by the patient or client.

EXERCISE 24.8 MULTIPLE CHOICE: COMPREHENSIVE

Instructions: Circle the one correct answer to each of the following questions.

1. Alternative medicine is used
   a. In conjunction with conventional medicine
   b. In place of conventional medicine
   c. In place of complementary medicine
   d. In conjunction with complementary medicine

2. Glucosamine provides which of the following?
   a. An inhibition of enzymes responsible for cartilage degradation
   b. Stimulation of glycosaminoglycans
   c. Enhancement of the production of hyaluronic acid
   d. A semi-synthetic product used to stimulate collagen production

3. Which of the following statements is true regarding medical herbs?
   a. Capsule and tablet delivery is best used for carnivores
   b. Bulk herbs are most commonly used in preparation for use in herbivores
   c. All medicinal herbs are not as safe as traditional medicines
   d. A and B are correct

4. An herb concentrated in alcohol or glycerin is known as a(n)
   a. Tea
   b. Poultice
   c. Liniment
   d. Extract

5. The most commonly practiced form of herbal medicine in veterinary medicine is
   a. Ayurvedic
   b. Chinese
   c. Western
   d. Native American

6. Western herbal medicine can be traced back to
   a. China
   b. Turkey
   c. Greece
   d. France

7. An Ayurvedic herb used to treat digestive disorders is which of the following?
   a. Boswellia
   b. Cinnamon
   c. Licorice
   d. Neem

8. Which of the following is a clinical indication for the use of *taracum officinale*?
   a. To increase mental alertness
   b. To support heart function
   c. As a diuretic
   d. To prevent anxiety

9. The Chinese herb used to treat nausea is which of the following?
   a. Red peony
   b. Ginger
   c. Maitake
   d. Coptis

10. The commonly used Western herb to treat skin irritation is
    a. Aloe
    b. Echinacea
    c. Hawthorne
    d. Milk thistle

11. A dermometer is used to
    a. Trigger a motor point
    b. Differentiate between type I and type II acupuncture points
    c. Locate acupuncture points
    d. Measure muscle resistance

12. Rehabilitation is primarily used to treat
    a. The physical aspects of a disability
    b. Lifestyle management and physical intervention
    c. The physical aspects of a disorder
    d. Pulmonary and cardiac disorders

13. Which of the following modalities would typically not be part of a comprehensive rehabilitation plan?
    a. Hydrotherapy
    b. Laser and ultrasound therapy
    c. Chiropractic
    d. Aromatherapy

14. The massage stroke most commonly used to loosen phlegm congestion in the lungs is
    a. Pétrissage
    b. Effleurage
    c. Tapotement
    d. Coupage

15. The massage stroke most commonly used to stimulate nerve endings is
    a. Pétrissage
    b. Effleurage
    c. Tapotement
    d. Coupage

16. Pneumo-acupuncture is used solely used to treat
    a. Muscle spasms
    b. Inflammation
    c. Atrophy
    d. Pain

17. It is felt that therapeutic ultrasound works by producing
    a. Sound waves
    b. A magnetic field
    c. Electrical impulses
    d. Vibration

18. A contraindication for cryotherapy is
    a. To reduce bruising
    b. To decrease enzyme activity
    c. An area of perfusion
    d. On surgical wounds

EXERCISE 24.9 FILL-IN-THE-BLANK: COMPREHENSIVE

Instructions: Fill in each of the spaces provided with the missing word or words that complete the sentence.

1. Information about herbs can be found in the publication called the _____ _____.

2. Cryotherapy causes _____.

3. In general, herbs tend to be less _____ than many drugs because the therapeutic substances are not as _____.

4. Today there are three styles of acupuncture: _____, _____, and _____.

5. The physiologic effects of acupuncture include both _____ and _____ effects as the therapy stimulates both the central and peripheral nervous systems.

6. There are _____ major acupuncture points in the horse and _____ points in the human.

7. _____ acupuncture points, which make up 67% of all points, are considered motor points.

8. _____ implantation provides long-term stimulation for chronic conditions.

9. Veterinary spinal manipulative therapy is similar to _____ in humans.

10. The hallmark or "triad" of signs that occurs with a subluxation includes _____, _____, and _____.

11. The first step in a VSMT appointment is _____.

12. _____ is particularly important for first-time VSMT patients because they are unsure about the process and may be nervous or frightened.

Chapter **24** **Physical Therapy, Rehabilitation, and Alternative Medical Nursing**

13. A _____ is used to measure the range of motion (both flexion and extension) of all distal joints, including the carpus, elbow, shoulder, tarsus, stifle, and hip.

14. Hippocrates used _____ as early as 400 BC to treat paralysis.

15. Whereas swimming strengthens muscle but not bone, exercises on a(n) _____ _____ strengthen both.

16. _____ is a massage technique in which finger pressure is applied to acupuncture points.

17. _____ is the most commonly used massage stroke in animals.

18. To loosen phlegm and relieve congestion in a patient's lungs, _____ can be used.

19. The length of one massage stroke is referred to as _____.

20. A voluntary muscle contraction involves slow-twitch, type _____ muscle fibers, whereas an electrically induced muscle contraction involves fast-twitch, type _____ fibers.

21. The technician's role in NMES is to shave and clean the skin with alcohol, apply gel, attach the pads, and use the NMES machine to obtain a strong, yet pain-free _____.

22. TENS is the use of electric current to relieve _____ and _____.

23. The three main therapeutic effects created with LLLT are _____, _____, and _____.

24. The most common indications for LLLT include treating pain associated with degenerative joint disease, intervertebral disc disease, _____ _____, and soft tissue injuries are _____, _____, _____, and _____.

EXERCISE 24.10 CASE STUDY #1: REHABILITATION AND COMPLEMENTARY MODALITIES

A Greyhound is being treated at your clinic for pain caused by trigger points. The veterinarian decides massage would be beneficial, and the owner has brought in her pet for its first massage session.

1. Explain to the owner the basic massage techniques you will perform on her pet.

   _____

   _____

   _____

A 7-year-old, spayed, female Dachshund presents with an inability to move her hindlimbs. She has normal reflexes in the front limbs but abnormal hindlimb reflexes and minimal response to a painful stimulus in the hindlimbs. The owner reports that the dog cries out when picked up or moved.

1. List the two most relevant physical dysfunctions you would associate with this case and explain why you feel they are most relevant.

   a. _____

   _____

   _____

   b. _____

   _____

   _____

2. This patient was diagnosed with intervertebral disc disease (IVDD) and underwent surgery to correct a compression at the lumbosacral junction. What general types of complementary modalities might be used as a part of holistic care of this patient, and what is the purpose of each modality?

   _____

   _____

   _____

   _____

   _____

   _____

   _____

   _____

   _____

EXERCISE 24.12 CASE STUDY #3: REHABILITATION AND COMPLEMENTARY MODALITIES

A 3-year-old, neutered, male Labrador returns to your practice for physical therapy 3 weeks after surgical repair of a ruptured cranial cruciate ligament. He is non-weight-bearing on the limb, and there is swelling of the stifle. The owner reports that the dog had been walking on the limb since the last therapy session 2 days ago, only exhibiting lameness this morning.

1. List the two most relevant physical dysfunctions you would associate with this case and explain why you feel they are most relevant.

   a. _____

   _____

   _____

   b. _____

   _____

   _____

EXERCISE 24.13 CASE STUDY #4: REHABILITATION AND COMPLEMENTARY MODALITIES

A 4-year-old, 65-pound German Shepherd is recovering from intervertebral disc disease (IVDD) and has minimal use of his hindlimbs. His owners are struggling with carrying him outside to urinate and defecate.

1. List two mobility aids that would benefit this patient, and discuss why each would be of benefit.

   a. _____

   _____

   _____

   b. _____

   _____

   _____

25 Fluid Therapy and Transfusion Medicine

LEARNING OBJECTIVES

When you have completed this chapter, you will be able to:

1. Pronounce, define, and spell all the key terms in this chapter.
2. Explain the indications for fluid therapy, and describe the body fluid compartments, including movement of fluids between these compartments.
3. Compare and contrast crystalloid and colloid fluids, and describe the uses for and characteristics of each.
4. Do the following regarding the administration of fluids and fluid therapy additives:
   - Discuss the objectives of each phase of fluid therapy and the specific products and administration rates used during each phase.
   - Compare and contrast the indications for and techniques used to administer fluids by the intravenous, subcutaneous, intraosseous, and enteral routes.
   - Explain the indications for and techniques used to administer potassium chloride, dextrose, and sodium bicarbonate.
5. Do the following regarding monitoring and complications of fluid therapy:
   - Describe the methods used to monitor the effectiveness of fluid therapy.
   - Discuss common complications of fluid therapy, including appropriate interventions.
6. Do the following regarding transfusion medicine:
   - Describe the indications for blood, plasma, and blood component transfusion.
   - Discuss the selection and care of blood donors.
   - Explain pretransfusion testing, including blood typing, antibody screening, and cross-matching.
7. Do the following regarding collection techniques, blood products, and product administration:
   - Describe the techniques used to collect blood from a dog, cat, or horse.
   - List blood products, including the indications for and benefits provided by each.
   - Describe the technique used to administer blood products to a patient, including calculating administration rates.
   - Discuss patient monitoring during blood transfusions and recognition and management of transfusion reactions.

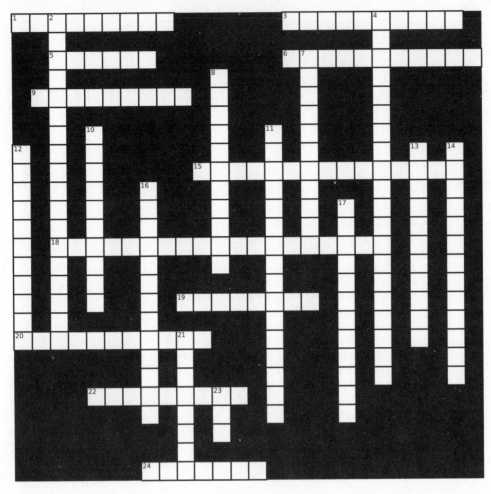

Across

1   The term used to describe a fluid with an osmolality of 154 mOsm/kg.
3   The term used to describe a fluid with an osmolality of 1026 mOsm/kg.
5   A condition that results from blood loss.
6   The most common general fluid type given during the replacement and the maintenance phases.
9   Destruction of red blood cells within the body.
15 A frozen plasma product.
18 A blood product processed from whole blood that must be stored at room temperature and used within 5 to 7 days. (2 words)
19 Canine albumin solution and hetastarch are two of these.
20 A serious hypersensitivity reaction to foreign proteins or drugs that may occur following transfusion of incompatible blood.
22 Tells you the specific erythrocyte antigens present in a donor or recipient. (2 words)
24 _____ pressure is the portion of total osmotic pressure contributed by albumin and like substances.

Down

2   A concentrated source of platelets prepared by centrifugation of fresh whole blood. (3 words)
4   TRALI and TACO are two types of these. (2 words)
7   The phase of fluid therapy intended to correct dehydration.
8   An abnormal depletion of body water.
10 A test for compatibility.
11 An exaggerated immune response to some source of stimulation.
12 A decreased circulating blood volume.
13 The _____ rate of fluid administration is needed to meet daily needs.
14 The phase of fluid therapy intended to reverse shock.
16 Sign of a donor-recipient incompatibility on a crossmatch.
17 A condition in which there is abnormal blood clotting.
21 The term used to describe a fluid with an osmolality of 308 mOsm/kg.
23 The percent of blood volume composed of red blood cells. (acronym)

Chapter **25 Fluid Therapy and Transfusion Medicine**

EXERCISE 25.2 MATCHING #1: BODY FLUID COMPARTMENTS

Instructions: Match each body fluid compartment term in column A with its corresponding statement in column B by writing the appropriate letter in the space provided.

Column A

1. _____ TBW

2. _____ Cell membrane

3. _____ ICF

4. _____ ECF

5. _____ Vascular endothelium

6. _____ ISF

7. _____ IVF

Column B

A. Separates the ISF and IVF

B. Approximately two-thirds of TBW

C. Approximately 60% of body weight

D. Approximately one-fourth of the ECF

E. Separates the ICF and ECF

F. Approximately three-fourths of ECF

G. Approximately one-third of TBW

EXERCISE 25.3 MATCHING #2: BODY TONICITY OF INTRAVENOUS FLUIDS

Instructions: Match each intravenous fluid in column A with its corresponding tonicity in column B by writing the appropriate letter in the space provided. (Note that responses may be used more than once.)

Column A

1. _____ Dextrose 5% in water

2. _____ 0.45% NaCl

3. _____ 7% NaCl

4. _____ Normosol M

5. _____ 0.9% Saline

6. _____ 0.45% Sodium chloride

7. _____ Lactated Ringer solution

8. _____ 3% NaCl

9. _____ Plasmalyte 148

10. _____ Plasmalyte 56

11. _____ Normosol R

Column B

A. Hypotonic

B. Isotonic

C. Hypertonic

EXERCISE 25.4 MATCHING #3: BLOOD GROUP FACTORS

Instructions: Match each species in column A with its corresponding blood group factors in column B by writing the appropriate letter in the space provided.

Column A

1. _____ Canine

2. _____ Equine

3. _____ Feline

4. _____ Bovine

Column B

A. Many, including Aa, Ca, Pa, Qa, and Ua

B. More than 70; negative for factor J

C. Many, including 1.1, 1.2, and 3 through 7

D. A, B, and AB

EXERCISE 25.5 MATCHING #4: IDEAL AND UNIVERSAL BLOOD DONORS

Instructions: Match each species donor in column A with its corresponding description in column B by writing the appropriate letter in the space provided. (Note that not all responses will be used.)

Column A

1. _____ Universal canine donor

2. _____ Ideal equine donor

3. _____ Universal feline donor

4. _____ Ideal bovine donor

Column B

A. 3, 5, and 7 negative

B. No universal donor for this species

C. J negative

D. A negative

E. Ca and Pa negative

F. Positive for only the DEA 4 antigen

G. J, M, and R negative

H. Aa and Qa negative

EXERCISE 25.6 MATCHING #5: BLOOD PRODUCTS

Instructions: Match each blood product in column A with the corresponding primary indication for its use in column B by writing the appropriate letter in the space provided.

Column A

1. _____ Washed RBCs

2. _____ Packed RBCs

3. _____ Fresh plasma or fresh-frozen plasma

4. _____ Platelet-rich plasma or platelet concentrate

5. _____ Cryoprecipitate

6. _____ Hyperimmune plasma

Column B

A. Thrombocytopenia

B. Neonatal foals with failure of passive transfer

C. Anemia

D. Replace some coagulation factors

E. Neonatal isoerythrolysis

F. von Willebrand disease

EXERCISE 25.7 TRUE OR FALSE: COMPREHENSIVE

Instructions: Read the following statements and write "T" for true or "F" for false in the blanks provided. If a statement is false, correct the statement to make it true.

1. _____ The circulating blood volume of a horse is approximately 40 to 60 mL/kg body weight.

2. _____ Both water and electrolytes are able to move freely across all fluid space barriers (the cell membrane and vascular endothelium) and so distribute throughout the total-body water.

3. _____ Colloids tend to remain in the vascular space.

4. _____ Dextrose 5% in water is an example of an isotonic fluid.

5. _____ Normosol R would be an appropriate fluid choice for a patient with severe acidemia.

6. _____ Administration of hypertonic saline IV will promote rapid and long-lasting expansion of the vascular volume.

7. _____ Hetastarch and 23.4% NaCl can be mixed in a 2:1 ratio to produce a combination fluid that reduces both the total dose of each and the side effects.

8. _____ Arterial blood pressure is an accurate indicator of response to fluid resuscitation.

9. _____ When calculating the ongoing losses so that the fluid administration rate can be increased appropriately, normal urinary losses should be included in this calculation.

10. _____ Pain or irritation when an IV catheter is flushed is a sign that the vein is inflamed.

11. _____ An advantage of subcutaneous fluid administration is that this route works well for resuscitation, replacement, or maintenance.

12. _____ Subcutaneous fluids can be given by a client at home.

13. _____ Only certain medications that are safe for IV administration can be given IO.

14. _____ Sodium bicarbonate is commonly used to treat a variety of conditions that lead to acidosis.

15. _____ Sodium bicarbonate can be used for severe cases of hyperkalemia to promote a shift of potassium into the cells.

16. _____ A normal blood pressure means everything is fine.

17. _____ If a patient has severe, acute hemorrhaging, the packed cell volume (PCV) will be decreased.

18. _____ The primary goal of blood transfusion is to improve oxygen delivery to the tissues.

19. _____ Dogs do not have naturally occurring antibodies to erythrocyte antigens and so a reaction is less likely following a transfusion of red blood cells.

20. _____ Like dogs, cats do not have naturally occurring antibodies to erythrocyte antigens, and so a reaction following a first transfusion is unlikely.

21. _____ Glass blood-collection bottles are preferred over bags because they preserve blood cells more effectively.

22. _____ To achieve optimal RBC viability during blood storage, blood bags should be weighed to ensure adequate fill (blood-to-anticoagulant ratio).

23. _____ Transfusion reactions will not occur as long as major and minor crossmatches indicate compatibility.

EXERCISE 25.8 MULTIPLE CHOICE: COMPREHENSIVE

Instructions: Circle the one correct answer to each of the following questions.

1. The circulating blood volume as a proportion of total body weight (mL/kg) is the lowest in a
   a. Dog
   b. Horse
   c. Cow
   d. Cat

2. When 0.9% saline solution is administered intravenously, within a short time, _____ will remain in the vascular space.
   a. One-quarter
   b. One-third
   c. One-half
   d. Most of it

3. Which of the following fluids is *not* a hypotonic fluid?
   a. 0.45% Saline
   b. Normosol M
   c. Plasmalyte 148
   d. D5W

4. Hypotonic fluids are used to treat
   a. Shock
   b. Hypernatremia
   c. Hypokalemia
   d. Metabolic acidosis

5. Which of the following fluids has an acidifying effect?
   a. LRS
   b. 0.9% Saline
   c. Normosol R
   d. Plasmalyte 148

6. 3% or 7% hypertonic saline is used to treat
   a. Heart failure
   b. Kidney failure
   c. Head trauma
   d. Hypernatremia

7. Which of the following fluids would increase intravascular oncotic pressure in a patient with hypoproteinemia?
   a. Hetastarch
   b. Normosol M
   c. Plasmalyte 148
   d. D5W

8. The shock dose of isotonic crystalloid fluids in a cat is (in mL/kg body weight)
   a. 2 to 4
   b. 10 to 15
   c. 40 to 60
   d. 80 to 90

9. What is the correct catheter placement for a patient requiring multiple blood samples to be taken over a period of time, or that needs multiple medications given by constant rate infusion?
   a. Cephalic
   b. Central line
   c. Butterfly
   d. Peripheral

10. Which of the following devices is often used to decrease the risk of fluid overload?
    a. Buretrol
    b. Administration line filter
    c. Carboy
    d. 10 drops/mL drip set

11. Fluids administered subcutaneously are usually absorbed in approximately
    a. 1 to 2 hours
    b. 2 to 4 hours
    c. 6 to 8 hours
    d. 12 to 24 hours

12. Even though it is isotonic, which of the following fluids can cause discomfort when given subcutaneously owing to its acidic pH?
    a. Lactated Ringer solution
    b. Plasmalyte 148
    c. Normosol R
    d. Dextrose 5% in water

13. Which of the following routes of fluid administration is used in neonates, because it has essentially the same effect as IV administration but does not require catheterization of a vein?
    a. Intramuscular
    b. Subcutaneous
    c. Enteral (via stomach tube)
    d. Intraosseous

14. Enteral fluids are often used to treat large-bowel impaction in
    a. Cattle
    b. Cats
    c. Dogs
    d. Horses

15. The combination of PU/PD, cardiac arrhythmias, and severe muscle weakness is very suggestive of
    a. Hypokalemia
    b. Hypoglycemia
    c. Lactic acidosis
    d. Dehydration

16. During the resuscitation phase of IV fluid therapy, arterial systolic blood pressure should be maintained at approximately
    a. 50 to 80 mm Hg
    b. 80 to 110 mm Hg
    c. 110 to 140 mm Hg
    d. 140 to 170 mm Hg

17. Normal central venous pressure is
    a. 0 to 10 cm H_2O
    b. 0 to 10 mm Hg
    c. 80 to 100 cm H_2O
    d. 80 to 100 mm Hg

18. A significant complication of fluid therapy is fluid overload. Of greatest concern in these patients is the possibility of
    a. Coagulation abnormalities
    b. Cavitary effusion
    c. Pulmonary edema
    d. Peripheral edema

19. During an acute bleeding episode, a blood transfusion is necessary if the PCV drops below
    a. 12% to 15%
    b. 15% to 20%
    c. 20% to 25%
    d. 25% to 30%

20. A blood plasma transfusion is not indicated for treatment of
    a. Low albumin
    b. A blood-clotting disorder
    c. Failure of passive transfer of immunity in foals
    d. Anemia

21. Canine blood-typing cards are used to detect
    a. DEA 1.1
    b. DEA 1.2
    c. DEA 4
    d. DEA 7

22. Which of the following statements regarding blood transfusions is most accurate?
    a. Transfusion of type A blood into a type B cat will result in decreased life span of transfused cells
    b. Transfusion of type B blood into a type A cat is expected to cause a severe, potentially fatal hemolytic reaction
    c. Transfusion of type B blood into a type AB cat is not expected to cause a reaction
    d. Transfusion of type AB blood into any cat should not cause a reaction, because this is the universal donor blood type in cats

23. A "major crossmatch" detects
    a. Reactions of a recipient's plasma with its own RBCs
    b. Reactions between donor RBCs and recipient plasma
    c. Reactions between donor plasma and recipient RBCs
    d. Reactions of a donor's plasma with its own RBCs

24. The maximum recommended blood donation for dogs expressed as a percent of the blood volume is
    a. 5% to 10%
    b. 10% to 15%
    c. 15% to 20%
    d. 20% to 25%

25. Donor blood plasma is considered to be fresh plasma if used within _____ hours of collection.
    a. 4
    b. 8
    c. 12
    d. 24

26. When transfusing blood, it is usually given concurrently with isotonic crystalloid fluids. Which of the following fluids should not be used for this purpose because it can result in activation of the coagulation cascade?
    a. Normosol R
    b. Plasmalyte 148
    c. 0.9% Saline
    d. Lactated Ringer solution

27. Using the rule of thumb provided, if you want to raise the PCV of a 25-kg patient by 10%, you should give approximately
    a. 250 mL of whole blood or packed RBCs
    b. 500 mL of whole blood or 250 mL of packed RBCs
    c. 250 mL of whole blood or 500 mL of packed RBCs
    d. 500 mL of whole blood or packed RBCs

EXERCISE 25.9 FILL-IN-THE-BLANK: COMPREHENSIVE

Instructions: Fill in each of the spaces provided with the missing word or words that complete the sentence.

1. The approximate circulating blood volume of a dog is estimated to be approximately _____ to _____ mL/kg body weight.

2. The two main categories of fluids based on the size of their solute molecules are _____ and _____.

3. A 23% saline solution must be _____ before giving it IV to avoid osmotic injury to the tissues.

4. The product "VetStarch" is a synthetic _____ that has a lesser negative effect on blood coagulation than hetastarch.

5. The maintenance fluid administration rate includes appropriate losses from the following three sources: (a) the _____ system, (b) the _____, and (c) the _____ tract.

6. A route of fluid administration used in small animals but not usually in large animals is _____. A route of fluid administration used in large animals but not in small animals is via a(n) _____ tube.

7. Subcutaneously administered fluids should have an osmotic pressure that is approximately _____ to extracellular fluid.

8. When tissues don't receive enough oxygen because of decreased tissue perfusion, the levels of _____ increase.

9. Central venous pressure (CVP) is the pressure inside the vena cava. This pressure is used to monitor fluid therapy because it approximates cardiac preload and thereby _____ volume.

10. Impaired blood coagulation is a possible side effect of administration of the synthetic colloid _____.

11. During severe, acute hemorrhage, the total protein (TP) will decrease before the packed cell volume (PCV) because of contraction of the _____.

12. The primary goal of blood transfusion is to increase the _____-carrying capacity of the blood.

13. The ideal equine blood donor is negative for factors _____ and _____.

14. The ideal bovine donor should be negative for factor _____.

15. If incompatible blood is given to a horse for a first transfusion, it takes approximately _____ to _____ days for RBC antibodies to form.

16. If a blood donation is taken from a dog in an amount equivalent to 20% of the blood volume, _____ to _____ mL/kg intravenous crystalloid fluids should be given to compensate for the fluid loss.

17. Concerning anticoagulants used for blood collection, if blood is going to be stored, either _____ or _____ anticoagulant should be used. If blood will be transfused immediately, _____ is acceptable. *(Note: The use of abbreviations is acceptable.)*

18. Donor blood plasma that is frozen within _____ hour(s) of collection and is less than _____ month(s) old is considered to be fresh-frozen plasma. Otherwise, it is considered to be frozen plasma.

19. When giving blood to hypothermic patients or those receiving large volumes of blood, refrigerated blood should be warmed to between _____° C and _____° C.

20. For patients with hemorrhage, the volume of blood to be transfused can be calculated based on the estimated blood _____, whereas for patients with chronic anemia, it can be calculated based on the _____ _____ _____.

A 4-year-old, 50-pound, neutered male Basset Hound presents for anorexia and vomiting. He is estimated to be 6% dehydrated. The attending veterinarian orders a diagnostic workup including blood work, urinalysis, and abdominal radiographs. She also orders intravenous lactated Ringer solution. She asks you to calculate the infusion and drip rates based on the sum of (a) the volume necessary to correct dehydration over the first 18 hours, (b) the standard maintenance rate, and (c) the amount necessary to replace ongoing losses.

1. Calculate the fluid deficit of this patient based on the estimated level of dehydration.

   _____ mL

2. Calculate the fluid infusion rate in mL/hour for replacement of this deficit over 18 hours.

   _____ mL/hour

3. Using the following formula, calculate the daily maintenance needs for this patient. **132*body weight (kg)$^{(3/4)}$**

   (Note: This is accomplished on a multifunction calculator by taking the body weight in kg, multiplying it by itself twice (wt*wt*wt), then pressing the square root button twice, and, finally, multiplying the result by 132.)

   _____ mL/day

4. Now calculate the hourly administration rate for maintenance.

   _____ mL/hour

5. Calculate this patient's infusion rate (in mL/hour) necessary for replacement of the deficit and for maintenance.

   _____ mL/hour

6. Calculate the drip rate in drops/second when using a drip set with a delivery rating of 10 drops/mL.

   _____ gtt/second

7. During the first 6 hours, the patient vomited several times into two absorbent pads. The pads by themselves weighed 160 grams each; including the vomitus, the two pads weighed 580 grams. Approximately how much volume (mL) did this patient lose through vomiting?

   _____ mL/hour

8. Adjust the infusion rate in mL/hour to replace this loss over the next 6 hours (as well as to replace the deficit and provide maintenance).

   _____ mL/hour

9. Finally calculate the drip rate in drops/second.

   _____ gtt/second

EXERCISE 25.11 CASE STUDY #2: IV FLUID THERAPY AND TRANSFUSION THERAPY

A 2-year-old, neutered male mix-breed dog weighing 20 kg is presented after being hit by a car. He is estimated to have lost approximately 30% of his blood volume and is shocky. The doctor has ordered a variety of interventions, including IV fluid therapy and a transfusion of whole blood.

1. Calculate the estimated volume of blood lost (in mL) by this patient.

   _____ mL

2. By this estimation, you determine that this patient needs about 1 unit of whole blood. During the first 10 to 20 minutes, there was no sign of a transfusion reaction. So the doctor would like you to administer the whole blood at a rate of 20 mL/kg/hour. Calculate the infusion rate (in mL/hour) for this patient.

   _____ mL/hour

3. Now calculate the drip rate in gtt/second. You are using a standard blood administration set rated at 10 gtt/mL.

   _____ gtt/second

4. The donor dog at your clinic weighs 70 pounds. Calculate the maximum amount of blood you can collect from this donor using the rule of thumb in the text, and determine if this will be enough blood to meet this patient's needs.

   _____ mL

   Yes, it will be enough to meet this patient's needs.   ❑

   No, it will not be enough to meet this patient's needs.   ❑

26 Emergency and Critical Care Nursing

1. Pronounce, define, and spell all the key terms in this chapter.
2. Triage a patient over the phone and upon arrival at the veterinary hospital.
3. Do the following regarding emergency and critical care assessment, initial diagnostics, and first aid:
   - Assess hydration, and recognize hypovolemia in critical care patients.
   - Identify the diagnostic tests most commonly used in emergency and critical care settings.
   - Explain the principles of basic first aid.
   - Identify the ideal location for an emergency care station and/or resuscitation area, and explain how to set up and stock a crash cart.
4. Compare and contrast the different types of shock, explain how each is treated, and identify and explain advanced emergency techniques most commonly performed on small animals.
5. Discuss disorders of the respiratory system seen in critically ill small animal patients.
6. Do the following regarding cardiopulmonary cerebral resuscitation:
   - List the common causes of cardiopulmonary arrest, and explain the principles of cardiopulmonary cerebral resuscitation (CPCR).
   - Describe the principles of basic and advanced life support in small animals and care of the post-arrest patient.
7. Describe methods used to monitor critically ill patients and the principles of effective patient monitoring.
8. Identify key aspects of recumbent patient care.
9. List common small animal emergencies, and discuss appropriate patient stabilization and treatment.
10. Do the following regarding canine and feline electrocardiography:
    - List the indications for and discuss the principles of electrocardiography.
    - Explain the processes used to acquire, analyze, and interpret an electrocardiogram.
    - Identify and explain the significance of common cardiac arrhythmias.
11. Describe initial management, assessment, diagnostic, and treatment procedures for common equine emergencies.
12. Describe initial management, assessment, diagnostic, and treatment procedures for common food animal emergencies.

EXERCISE 26.1 CROSSWORD PUZZLE: TERMS AND DEFINITIONS

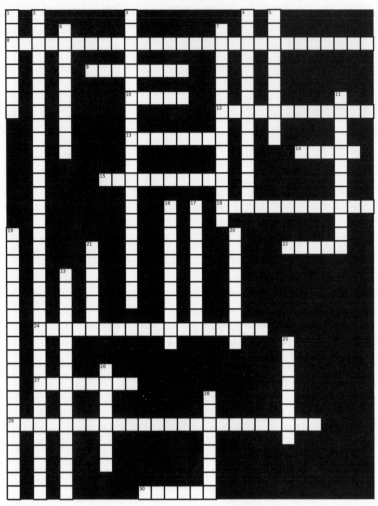

Across

8 A syndrome also known as SIRS. (3 words)
9 Inflammation of the uterus.
10 An esophageal obstruction from a foreign body (seen most commonly in cows).
12 Air within the pleural space.
13 A cardiac arrhythmia associated with a "flatline" appearance to the ECG tracing.
14 Any condition causing severe abdominal pain; common in horses.
15 A fracture of two or more ribs resulting in a freely moveable segment of chest wall. (2 words)
18 A condition in cows commonly referred to as bloat. (2 words)
22 A loss of intestinal motility.
24 A fast irregularly irregular cardiac arrhythmia identified by fibrillatory (f) waves instead of P waves. (2 words)
27 An abnormally low pH of the blood or tissue.
29 The syndrome that is a serious complication of shock involving failure of multiple organs. (3 words)
30 A state of systemic inflammation caused by infection.

Down

1 Difficult birth.
2 A serious complication of shock that involves a pattern of generalized concurrent intravascular thrombosis and bleeding. (3 words)
3 A run of four or more VPCs in succession. (2 words)
4 Blood clot formation with obstruction of blood flow.
5 An abnormal heart rhythm.
6 Blood in the pleural space.
7 QRS complexes originating from the atrial myocardium that occur early but are otherwise normal. (2 words)
11 The presence of urinary stones.
16 Decreased circulating blood volume.
17 The term for a cow that cannot stand. (2 words)
19 An early, wide, and bizarre QRS complex. (2 words)
20 Low blood oxygen.
21 Low tissue oxygen.
23 Tissue damage resulting from the reestablishment of blood flow following a period of oxygen deprivation. (2 words)
25 Excess of nitrogenous wastes in the blood because of kidney insufficiency.
26 Deficient blood supply to a body part.
28 Inflammation of the mammary gland.

EXERCISE 26.2 DEFINITIONS: KEY TERMS

Instructions: Define each term in your own words.

1. Borborygmi: _____

_____

2. Capillary refill time: _____

_____

3. Eructation: _____

_____

4. Stridor: _____

_____

5. Syncope: _____

_____

6. Tachycardia: _____

_____

7. Tachypnea: _____

_____

8. Tympany: _____

_____

9. Toxin: _____

_____

10. Urethral process: _____

_____

11. Uterine prolapse: _____

_____

12. Uterine torsion: _____

_____

13. Endometrial: _____

_____

14. Jugular vein: _____

_____

15. Perineal area: _____

_____

EXERCISE 26.3 MATCHING #1: TERMS AND DEFINITIONS RELATED TO PROCEDURES

Instructions: Match each term in column A with its corresponding definition in column B by writing the appropriate letter in the space provided.

Column A

1. _____ Abdominocentesis
2. _____ Cardiopulmonary resuscitation
3. _____ Chest tube
4. _____ Defibrillation
5. _____ Electrocardiogram
6. _____ Fetatome
7. _____ Fetotomy
8. _____ Pericardiocentesis
9. _____ Pulse oximeter
10. _____ Regional nerve block
11. _____ Rumenostomy
12. _____ Thoracocentesis
13. _____ Tracheostomy
14. _____ Tracheotomy
15. _____ Transfaunation
16. _____ Triage
17. _____ Tube cystostomy
18. _____ Urethrostomy

Column B

A. The transfer of beneficial microorganisms from the rumen of one individual to another.

B. A procedure in which a relatively small amount of local anesthetic is injected near a nerve causing desensitization of a larger area of the body.

C. A tube inserted into the pleural space.

D. A device that is used to cut a fetus into smaller parts that can be extracted vaginally more easily.

E. Aspiration of fluid by inserting a needle in the pleural space.

F. Creation of a permanent opening from the skin into the urethra.

G. A response to cardiac arrest.

H. Aspiration of fluid by inserting a needle into the sac around the heart.

I. Creation of a permanent opening from the skin to the trachea.

J. Aspiration of fluid by inserting a needle in the peritoneal cavity.

K. Placement of a catheter through the abdominal wall and into the bladder.

L. A procedure in which a dead fetus is cut into smaller pieces so that it can be extracted vaginally.

M. The treatment for ventricular fibrillation.

N. Sorting patients according to the severity of an injury.

O. A visual representation of the electrical activity of the heart.

P. Creation of a temporary opening from the skin to the trachea.

Q. Creation of the permanent opening from the skin to the rumen.

R. A monitor used to measure oxygen saturation of hemoglobin.

EXERCISE 26.4 MATCHING #2: BREATHING PATTERNS

Instructions: Match each breathing pattern in column A with its corresponding description in column B by writing the appropriate letter in the space provided.

Column A

1. _____ Restrictive breathing

2. _____ Apneustic breathing

3. _____ Labored breathing

4. _____ Cheyne-Stokes breathing

5. _____ Kussmaul breathing

Column B

A. Alternating tachypnea and bradypnea.

B. Deep inhalation with an abnormally long pause before exhalation.

C. A slow, deep, regular respiratory pattern.

D. Fast, short, and shallow breaths.

E. Prolonged and deep respirations.

EXERCISE 26.5 MATCHING #3: MENTATION

Instructions: Match each term used to describe mentation in column A with its corresponding description in column B by writing the appropriate letter in the space provided.

Column A

1. _____ Normal

2. _____ Dull

3. _____ Obtunded

4. _____ Stuporous

5. _____ Comatose

Column B

A. Only reacts to noxious stimuli.

B. Not eager to interact with the environment.

C. Interacts with the environment and is alert.

D. Unresponsive to any stimuli.

E. Reacts to stimuli more slowly than normal.

EXERCISE 26.6 MATCHING #4: EVALUATION OF PUPILS AND POSTURE

Instructions: Match each pupillary assessment or postural finding in column A with its corresponding significance in column B by writing the appropriate letter in the space provided.

Column A

1. _____ Fixed and dilated pupils

2. _____ Rigid forelimbs and flexed hindlimbs with normal mentation

3. _____ Anisocoria

4. _____ Rigid forelimbs and flaccid hindlimbs when in lateral recumbency is typical

5. _____ Unresponsive midrange pupils

6. _____ Extreme rigidity of all four limbs with arching of the neck and back

Column B

A. A lack of connection between the forebrain and brainstem.

B. Irreversible midbrain lesion.

C. Schiff-Sherrington, associated with a T3 to L3 spinal lesion.

D. Lesion in the medulla supporting brain injury.

E. Injury to the cerebellum.

F. Injury of the cerebrum.

EXERCISE 26.7 MATCHING #5: TYPES OF SHOCK

Instructions: Match each type of shock in column A with its corresponding cause in column B by writing the appropriate letter in the space provided.

Column A

1. ____ Septic shock

2. ____ Distributive shock

3. ____ Hypovolemic shock

4. ____ Cardiogenic shock

5. ____ Obstructive shock

Column B

A. Impaired venous return to the heart.

B. Decreased circulating blood volume.

C. Severe infection.

D. Vasodilation and pooling of blood in the capillaries.

E. Decreased cardiac output.

EXERCISE 26.8 MATCHING #6: ABNORMAL RHYTHMS ASSOCIATED WITH CARDIAC ARREST

Instructions: Match each abnormal rhythm associated with cardiac arrest in column A with the drug(s) used to treat the abnormality in column B by writing the appropriate letter(s) in the space provided. (Note that there may be more than one correct response and that responses may be used more than once.)

Column A

1. ____ Ventricular tachycardia

2. ____ Asystole

3. ____ PEA

4. ____ Bradycardia

5. ____ Vagally mediated arrest or AV block

6. ____ Refractory, unstable ventricular tachycardia

Column B

A. Epinephrine

B. Atropine

C. Vasopressin

D. Lidocaine

E. Magnesium sulfate

F. Amiodarone

EXERCISE 26.9 MATCHING #7: DRUGS USED DURING CPCR

Instructions: Match each abnormality seen in patients that arrest in column A with the drug(s) used to treat the abnormality in column B by writing the appropriate letter(s) in the space provided. (Note that there may be more than one correct response.)

Column A

1. ____ Hypotension

2. ____ Pulmonary edema

3. ____ Cerebral edema

4. ____ Low cardiac output

5. ____ Hyperkalemia

Column B

A. Furosemide

B. Dobutamine

C. Mannitol

D. Vasopressin

E. Dopamine

F. Calcium gluconate

EXERCISE 26.10 MATCHING #8: ELECTROCARDIOGRAPHIC WAVEFORMS

Instructions: Match each waveform in column A with its corresponding significance in column B by writing the appropriate letter in the space provided.

Column A

1. ____ P wave

2. ____ PR interval

3. ____ QRS complex

4. ____ ST segment

5. ____ T wave

Column B

A. Time interval from ventricular depolarization to repolarization.

B. Ventricular depolarization.

C. Time it takes for the impulse to conduct through the AV node.

D. Ventricular repolarization.

E. Atrial depolarization.

EXERCISE 26.11 PHOTO QUIZ: ECG TRACINGS

Instructions: Match each ECG tracing with the name corresponding to the cardiac rhythm by writing the name in the space provided. Then summarize the significance of each rhythm.

A. Normal sinus rhythm

B. Sinus arrhythmia

C. Atrial premature complexes (APCs)

D. Atrial tachycardia

E. Atrial fibrillation

F. Ventricular premature complexes (VPCs)

G. Ventricular tachycardia

H. Ventricular fibrillation

I. Atrial standstill

J. Second-degree AV block

K. Third-degree (complete) AV block

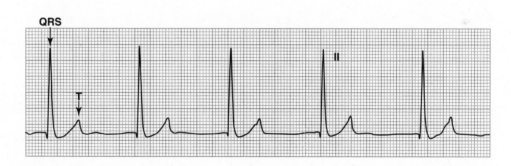

1. Name, reading summary, and significance of this rhythm: _____

_____

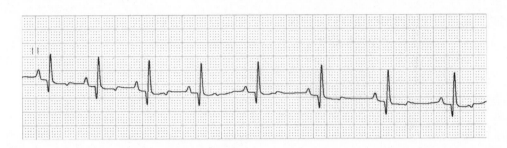

2. Name, reading summary, and significance of this rhythm: _____

_____

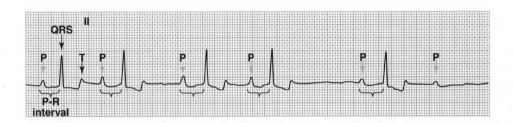

3. Name, reading summary, and significance of this rhythm: _____

_____

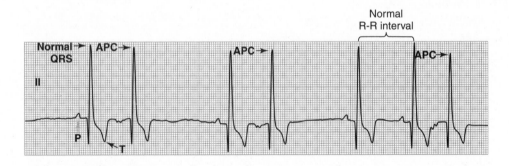

4. Name, reading summary, and significance of this rhythm: _____

_____

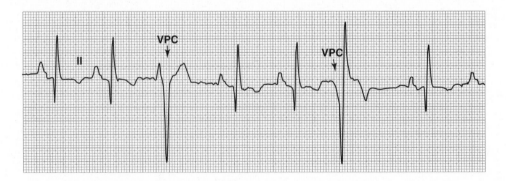

5. Name, reading summary, and significance of this rhythm: _____

_____

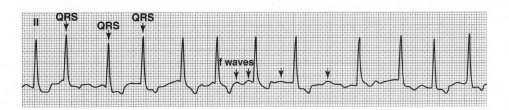

6. Name, reading summary, and significance of this rhythm: _____

_____

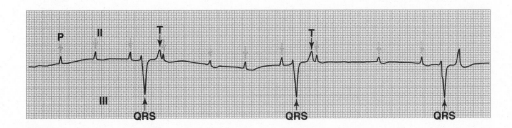

7. Name, reading summary, and significance of this rhythm: _____

_____

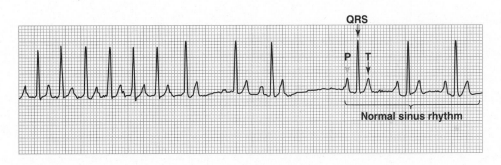

8. Name, reading summary, and significance of this rhythm: _____

_____

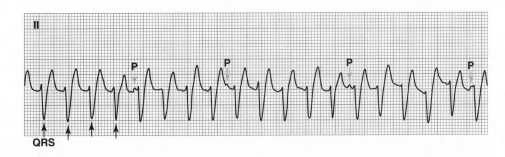

9. Name, reading summary, and significance of this rhythm: _____

_____

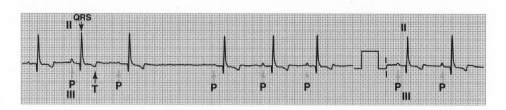

10. Name, reading summary, and significance of this rhythm: _____

_____

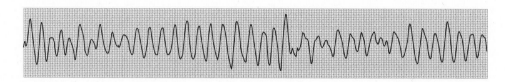

11. Name, reading summary, and significance of this rhythm: _____

_____

EXERCISE 26.12 TRUE OR FALSE: COMPREHENSIVE

Instructions: Read the following statements and write "T" for true or "F" for false in the blanks provided. If a statement is false, correct the statement to make it true.

1. _____ Orthopnea refers to a posture assumed by animals to ease breathing.

2. _____ When evaluating mucous membrane color, blue means something is wrong, whereas mottled pink means things are fine.

3. _____ Animals that are 3% to 4% dehydrated have decreased skin turgor.

4. _____ Kussmaul breathing indicates respiratory compensation for a metabolic acidosis, such as diabetic ketoacidosis.

5. _____ When blood is aspirated during abdominocentesis, abdominal bleeding can be differentiated from fresh blood by looking at the color.

6. _____ The ventral neck should be aseptically prepared when performing a tracheostomy tube placement.

7. _____ Animals with respiratory distress should have chest radiographs taken immediately upon presentation to diagnose the cause quickly.

8. _____ Animals with hypoxia caused by severe anemia can have normal pulse oximeter readings.

9. _____ The partial pressure of oxygen in arterial blood (PaO_2) can be used to assess pulmonary function.

10. _____ An ECG tracing is a reliable method of determining cardiac activity following cardiopulmonary arrest.

11. _____ An Ambu bag is used to provide ventilatory support.

12. _____ When performing defibrillation, electrical conduction should be enhanced by wetting the hair with 70% isopropyl alcohol.

13. _____ The overall survival rate for all causes of witnessed in-hospital cardiopulmonary arrest patients is good, as long as treatment is initiated quickly.

14. _____ A single increased central venous pressure (CVP) measurement is an accurate indicator of fluid overload.

15. _____ Doppler blood pressure monitoring is only reliable for detecting systolic arterial blood pressure.

16. _____ The life-threatening condition gastric dilation volvulus (GDV) can be readily ruled out as long as the patient doesn't have visible abdominal distention.

17. _____ The "P" wave on an ECG tracing corresponds to propagation of the electrical impulse through the atrial heart muscle.

18. _____ The horizontal axis on an ECG tracing represents the strength of the electrical impulse measured in mV.

19. _____ NSR is a normal rhythm in both the dog and the cat.

20. _____ Atrial standstill is a cardiac arrhythmia that has hyperkalemia as its most common cause.

21. _____ A second-degree AV block is a rhythm characterized by a prolonged PR interval on the ECG.

22. _____ Horses that have colic can be divided into two main categories: a small number that resolve with minimal or no treatment, and many more that require aggressive treatment.

23. _____ Abrasions around the head and the presence of dirt, mud, and hay in the hair coat of a horse experiencing colic are signs that it was in severe pain prior to arrival at the hospital.

24. _____ Nasogastric intubation in colic patients is important, because horses with excessive accumulation of stomach gas and fluid will often vomit and aspirate.

25. _____ After passing a nasogastric tube in a colic patient, the tube should be removed immediately if no fluid is obtained to avoid further damage to the stomach.

26. _____ When managing a colic patient, the body temperature should always be taken prior to performing a rectal examination.

27. _____ Endoscopic examination of the airways can be used to evaluate the pharynx, guttural pouches, and trachea in horses, but cannot be used to evaluate deeper structures like the bifurcation of the bronchi.

28. _____ When performing a thoracocentesis, the caudal aspect of the rib should be avoided with the needle.

29. _____ The location most often used to perform a tracheotomy in an equine patient is the ventral midline between the middle and caudal third of the neck.

30. _____ Splint stabilization of an equine elbow fracture is not necessary if the patient can extend, plant, and move the leg.

31. _____ A scapula plantar splint is applied up to the point of the calcaneus to stabilize a distal to mid-hindlimb fracture.

32. _____ The size of the area around a wound that should be clipped is most closely associated with the presence or absence of infection.

33. _____ When checking a wound for joint involvement by tapping the joint, the needle should always be introduced at a site distant from the wound.

34. _____ Food animals seldom need emergency care because, with few exceptions, their value is seen as economic.

35. _____ Farm animals are frequently presented to emergency service because of complications of gastrointestinal parasitism.

36. _____ Choke is a gastrointestinal condition commonly seen in camelids.

37. _____ The ruminal contents of a cow can be used to perform ruminal transfaunation of a goat.

38. _____ A veterinarian can usually diagnose urethral obstruction form a good history and physical examination.

39. _____ The rapidity with which joint luxations are treated is an important determinant of the likelihood of success.

40. _____ Sheep and goats that are targets of dog attacks often suffer puncture wounds, which, although potentially serious, usually involve only superficial structures.

41. _____ By using proper equipment, dystocias of food animals can usually be managed by the vet without additional help.

42. _____ When replacing a prolapsed uterus, a large plastic bag can be used to prevent further contamination and trauma of the prolapsed organ.

43. _____ When faced with a small ruminant with an inability to urinate, urethral stones can easily be ruled out by taking radiographs.

44. _____ General anesthesia is required to perform a urethrostomy in a goat.

EXERCISE 26.13 MULTIPLE CHOICE: COMPREHENSIVE

Instructions: Circle the one correct answer to each of the following questions.

1. Laryngeal paralysis and other extrathoracic airway obstructions are characterized by
   a. Fast, short, and shallow breaths
   b. Prolonged and deep breaths
   c. Long, slow inspirations and short exhalations
   d. Expiratory dyspnea with increased abdominal effort

2. Increased bronchovesicular sounds indicate
   a. Diaphragmatic hernia
   b. Pulmonary edema
   c. Pneumothorax
   d. Pleural effusion

3. A weak, thready arterial pulse can indicate
   a. Decompensated shock
   b. Anemia
   c. Compensated shock
   d. Aortic regurgitation

4. A patient with pronounced loss of skin turgor, dry mucous membranes, tachycardia, weak pulses, and sunken eyes, but not in shock or comatose, is approximately _____ dehydrated.
   a. 5%
   b. 7%
   c. 10%
   d. >10%

5. An elevated blood lactate indicates
   a. Overhydration
   b. Brain injury
   c. Poor tissue perfusion
   d. Urinary blockage

6. Which of the following is a sign of compensated shock, but not a sign of decompensated shock?
   a. Pale mucous membrane color
   b. Tachycardia
   c. Hypotension
   d. Increased pulse pressure

7. A complication of shock that is characterized by widespread inflammation of tissues resulting from lack of oxygen is known as
   a. MODS
   b. DIC
   c. BAR
   d. SIRS

8. When performing a thoracentesis to diagnose or treat pneumothorax, prepare the area around the
   a. Fourth to fifth intercostal space between the top one-third and bottom two-thirds of the thorax
   b. Fourth to fifth intercostal space between the top two-thirds and bottom one-third of the thorax
   c. Seventh to ninth intercostal space between the top one-third and bottom two-thirds of the thorax
   d. Seventh to ninth intercostal space between the top two-thirds and bottom one-third of the thorax

9. Cats with asthma will usually have
   a. Deep, slow breaths
   b. Rapid, shallow breaths
   c. Crackles heard during inspiration and expiration
   d. Increased respiratory effort and wheezing

10. Increased end-tidal carbon dioxide levels occur with
    a. Hypoventilation
    b. A leak in the anesthetic system
    c. An incompletely inflated endotracheal tube cuff
    d. Decreased cardiac output

11. PaO_2 is measured with
    a. End-tidal CO_2 monitoring
    b. Pulse oximetry
    c. Arterial blood-gas monitoring
    d. Oscillometry

12. The first priority when performing CPCR is considered by many critical care veterinarians to be
    a. Providing breaths
    b. Chest compressions
    c. Placing an endotracheal tube
    d. Running an ECG tracing

13. During cardiopulmonary arrest and subsequent CPCR, which of the following end-tidal carbon dioxide monitor values indicate that chest compressions are adequate?
    a. 0 mm Hg
    b. 5 to 10 mm Hg
    c. 10 to 15 mm Hg
    d. 20 to 30 mm Hg

14. Closed-chest compressions are often not effective in
    a. Animals with pneumothorax
    b. Small dogs
    c. Cats
    d. Animals that arrest because of anesthetic complications

15. During CPCR, stimulation of the Governor Vessel 26 acupuncture point is used to
    a. Stimulate the heart
    b. Increase tissue perfusion
    c. Increase blood oxygen
    d. Stimulate respirations

16. The drug most commonly used to treat asystole during CPCR is
    a. Lidocaine
    b. Naloxone
    c. Epinephrine
    d. Calcium gluconate

17. When administering advanced life support during CPCR, some drugs may be given via the endotracheal tube. Which drug cannot be given this way?
    a. Naloxone
    b. Vasopressin
    c. Epinephrine
    d. Sodium bicarbonate

18. Marked increased central venous pressure (CVP) is caused by
    a. Dehydration
    b. Heart failure
    c. Hypovolemia
    d. Venodilation

19. Hyperkalemia is often a feature of which emergency disease?
    a. Urethral obstruction
    b. Gastric dilation volvulus
    c. Heart failure
    d. Respiratory distress

20. The ECG electrode that should be placed on the right rear limb is
    a. Black
    b. Green
    c. White
    d. Red

21. Arrhythmias that originate from below the AV node are classified as
    a. Tachyarrhythmias
    b. Supraventricular arrhythmias
    c. Bradyarrhythmias
    d. Ventricular arrhythmias

22. A sinus arrhythmia is
    a. Normal in the dog and cat
    b. Normal in the dog, but not the cat
    c. Normal in the cat, but not the dog
    d. An abnormal rhythm in both cats and dogs

23. Which of the following cardiac rhythms commonly occurs in normal animals as a response to pain, excitement, stress, or anxiety?
    a. Sinus arrhythmia
    b. Atrial fibrillation
    c. Sinus tachycardia
    d. Atrial tachycardia

24. Which of the following is a QRS complex that occurs too soon and is of identical or nearly identical shape as a normal QRS complex?
   a. Atrial premature complex
   b. Junctional escape beat
   c. Ventricular premature complex
   d. Ventricular escape beat

25. A cardiac arrhythmia that appears on an ECG tracing as a flat line is called
   a. Atrial standstill
   b. Third-degree AV block
   c. Pulseless electrical activity
   d. Ventricular asystole

26. In equine medicine, emergencies involving three major organ systems make up a large part of the caseload. Which organ system is typically not involved?
   a. Gastrointestinal system
   b. Genitourinary system
   c. Musculoskeletal system
   d. Respiratory system

27. The 10-cm × 10-cm location that should be clipped and surgically prepared prior to performing an abdominocentesis in colic patients is usually located
   a. 3 to 5 cm caudal to the umbilicus and 3 to 5 cm to the left of the midline
   b. 3 to 5 cm caudal to the xiphoid and 3 to 5 cm to the left of the midline
   c. 3 to 5 cm caudal to the umbilicus and 3 to 5 cm to the right of the midline
   d. 3 to 5 cm caudal to the xiphoid and 3 to 5 cm to the right of the midline

28. The most common reason for surgical intervention in a colic patient is to
   a. Investigate a total absence of borborygmi
   b. Repair a rectal tear
   c. Investigate pain that is unresponsive to sedation
   d. Repair an intussusception

29. An upper respiratory tract obstruction in an equine patient is generally characterized by
   a. Rapid, shallow breathing and absent lung sounds
   b. Severe distress, inspiratory stridor, and normal lung sounds
   c. Abnormal lung sounds, including crackles and wheezes
   d. Rapid, shallow breathing with abnormal lung sounds

30. Effective treatment of equine pneumonia may require a bacterial culture and cytologic evaluation of respiratory secretions. Samples for these tests are best obtained by
   a. Thoracocentesis
   b. Lower-airway endoscopy
   c. Transtracheal wash
   d. Tracheotomy

31. A bandage designed to stabilize a fracture of the proximal metacarpus of the horse must extend from the coronary band to the
   a. Highest point of the elbow
   b. Top of the metacarpus
   c. Top of the carpus
   d. Highest point of the shoulder

32. Equine patients with _____ should always be assessed for blood loss, which is commonly associated with this condition.
   a. Colic
   b. An upper respiratory obstruction
   c. A wound
   d. Heaves

33. A nonviable segment of bone that acts as a foreign body and frequently prevents full wound healing until it is removed is called a(n)
   a. Osteoblast
   b. Chondrocyte
   c. Bone fragment
   d. Sequestrum

34. A cow in hypovolemic shock should receive a rapid 1-L IV infusion of
   a. Normal (0.9%) saline
   b. Lactated Ringer solution
   c. Hypertonic (7%) saline
   d. Ringer solution

35. The area that must be prepared prior to abdominal surgery in cattle to correct GI abnormalities such as an abomasal volvulus or cecal volvulus is typically
   a. The right paralumbar fossa
   b. The left paralumbar fossa
   c. The ventral midline
   d. The paramedian region

36. A large-bore tube used to remove ingesta, liquid, and gas from the rumen of a cow is called a
   a. Nasoesophageal tube
   b. Kingman tube
   c. Rumenostomy tube
   d. Urethrostomy tube

37. The term *down animal* or *downer* is typically used to describe
    a. Animals that need to be removed from the herd
    b. Animals in a downward posture as the result of an infection
    c. Animals that cannot stand
    d. Animals experiencing gastrointestinal distress in the evening

38. The best option for supporting cows that can't stand for long periods of time is
    a. Hydroflotation
    b. Slings
    c. Hip lifters
    d. Water beds

39. A Krey hook is a device used to
    a. Support downer cows
    b. Correct a uterine torsion
    c. Retrieve foreign objects
    d. Perform a fetotomy

40. A "breech" presentation of a fetus during parturition is one in which
    a. The head presents first
    b. The front legs present first
    c. The rump presents first
    d. The hind legs present first

41. The "plank-in-the-flank" method is a technique used to correct a
    a. Uterine torsion in a cow
    b. Cecal impaction in a horse
    c. Uterine prolapse in a ewe
    d. Dystocia in a camel

42. Urolithiasis is a condition most often seen in
    a. Cows
    b. Bulls
    c. Male sheep and goats
    d. Female sheep and goats

43. The most common place for a urinary stone to lodge in a goat is the
    a. Sigmoid flexure of the urethra
    b. Neck of the bladder
    c. Prostatic urethra
    d. Urethral process

44. The procedure used to create a permanent opening from the skin into the bladder is called a
    a. Bladder marsupialization
    b. Cystocentesis
    c. Tube cystotomy
    d. Cystoscopy

45. To minimize the likelihood of development of urolithiasis in goats, it is important to
    a. Decrease salt intake
    b. Limit hay intake
    c. Alkalinize the urine
    d. Eliminate grain from the diet

EXERCISE 26.14 FILL-IN-THE-BLANK: COMPREHENSIVE

Instructions: Fill in each of the spaces provided with the missing word or words that complete the sentence.

1. During an initial triage examination, the _____, _____, and _____ organ systems should be systematically and carefully evaluated.

2. Dogs that are in shock often have an abnormally fast heart rate (HR), also known as _____, whereas cats often have an abnormally slow HR, also known as _____.

3. A nonpalpable dorsal metatarsal arterial pulse in a dog indicates a mean arterial pressure (MAP) lower than _____ mm Hg, whereas a nonpalpable femoral pulse in a dog or cat indicates a MAP lower than _____ mm Hg.

4. The clip-like probe of a pulse oximeter is designed to attach to a _____, poorly haired area.

5. Shock occurs as a result of altered blood flow, and ultimately impaired delivery of _____ to the tissues.

6. Normal arterial blood pressure values for dogs and cats are in the range of _____-_____ mmHG systolic and _____-_____ mmHg (diastolic).

7. The heart, lungs, _____, and _____ are the organs most often affected by MODS.

8. A pulse oximeter measures the percentage of hemoglobin that is saturated with _____, as well as the _____ rate.

9. During CPCR, when performing chest compressions and interposed abdominal compressions, the abdomen is compressed during the _____ phase of the chest compression.

10. When providing ventilation during CPCR with an anesthetic machine, a rate of approximately _____ to _____ respirations per minute should be used.

11. Central venous pressure (CVP) is the pressure in the cranial _____ _____. In normal dogs, CVP is _____ to _____ cm H_2O.

12. Regarding arterial blood pressure, in dogs and cats, normal _____ pressure is 80 to 140 mm Hg, normal _____ pressure is 60 to 100 mm Hg, and normal _____ pressure is 50 to 80 mm Hg.

13. A blood pressure cuff is properly sized if the _____ of the cuff is approximately 40% of the _____ of the limb.

14. Patients with emergency respiratory disease are often treated with particular drugs related to the primary problem. For instance, patients in respiratory distress benefit from sedation with an opioid drug such as _____, cats suspected to have asthma should receive the drug _____ by inhalation, and patients suspected to be in heart failure should receive _____.

15. The most commonly used electrocardiographic leads are I, II, III, aVR, aVL, and aVF. I, II, and III are known as _____ leads, and aVR, aVL, and aVF are known as _____ leads.

16. When acquiring an ECG, the tracing should be recorded at a paper speed of _____ or _____ mm/sec, and a calibration of _____ mm/mV.

17. On a diagnostic ECG tracing, the QRS wave is made up of three separate waveforms. The first negative deflection represents the _____ wave, the first positive deflection represents the _____ wave, and the first negative wave following the first positive wave is the _____ wave.

18. When a QRS complex is normal in shape, this suggests that it is _____ in origin, but if it is wide and bizarre in shape, this suggests that it is _____ in origin.

19. In a patient with a sinus arrhythmia, the HR typically increases during _____ and decreases during _____.

20. Ventricular premature complexes (VPCs) may occur in groups of two, three, four, or more, and may occur in patterns. A group of two sequential VPCs is called a _____, and a group of three sequential VPCs is called a _____. A _____ is a rhythm in which every other beat is a VPC, and a _____ is a rhythm in which every third beat is a VPC.

21. Nasogastric intubation is typically performed in colic patients to remove excess gas and fluid from the stomach. This excess fluid is called _____ _____.

22. On physical examination, mucous membrane color is an important indicator of various conditions. For instance, an animal that presents with blue mucous membranes, also known as _____, should immediately be provided with _____.

23. In horses, thoracic problems, such as diaphragmatic hernia and pneumothorax, can lead to signs of respiratory distress or _____ (a disease of the gastrointestinal system).

24. _____ supplementation is required in patients with respiratory distress when the PaO_2 is less than 100 mm Hg.

25. When supplementing oxygen to an adult equine patient, a flow rate of at least _____ L/min should be used, whereas foals and miniature horses may require as little as _____ L/min.

26. Bovine patients with bloat may have respiratory compromise because the rumen becomes distended and cranially pushes on the _____.

27. Microbial function of the ruminal contents can be determined by a methylene blue reduction test. If rumen flora is normal, the ruminal contents will change from a _____ color to a _____ color within 5 minutes.

28. In a ruminant, the incision for a C-section is usually made in the _____ _____ with the animal awake.

29. Cattle with metritis and mastitis can develop endotoxemia and may present with signs of _____ _____, which include tachycardia and tachypnea.

30. Animals with urinary obstructions frequently have serious electrolyte abnormalities. The most dangerous of these is _____ because it may lead to fatal _____ _____.

31. The surgical procedure performed to create an opening in the urethra proximal to an obstruction is called a _____.

EXERCISE 26.15 CASE STUDY: MANAGEMENT OF RECUMBENT PATIENTS

Leslie, a 10-year-old, spayed female Shepherd mix is presented for management of recumbency caused by paralysis secondary to a rupture of an intervertebral disc. She has not been eating well and has disturbed fluid balance. She is also in pain secondary to the disc rupture and has developed several open ulcers over her elbows and other bony prominences. Because she is panting a lot, she has dry oral mucous membranes, and she also has red and irritated skin around her rear quarters because she is often lying in a pool of her own urine. In addition to these problems, if her recumbency is prolonged, she will be prone to loss of muscle mass, and contracture and edema of her limbs.

Recumbent patients may also require placement of an endotracheal tube or tracheostomy tube, may be on mechanical ventilation, and, in some cases, may develop corneal damage. For the problems Leslie is facing, as well as the additional problems common to recumbent patients, indicate the reasons that each occurs and then summarize the care that must be provided to manage each problem appropriately and effectively.

1. Inadequate nutritional intake

   Reasons: _____

   _____

   Management: _____

   _____

   _____

   _____

   _____

   _____

   _____

2. Dehydration or overhydration

   Reasons: _____

   _____

   Management: _____

   _____

   _____

   _____

   _____

   _____

3. Pain

   Reasons: _____

   _____

   Management: _____

   _____

   _____

_____

_____

_____

4. Development of decubital ulcers

Reasons: _____

_____

Management: _____

_____

_____

_____

_____

_____

_____

5. Dry oral mucous membranes and other oral problems

Reasons: _____

_____

Management: _____

_____

_____

_____

_____

_____

_____

6. Peripheral edema, muscle wasting, and contracture

Reasons: _____

_____

Management: _____

_____

_____

_____

_____

_____

7. Urine scald

   Reasons: _____

   _____

   Management: _____

   _____

   _____

   _____

   _____

   _____

   _____

8. Placement of an endotracheal tube or tracheostomy tube and/or mechanical ventilation

   Reasons: _____

   _____

   Management: _____

   _____

   _____

   _____

   _____

   _____

   _____

9. Corneal damage

   Reasons: _____

   _____

   Management: _____

   _____

   _____

   _____

   _____

   _____

27 Toxicology

LEARNING OBJECTIVES

When you have completed this chapter, you will be able to:
1. Pronounce, define, and spell all of the key terms in this chapter.
2. Assess and stabilize a patient presenting with a toxicologic emergency.
3. Use appropriate decontamination techniques for ocular, dermal, and GI toxin exposure in order to prevent absorption and/or remove the toxin from the body.
4. Provide supportive care to a patient being treated for toxicosis.
5. Do the following regarding common household hazards, including dangerous food items, household cleaning agents, and miscellaneous household items:
    - Identify the toxic component of the item or product.
    - Describe clinical signs expected with toxicosis.
    - Describe specific decontamination techniques used to prevent absorption and/or remove the toxin from the body.
6. Do the following regarding dangerous plants, including Rhododendron species, cardiac glycoside – containing plants, castor beans, cycad palms, lilies, and insoluble calcium oxalate – containing plants:
    - Identify the toxic component of the item or product.
    - Describe clinical signs expected with toxicosis.
    - Describe specific decontamination techniques used to prevent absorption and/or remove the toxin from the body.
7. Do the following regarding pesticides, including ant and roach baits, flea/tick products, methomyl, metaldehyde, and rodenticides:
    - Identify the toxic component of the item or product.
    - Describe clinical signs expected with toxicosis.
    - Describe specific decontamination techniques used to prevent absorption and/or remove the toxin from the body.
8. Do the following regarding antifreeze products, including methanol, propylene glycol, and ethylene glycol:
    - Identify the toxic component of the item or product.
    - Describe clinical signs expected with toxicosis.
    - Describe specific decontamination techniques used to prevent absorption and/or remove the toxin from the body.
9. Do the following regarding human medications, including acetaminophen, nonsteroidal anti-inflammatory drugs, aspirin, pseudoephedrine and amphetamines, isoniazid, calcipotriene, and 5-fluorouracil:
    - Identify the toxic component of the item or product.
    - Describe clinical signs expected with toxicosis.
    - Describe specific decontamination techniques used to prevent absorption and/or remove the toxin from the body.
10. Do the following regarding drugs of abuse, including marijuana, cocaine, ethanol, and methamphetamine:
    - Identify the toxic component of the item or product.
    - Describe clinical signs expected with toxicosis.
    - Describe specific decontamination techniques used to prevent absorption and/or remove the toxin from the body.

Instructions: Match each term in column A with its corresponding definition in column B by writing the appropriate letter in the space provided.

Column A

1. _____ Alkalis
2. _____ Anionic detergent
3. _____ Toxin
4. _____ Cationic detergents
5. _____ Decontamination
6. _____ Acids
7. _____ Toxicosis

Column B

A. Any disease of toxic origin

B. A poisonous substance

C. Neutralization of injurious agents

D. Produce(s) an initially nonpainful, deep and penetrating wound

E. Produce(s) an initially painful wound

F. Found in shampoos

G. Found in fabric softeners

EXERCISE 27.2 MATCHING #2: CLASSIFICATION OF TOXINS

Instructions: Match each toxic substance in column A with its corresponding toxin category in column B by writing the appropriate letter in the space provided. (Note that responses may be used more than once.)

Column A

1. _____ St. John's wort
2. _____ Tobacco
3. _____ Yew
4. _____ Lantana
5. _____ Raisins
6. _____ Marijuana
7. _____ Cocklebur
8. _____ Avocado
9. _____ White and yellow sweet clover
10. _____ Bermuda grass
11. _____ Cotton
12. _____ Milkweed
13. _____ Buckwheat
14. _____ Shamrock
15. _____ Agave
16. _____ Fescue
17. _____ Rhubarb
18. _____ Common juniper
19. _____ Queen Anne's lace
20. _____ Amanita mushrooms

Column B

A. Neurotoxic

B. Hepatotoxic

C. Nephrotoxic

D. Dermal

E. Fungal

F. Reproduction

G. Cardiotoxic

EXERCISE 27.3 COMPLETING TREATMENT OPTIONS: ORALLY INGESTED TOXINS

Instructions: Complete the chart by supplying the missing information for each treatment/agent identified.

Treatment/Agent	Indication	Dose	Contraindications/Exceptions
Dilution—Milk or water			
Emesis—Hydrogen peroxide			
Activated Charcoal			
Enemas—Plain warm or soapy water			
Gastric Lavage			
Enterogastric Lavage			

EXERCISE 27.4 FILL-IN-THE-BLANK

Instructions: Fill in each of the spaces provided with the missing word or words that complete the sentence.

1. Toxicity is dependent upon the _____ and _____ dose, as well as the _____ and _____ of the animal.

2. The general rule of toxicology is to _____.

3. _____ _____ is the preferred emetic agent for dogs.

4. Sedation that can result from the use of apomorphine hydrochloride can be reversed with _____.

5. _____ should never be used as an emetic.

6. A _____ % solution of hydrogen peroxide has been shown to be an effective emetic for dogs, ferrets, and _____.

7. As a general rule, the _____ and more _____ the chocolate, the more toxic it likely is.

8. Members of the *Allium* family that can be harmful to all animals include onions, _____, _____, and _____.

9. _____ _____ is recommended in patients with hemoglobinuria.

10. Grapes and raisins have shown to cause _____ _____ in some dogs when eaten.

11. _____ is the only toxin that will cause imminent seizures.

12. _____ and _____ _____ _____ are effective chelating agents that can be administered in the case of lead poisoning.

13. Signs of nicotine poisoning usually occur within _____ to _____ minutes of ingestion.

14. _____ is commonly found in snail or slug bait and are highly toxic.

15. Anticoagulant rodenticides act by competitive inhibition of vitamin _____.

16. _____ _____ is the most dangerous type of antifreeze.

17. _____ are more sensitive to acetaminophen than dogs.

18. Initial signs of marijuana toxicity in dogs include _____ and _____ that can progress into _____.

19. An ataxic animal dribbling urine is considered to be intoxicated by _____ until proven otherwise.

20. Ingestion of members of the Rhododendron family can lead to _____ _____.

EXERCISE 27.5 TRUE OR FALSE: COMPREHENSIVE

Instructions: Read the following statements and write "T" for true or "F" for false in the blanks provided. If a statement is false, correct the statement to make it true.

1. _____ The best way to prevent serious problems from toxicosis is to have emetics and activated charcoal on hand.

2. _____ Taking a good history will be critical for preparation for the toxicologic emergency.

3. _____ The general rule of toxicology is to "treat the patient, not the poison."

4. _____ Decontamination is performed to prevent other animals from similar ingestion.

5. _____ With any ocular exposure, the eyes should be flushed repeatedly with tepid water or saline solution for a minimum of 20 to 30 minutes.

6. _____ To remove sticky substances from birds, work a small amount of vegetable oil, mineral oil, mayonnaise, or peanut butter through the rest of the substance until it breaks down into "gummy balls."

7. _____ Hypothermia is rarely encountered when treating a patient for toxicosis.

8. _____ Emesis is contraindicated in rodents, rabbits, birds, horses, and ruminants.

9. _____ Emesis is more likely to be productive if the animal is fed a large, moist meal before inducing vomiting.

10. _____ Food grade hydrogen peroxide is an acceptable grade for animal use.

11. _____ Salt water should be administered within 10 minutes of arrival to the clinic when ingestion of a caustic agent is suspected.

12. _____ Chocolate contains theobromine and caffeine, which are both classified as methylxanthines.

13. _____ If ingested by dogs, macadamia nuts may cause weakness, depression, vomiting, ataxia, tremors, and hyperthermia.

14. _____ Grapes and raisins, when eaten, cause cardiovascular episodes in cats.

15. _____ Alkali burns are initially nonpainful.

16. _____ Acid and alkali burns are treated the same.

17. _____ Bathing and dilution are the cornerstones in treating contact with bleach.

18. _____ The treatment for zinc ingestion is dilution.

19. _____ Lead must be in an acidic environment to be absorbed into the bloodstream.

20. _____ Toxicity risks for the ingestion of dangerous plants are similar for all plant types.

21. _____ One of the most potent plant toxins is contained in the castor bean, for which there is no anecdote.

22. _____ Delaying treatment for the ingestion of an Easter lily in a cat beyond 18 hours frequently results in death.

23. _____ Outdoor plants contain calcium oxalate crystals; common houseplants do not.

24. _____ Cats are extremely sensitive to concentrated permethrin.

25. _____ The first step in treating symptomatic cats exposed to permethrin compounds is emesis.

26. _____ Cats are very sensitive to bromethalin; dogs are more resistant.

27. _____ Vitamin B12 increases the absorption of calcium, stimulates bone resorption, and enhances kidney reabsorption of calcium.

28. _____ The smell of rotten fish in the air could signal a phosphine gas, dangerous to both humans and animals.

29. _____ Large ingestions of methanol require monitoring for acidosis.

30. _____ The ingestion of ethylene glycol can cause acute renal failure.

EXERCISE 27.6 SHORT ANSWER: COMPREHENSIVE

Instructions: Each of the following is a TRUE statement. In the space provided, please provide a short answer as to WHY the statement is true.

1. Apples and cherries can cause problems in grazing animals.

   _____

2. The ingestion of certain grasses (Dallis, Perennial ryegrass, Bermuda, Phalaris) can cause grass staggers and tremors.

   _____

3. Aspiration is a concern with the ingestion of ethanol.

_____

4. In treating cocaine ingestion, emesis should only be induced within 15 minutes of ingestion.

_____

5. Aspirin can be used therapeutically in both dogs and cats but must be used cautiously in cats.

_____

6. The appropriate dose of acetaminophen is significantly lower in cats than in dogs.

_____

7. The test kit for EG poisoning must be used very carefully with consultation of the package insert and directions.

_____

8. When managing a zinc phosphide case, if any staff members have a headache or shortness of breath, they should seek medical attention.

_____

9. Guinea pigs are not affected by bromethalin.

_____

10. A drooling cat should be evaluated for ingestion of topical insecticides or sprays.

_____

11. Clinical signs associated with the ingestion of calcium oxalate – containing plants include oral irritation; intense burning and irritation of the mouth, lips, and tongue; excessive drooling; vomiting; and difficulty in swallowing.

_____

12. Ingestion of raw yeast bread dough can be life-threatening to dogs.

_____

13. Onions and other members of the *Allium* family can be harmful to all animals.

_____

14. Cats are considered to be at higher risk for onion toxicity.

_____

15. The veterinary staff should take extra steps to keep the bladder empty either through catheterization or frequent walking in a patient who has ingested chocolate.

_____

16. As a general rule, the darker and more bitter the chocolate, the more toxic it likely is.

_____

17. Samples collected should always be kept and properly labeled.

_____

18. It is extremely important to maintain nutritional requirements in a cat undergoing treatment.

_____

19. A 3% hydrogen peroxide solution has been shown to be an effective emetic for dogs, ferrets, and pigs.

_____

20. The use of hydrogen peroxide as an emetic in the cat is not recommended.

_____

21. Emesis should be induced on a hard surface where the vomitus can be examined.

_____

22. It is especially important to make sure young animals are kept warm after a bath.

_____

23. When dealing with sticky substances (e.g., gum, glue traps, tar), the use of solvents should be avoided.

_____

24. For birds, do not follow all the same instructions for the removal of sticky substances as for other animals.

_____

28 Wound Management and Bandaging

When you have completed this chapter, you will be able to:

1. Pronounce, define, and spell all of the key terms in this chapter.
2. Identify the phases of wound healing, and describe patient, wound, and treatment factors that adversely affect wound healing.
3. Do the following regarding wound management in the small animal:
   - Describe the objectives of and principles of immediate wound care, including wound lavage.
   - Describe the goals and methods of wound debridement.
   - Differentiate among primary, delayed primary, and secondary wound closure, and among primary, second, and third intention healing.
   - Compare and contrast methods of managing wound drainage and wound infection.
   - Explain the nature of and appearance of abrasions, lacerations, degloving injuries, bite wounds, burns, decubitus ulcers, and pressure sores, and discuss the methods used to treat each.
4. Identify the principles of bandaging, and discuss the purpose of the primary, secondary, and tertiary layers of a bandage, including the specific materials used for each.
5. Discuss the uses for and characteristics of the following external coaptation methods in small animals, as well as their application technique:
   - Robert Jones bandage and modified Robert Jones bandage.
   - Casts and splints.
   - Ehmer, 90/90 flexion, Velpeau, Spica sling, and hobbles.
   - Bandages for the head, chest, abdomen, tail, and areas that are difficult to bandage such as the pelvis and the axilla.
6. Explain aftercare of bandages, splints, casts, and slings, including complications that may occur.
7. Discuss the principles of equine wound care, including treatment of exuberant granulation tissue.
8. Do the following regarding application of bandages, splints, and casts in horses:
   - Discuss uses for, characteristics of, and the technique used to place a lower limb wound bandage or a support bandage on an equine limb.
   - Discuss uses for and characteristics of equine casts and splints and techniques used to place a cast or a splint on an equine limb.
   - Describe the technique used to remove a cast.
9. Discuss uses for and characteristics of bandages, splints, and casts used for cattle and describe techniques used to place a claw block and a modified Thomas splint on a ruminant limb.

EXERCISE 28.1 CROSSWORD PUZZLE: TERMS AND DEFINITIONS

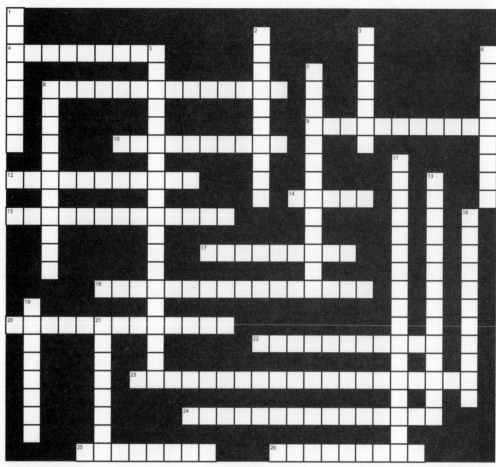

Across

4 A wound dressing that is a primary layer impermeable to moisture.
8 Wound caused by pressure on skin over bony prominences. (2 words)
9 Cells recruited into a wound during the proliferative phase that help form granulation tissue.
10 Sharp cut or tear of skin.
12 Having an affinity for water.
14 Wound healing involving treatment that does not allow the wound to dry out.
15 A primary wound dressing that allows air and moisture to move through.
17 Closure of a wound by apposing the skin over healthy granulation tissue.
18 Healing of a wound across a surgically closed incision. (2 words)
20 The opposite side.
22 Vascularized fibrous tissue that covers a wound if left to heal by second intention.
23 Tissue also known as proud flesh. (2 words)
24 Healing of a wound by granulation tissue formation, epithelialization and contraction. (2 words)
25 Pertaining to the groin area.
26 Type of injury that features a large section of skin torn off the underlying tissue in a glove-like fashion.

Down

1 Having an osmotic pressure equivalent to that of blood plasma.
2 Having an osmotic pressure greater than that of blood plasma.
3 Surgical closure of a wound.
5 Meshwork-like substance in a wound, attached to the outer cell surface that provides support and anchorage. (2 words)
6 Space between tissues allowing accumulation of fluid. (2 words)
7 A cell with contractile properties that is responsible for wound contraction.
8 Removal of foreign matter and dead tissue from a wound.
11 The process in which skin cells advance in a single layer across the wound.
13 Wound healing by secondary closure after allowing granulation tissue to form. (2 words)
16 A Teflon pad is one example of this type of wound dressing.
19 Deposited into a wound by fibroblasts during the proliferative phase of healing.
21 An area of skin that has been superficially scraped.

EXERCISE 28.2 MATCHING #1: WOUND CLASSIFICATIONS

Instructions: Match each wound type in column A with its corresponding classification in column B by writing the appropriate letter in the space provided. (Note that responses may be used more than once.)

Column A

1. _____ A wound with a high bacterial count.
2. _____ Surgical wound that enters a hollow viscus.
3. _____ Surgical wound.
4. _____ An open traumatic wound.
5. _____ An old traumatic wound.
6. _____ A surgical wound with a minor break in sterile technique.
7. _____ A surgical wound into the colon.
8. _____ A natural wound with minor contamination.
9. _____ A surgical wound with a major break in sterile technique.

Column B

A. Clean wound

B. Clean-contaminated wound

C. Contaminated wound

D. Dirty and infected wound

EXERCISE 28.3 MATCHING #2: BANDAGES, SLINGS, SPLINTS, AND CASTS

Instructions: Match each device in column A with its corresponding description in column B by writing the appropriate letter in the space provided.

Column A

1. _____ Carpal flexion sling
2. _____ Cast
3. _____ Ehmer sling
4. _____ Modified Thomas splint
5. _____ Modified Robert Jones bandage
6. _____ Robert Jones bandage
7. _____ Schroeder-Thomas splint
8. _____ Spica splint
9. _____ Velpeau sling
10. _____ 90/90 Flexion sling
11. _____ Hobbles

Column B

A. A traction splint constructed of rods used for stabilizing long bone fractures in large animals.

B. Maintains the limb in extension. Includes a lateral splint that reaches over the shoulder or hip.

C. Prevents abduction of the pelvic limbs. Primarily used after reduction of ventral hip luxations.

D. Used for the forelimb in any situation where weight bearing should be avoided but some movement of the elbow and shoulder joints is acceptable.

E. A very bulky bandage used to immobilize a limb distal to the elbow or stifle joint.

F. A device that prevents weight bearing of the pelvic limb. Frequently used after closed reduction of craniodorsal hip luxations.

G. A device that prevents weight bearing of the thoracic limb. Primarily used after reduction of medial shoulder luxations.

H. A device used to immobilize fractures that is most often made of fiberglass material.

I. Used in puppies after repair of distal femoral fractures to prevent quadriceps tie-down or contracture.

J. Also known as a "soft-padded bandage." The most commonly used distal limb bandage in small animals.

K. An immobilization device with a rigid metal frame. No longer recommended.

EXERCISE 28.4 MATCHING #3: WOUND CLOSURE AND HEALING

Instructions: Match each bandage material in column A with the corresponding type of wound healing that will follow in column B by writing the appropriate response in the space provided.

Column A

1. No closure of a wound will lead to _____.

2. Primary closure of a wound will lead to _____.

3. Secondary closure of a wound will lead to _____.

Column B

A. Primary intention healing

B. Third intention healing

C. Second intention healing

EXERCISE 28.5 MATCHING #4: BURNS

Instructions: Match each type of burn in column A with its corresponding description in column B by writing the appropriate letter in the space provided.

Column A

1. _____ First-degree burn

2. _____ Second-degree burn

3. _____ Third-degree burn

4. _____ Fourth-degree burn

Column B

A. Skin that is thick, leathery, and often black.

B. A burn with the presence of fluid-filled blisters.

C. A burn that involves tissues deep to the skin.

D. Skin is red and painful.

EXERCISE 28.6 MATCHING #5: BANDAGE MATERIALS

Instructions: Match each bandage material in column A with its corresponding characteristics in column B by writing the appropriate letter in the space provided. (Note that responses may be used more than once.)

Column A

1. _____ Elastikon elastic adhesive tape (Johnson & Johnson Medical, Arlington, TX)
2. _____ Curagel hydrogel (Kendall/Covidien, Mansfield, MA)
3. _____ Cotton sheets
4. _____ NU-GEL hydrogel (Johnson & Johnson Medical, Arlington, TX)
5. _____ Cast padding (3M Skin and Wound Care, St. Paul, MN)
6. _____ 20% sodium chloride dressing
7. _____ Vetrap elastic bandage (3M Animal Care Products, St. Paul, MN)
8. _____ Hydrosorb Plus Foam (Kendall/Covidien, Mansfield, MA)
9. _____ Military field bandage
10. _____ Petrolatum-impregnated gauze
11. _____ Ultec hydrocolloid dressing (Kendall/Covidien, Mansfield, MA)
12. _____ Flannel track wrap
13. _____ Kling conforming gauze (Johnson & Johnson Medical, Arlington, TX)
14. _____ Honey
15. _____ Bioclusive polyurethane film (Johnson & Johnson Medical, Arlington, TX)
16. _____ Rolled cotton (Johnson & Johnson Medical, Arlington, TX)
17. _____ Teflon pads
18. _____ Tegaderm transparent dressing (3M Skin and Wound Care, St. Paul, MN)
19. _____ Quilted leg wraps
20. _____ Sterile wide-mesh gauze
21. _____ Tegaderm hydrocolloid (3M Skin and Wound Care, St. Paul, MN)
22. _____ Ace bandage
23. _____ Granulated sugar

Column B

A. Primary layer adherent
B. Primary layer nonadherent nonocclusive
C. Primary layer nonadherent semiocclusive
D. Primary layer nonadherent occlusive
E. Primary layer hypertonic or hyperosmolar
F. Secondary layer
G. Tertiary layer

306

Chapter 28 **Wound Management and Bandaging**

Copyright © 2018, Elsevier Inc. All Rights Reserved.

Instructions: Match each bandage, cast, or sling with its corresponding photo by writing the name in the space provided. Then list the primary indication(s) for each bandage, cast, or sling.

A. Hobbles

B. Modified Robert Jones bandage

C. Robert Jones bandage

D. Fiberglass cast

E. Velpeau sling

F. Carpal flexion sling

G. Ehmer sling

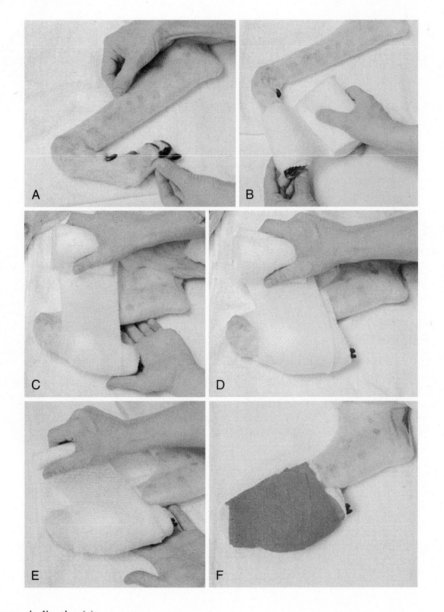

1. Name and primary indication(s): _____

_____

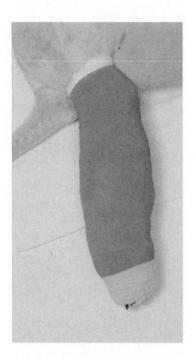

2. Name and primary indication(s): _____

_____

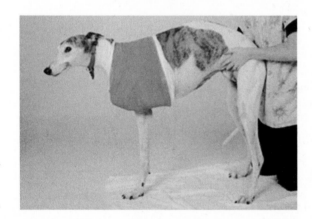

3. Name and primary indication(s): _____

_____

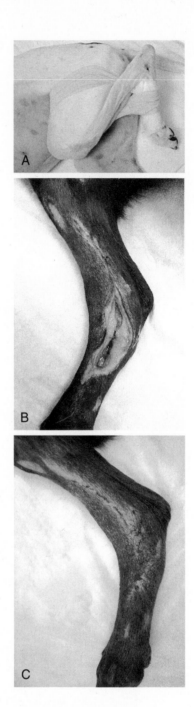

4. Name and primary indication(s): _____

_____

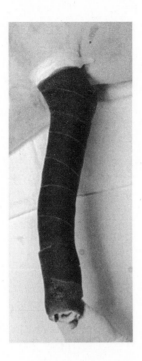

5. Name and primary indication(s): _____

_____

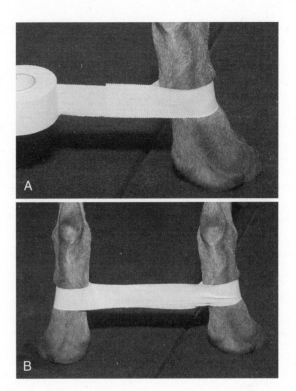

A

B

6. Name and primary indication(s): _____

_____

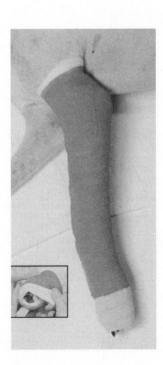

7. Name and primary indication(s): _____

_____

Chapter **28** **Wound Management and Bandaging**

EXERCISE 28.8 ORDERING: APPLYING A CAST TO A HORSE'S LIMB

A cast is the external coaptation most frequently used to manage various orthopedic injuries or problems in horses when maximum support and immobilization are required. Collecting all necessary materials is the first step when applying a cast. A number of other specific steps must be performed in the correct order to apply the cast properly.

Instructions: Place the steps of applying a cast to a horse's limb in the proper order from first to last by writing the appropriate number (2 through 15) in the space provided. The first step has already been completed.

A. ___1___ Collect all necessary materials.

B. _____ Place wire traction loops through the hoof.

C. _____ Place a wooden wedge underneath the heel.

D. _____ Induce general anesthesia.

E. _____ Cover the limb with a double layer of stockinette.

F. _____ Clean the sole, remove the shoe, and trim the hoof.

G. _____ Cap the bottom of the cast with hard acrylic.

H. _____ Twist ends of the wire together to form a loop.

I. _____ Apply two layers of 3-inch plaster material.

J. _____ Dry the skin and powder it with talcum or boric acid.

K. _____ Seal the top of the cast with stockinette and/or adhesive tape.

L. _____ Apply orthopedic felt at points of pressure.

M. _____ Apply two to three layers of 4- to 5-inch fiberglass material.

N. _____ Apply support foam.

O. _____ Apply two layers of 3-inch fiberglass material.

EXERCISE 28.9 TRUE OR FALSE: COMPREHENSIVE

Instructions: Read the following statements and write "T" for true or "F" for false in the blanks provided. If a statement is false, correct the statement to make it true.

1. _____ During the maturation phase of wound healing, the tissue regains normal strength.

2. _____ Multiplication of bacteria beyond 10^5 organisms per gram of tissue will stop wound healing.

3. _____ When lavaging a highly contaminated wound for initial removal of debris and contamination, the type of fluid is more important than the amount you use.

4. _____ Fluid drainage from a wound is a reliable sign of infection and warrants antimicrobial therapy.

5. _____ Healthy granulation tissue is naturally resistant to infection and therefore does not require routine antimicrobial therapy.

6. _____ Bite wounds are usually relatively easy to assess because the extent of the damage is visually apparent.

7. _____ Bite wounds should always be considered contaminated.

310

8. _____ Most burns in domestic animals are a result of accidental or deliberate injury from things like barn fires, car mufflers, electrical cords, or hot liquids.

9. _____ The best treatment for pressure sores arising from splints or casts is the use of occlusive, nonadherent dressings.

10. _____ The wet-to-dry bandage technique has largely been replaced by the nonadherent dressing.

11. _____ The Robert Jones bandage is a frequently used bandage for small animal patients.

12. _____ In general, small animals cannot tolerate excessive bandage tightness as easily as large animals unless a thick secondary layer is used.

13. _____ As long as the device has been applied correctly, dogs with bandages, slings, and casts can be permitted to play in a fenced-in yard.

14. _____ To keep a bandage dry, it should be covered with a plastic bag or an empty fluid IV bag at all times.

15. _____ Basic wound management in horses is very similar to that of small companion animals.

16. _____ Horses with open wounds on a limb below the carpus or tarsus are at risk for development of exuberant granulation tissue.

17. _____ Full limb casts can easily be applied to a horse under standing sedation.

18. _____ Fiberglass casting tape is the preferred material to use, due to its rigid, lightweight properties.

19. _____ Stall confinement is mandatory after equine cast application.

20. _____ The management of lameness in cattle is aided by the number of weight-bearing digits on each foot.

EXERCISE 28.10 MULTIPLE CHOICE: COMPREHENSIVE

Instructions: Circle the one correct answer to each of the following questions.

1. The inflammatory phase of wound healing is also known as the
   a. Lag phase
   b. Second phase
   c. Final phase
   d. Contraction phase

2. All of the following treatments but one negatively impact wound healing. Which one does not negatively affect wound healing?
   a. Chemotherapy
   b. Corticosteroids
   c. Antimicrobials
   d. Radiation

3. The preferred antiseptic for wound lavage is
   a. 1:40 (0.05%) dilution of chlorhexidine solution and water
   b. Warm isotonic crystalloid fluid
   c. 1% Povidone-iodine solution
   d. 2% Chlorhexidine gluconate surgical scrub

4. Wound débridement by use of a wet-to-dry bandage causes débridement that is classified as
   a. Débridement "en bloc"
   b. Selective biologic débridement
   c. Staged selective surgical débridement
   d. Nonselective débridement

5. Surgical wounds closed by direct apposition heal by
   a. Moist wound healing
   b. Primary intention healing
   c. Second intention healing
   d. Third intention healing

6. Wound drains should be removed when the amount of fluid decreases. This is often after approximately
   a. 1 to 2 days
   b. 3 to 5 days
   c. 5 to 7 days
   d. 7 to 10 days

7. Patients with a severely infected wound and systemic signs (such as lethargy, pain, and decreased appetite) often require that antimicrobials be given
   a. Topically
   b. Orally
   c. Intramuscularly
   d. Intravenously

8. Burn wounds are classified based on
   a. The depth and size
   b. The size and duration
   c. The duration and location
   d. The location and depth

9. A partial-thickness burn that is characterized by blisters and discoloration would be classified as
   a. First degree
   b. Second degree
   c. Third degree
   d. Fourth degree

10. A full-thickness burn that is characterized by tough, discolored skin, but without involvement of deep tissues, would be classified as
    a. First degree
    b. Second degree
    c. Third degree
    d. Fourth degree

11. Splints, casts, and slings can be used only to immobilize injuries below the
    a. Metacarpus and metatarsus
    b. Carpus and tarsus
    c. Elbow and stifle
    d. Hip and shoulder

12. There is a relatively low risk of complications from tightening the tertiary layer of a
    a. Modified Robert-Jones bandage
    b. Chest bandage
    c. Head bandage
    d. Robert-Jones bandage

13. In small animals, the most commonly used device for treatment of the distal limb is the
    a. Modified Robert-Jones bandage
    b. Fiberglass cast
    c. Schroeder-Thomas splint
    d. Robert-Jones bandage

14. When applying cast padding and conforming gauze that comes on a roll, often it should be overlapped by approximately
    a. 30%
    b. 50%
    c. 70%
    d. It should not be overlapped

15. Most forelimb splints should be applied to the
    a. Cranial surface
    b. Lateral surface
    c. Medial surface
    d. Caudal surface

16. Most rear limb splints (with the exception of metatarsal and foot splints) should be applied to the
    a. Cranial surface
    b. Lateral surface
    c. Medial surface
    d. Caudal surface

17. Non-weight-bearing slings, like the Ehmer and the Velpeau, should not be maintained for more than
    a. 7 to 10 days
    b. 1 to 2 weeks
    c. 2 to 3 weeks
    d. 4 to 6 weeks

18. The toes of an animal with a distal limb bandage must be monitored for complications daily. An increased distance between the toenails of a foot is a sign of
    a. Decreased viability
    b. Nothing (It is normal)
    c. Swelling
    d. Skin maceration

19. Horses can get proud flesh in wounds on the distal limb. The term *proud flesh* refers to
    a. An infected wound
    b. Excessive granulation tissue
    c. A healthy looking wound bed
    d. A nonhealing open wound

20. Casting material used in horses may include
    a. Polyvinyl chloride (PVC) pipe
    b. Wooden slats
    c. Metal bars
    d. All of the above

21. When applying a cast to a limb, for optimal effectiveness, the cast must immobilize
    a. The joints proximal and distal to the injury
    b. All the joints of the limb
    c. Only the joint proximal to the injury
    d. Only the bone that is fractured

22. Application of excessive padding under a cast will
    a. Cause it to get wet
    b. Cause pressure necrosis of the skin
    c. Result in cast sores
    d. Not be a problem in most cases

23. When removing an equine distal limb cast, it should be split on
    a. The medial and lateral surfaces
    b. The cranial and caudal surfaces
    c. The diagonal surfaces
    d. All four surfaces

24. The best method for controlling proud flesh in horses is usually
    a. Cryotherapy
    b. Electrocautery
    c. Topical treatment
    d. Surgical removal

25. Despite advances in external and internal skeletal fixation, modified Thomas splints are still often used in
    a. Horses
    b. Dogs
    c. Cattle
    d. Cats

26. A "beehive" and aluminum rod are used to construct a
    a. Coaptation splint
    b. Fiberglass cast
    c. Modified Thomas splint
    d. Robert-Jones bandage

EXERCISE 28.11 FILL-IN-THE-BLANK: COMPREHENSIVE

Instructions: Fill in each of the spaces provided with the missing word or words that complete the sentence.

1. Wound strength is lowest during the _____ phase of healing.

2. Concerning the proliferative phase of wound healing, granulation tissue begins to form approximately _____ to _____ days after the injury, epithelialization begins approximately _____ to _____ days after the injury, and contraction of the wound begins approximately _____ days after the injury.

3. Healthy granulation tissue is _____ in color, but if it is unhealthy, it is _____ in color.

4. When caring for a wound in a patient first presented for treatment, the first objective is always to prevent further _____ of the wound.

5. _____-intention healing is often used on the distal limb in situations where there is little available skin.

6. When treating patients with wound infections, antimicrobials are often chosen _____ (i.e., based on experience or observation). If the correct medication was chosen, the infection should generally resolve within _____ to _____ days of initiation of treatment.

7. Gunshot wounds and wounds caused by sticks are often treated in a similar manner to _____ wounds.

8. You might know that a pressure sore is starting to form if you see _____ of the skin with _____ _____.

9. When treating wounds, once granulation tissue has formed and epithelialization begins, a _____ primary layer must be used to promote second-intention healing.

10. A cast that has been cut on both sides to create a top and bottom half is said to have been _____.

11. A properly applied Ehmer sling will internally _____ and _____ the femur.

12. After placing a tail bandage, a _____ _____ should be used to provide additional protection for the tip of the tail.

13. Bandages covering wounds with a lot of exudate should be replaced _____ to _____ times a day, whereas support bandages should be changed about every _____ days to check for complications.

14. A lower-limb wound bandage on a horse is defined as a bandage distal to the _____ in the forelimb, or the _____ in the rear limb.

15. When applying an equine cast to the forelimb, orthopedic felt must be placed over pressure points. These points include the most _____ limit of the cast, and the _____ _____ bone.

EXERCISE 28.12 CASE STUDY: WOUND CARE

Signalment: Mindy, a 2-year-old, female, Spaniel mix.
History: The owner reported that Mindy jumped over the fence and disappeared from the yard 2 days ago. This morning, they found her lying on the front porch. She was covered with burs and had a large laceration on her left forelimb. The owner is not sure what happened, but it appears that she may have gotten caught on the fence and torn the skin as she jumped over.
Physical examination: Other than the laceration and mats and burs in her hair, Mindy appears normal. The wound is approximately 10 cm long; there is a 1 to 2 cm gap between the edges of the wound; and the wound is visibly dirty, appears to have some dead tissue around the edges, and is covered with a thick discharge. It appears that some skin was torn away, and it does not appear that there will be enough skin to completely cover the wound. After talking with the doctor, the owner elected to treat it as an open wound and let it heal by second intention. Answer the following questions regarding management of this case.

1. What type of bandage could be used to nonselectively débride this wound?

   _____

   a. Summarize the steps used to apply this bandage.

   _____

   _____

   _____

   _____

   _____

   b. Briefly explain how this bandage works to débride the wound.

   _____

   _____

   _____

   _____

   _____

   _____

c. What precautions must you take when using this type of bandage?

_____

_____

_____

_____

_____

_____

_____

_____

d. How often do you estimate this bandage would have to be changed?

_____

_____

_____

_____

_____

2. What type of primary layer is often preferred to prevent destruction of granulation tissue and other healthy tissue? Give a few examples of the specific types of materials that can be used for this alternative type of primary layer.

_____

_____

_____

_____

_____

_____

3. Mindy was kept for the day while the wound was treated and the bandage was applied. The attending veterinarian has now asked you to discharge Mindy from the hospital and speak with her owner about care of the bandage.

a. What instructions would you need to give Mindy's owner regarding care of this bandage?

_____

_____

_____

_____

_____

_____

b. What signs should Mindy's owner watch for that would alert her of a complication that would need to be addressed?

_____

_____

_____

_____

_____

_____

_____

Pharmacology and Pharmacy

LEARNING OBJECTIVES

When you have completed this chapter, you will be able to:

1. Pronounce, define, and spell all the key terms in this chapter.
2. Do the following related to types of drugs:
   - List approval categories of drugs, and compare and contrast prescription drugs and over-the-counter drugs.
   - Explain the concept of a valid veterinary-client-patient relationship, and explain how it affects the use of prescription drugs.
   - Discuss laws affecting the use of controlled substances, and list commonly used drugs that are classified as controlled substances.
3. List the dosage forms of medications, the routes by which medications may be administered, and factors that affect route selection and discuss dosage terminology.
4. Do the following related to pharmacokinetics and pharmacodynamics:
   - Describe the principles of basic pharmacokinetics, including drug absorption, distribution, metabolism, and elimination.
   - Describe the principles of basic pharmacodynamics, including mechanism of action, side effects, and adverse drug reactions.
   - Discuss the impact of disease (specifically cardiovascular, kidney, and liver diseases) on drug pharmacokinetics.
   - Discuss aging and drug pharmacokinetics.
5. Do the following regarding drug nomenclature and the systemic approach to drug classification:
   - Discuss the different ways drugs can be identified.
   - List the main drug classes used to treat major animal diseases and give examples of drugs in each class, including their mechanism of action and common side effects.
6. Do the following regarding regulatory pharmacology:
   - List state and federal agencies regulating drug use and explain how they work together to ensure that available drugs are safe and effective and are used appropriately to treat and prevent animal diseases.
   - Define extra-label drug use and discuss circumstances under which drugs may or may not be used in this manner, including special restrictions on extra-label drug use in food-producing animals.
   - Discuss the significance of drug residues in food producing animals and the importance of observing withdrawal times to keep the human food supply safe.
   - Define drug compounding and explain legal issues related to compounding of medications.
7. Describe regulatory issues related to procurement, storage, and disposal of pharmacologic agents.
8. Do the following regarding prescribing and dispensing drugs:
   - Correctly describe how to write a prescription and explain the parts of a prescription label.
   - Perform dosage calculations required to dispense drugs and to administer drugs to patients.

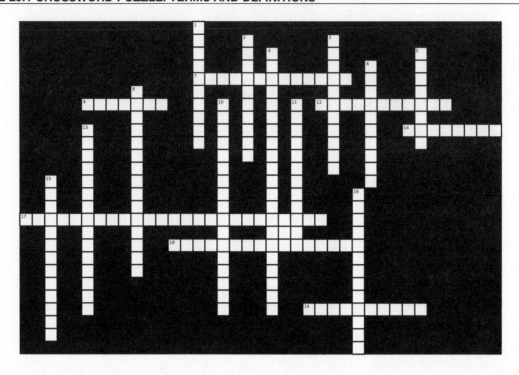

Across

7   A nondrug substance administered orally to provide substances required for normal body structure and function.

9   A drug that activates a receptor, producing the same action as an endogenous substrate.

12 Soluble in water.

14 A drug's capacity, once bound to its receptor, to produce an effect.

17 The periodic measurement of the amount of a drug in the blood. (3 words)

18 A term summarized by the phrase "what the drug does to the body."

19 Use of a formulation of human insulin to treat type I diabetes in a dog is an example of this drug use. (2 words)

Down

1   The term for administration of a drug by injection.

2   Naloxone is one of these within the opioid family of drugs.

3   When the amount of drug administered equals the amount of drug eliminated, the blood level is said to have reached _____. (2 words)

4   A drug will be expected to have the desired effect when the concentration in the bloodstream is within this level. (3 words)

5   The time required for the amount of a drug in the body to decrease by 50%; used to estimate the dosing interval. (2 words)

6   Absorption across cell membranes is more efficient for these drugs, than for hydrophilic drugs.

8   A measure of the percentage of a drug dose that reaches the bloodstream.

10 The chemical modification of a drug by the body.

11 Another name for an Rx drug.

13 Preparation of a flavored suspension of metronidazole to facilitate accurate oral dosing in a cat is a form of this. (2 words)

15 A predictable reaction to a drug, the likelihood of which increases as the drug dose increases. (2 words)

16 An unpredictable reaction to a drug that does not occur immediately, but after several days of treatment, and that is often associated with an immune system response.

EXERCISE 29.2 MATCHING #1: TERMS RELATED TO REGULATORY ISSUES

Instructions: Match each term related to regulatory issues in column A with its corresponding definition in column B by writing the appropriate letter in the space provided.

Column A

1. _____ Animal Medicinal Drug Use Clarification Act (AMDUCA)

2. _____ Center for Veterinary Medicine (CVM)

3. _____ Drug Enforcement Agency (DEA)

4. _____ Environmental Protection Agency (EPA)

5. _____ Federal Food, Drug, and Cosmetic Act (FFD&C Act)

6. _____ Food and Drug Administration's Center for Veterinary Medicine (FDA CVM)

7. _____ U.S. Department of Agriculture (USDA)

8. _____ U.S. Pharmacopoeia (USP)—National Formulary (NF)

9. _____ Veterinarian-client-patient relationship (VCPR)

10. _____ Compendium of Veterinary Products (CVP)

Column B

A. A set of requirements that must be met in order for a veterinarian to prescribe a drug for a patient.

B. The federal law regulating drug approval, use, safety, and efficacy.

C. The governing body that regulates the manufacture and distribution of drugs, food additives, and medical devices used in veterinary species under the FFD&C Act.

D. The government agency that regulates veterinary biologics.

E. An amendment of the FFD&C Act that allows extralabel drug use for the treatment of veterinary species, provided specific conditions are met.

F. The organization through which adverse drug events can be reported in order to identify post-approval drug risks.

G. A compilation of information about veterinary drugs and biologics.

H. The government agency charged with overseeing and regulating pesticides.

I. The official legal drug compendium for the United States. A compilation of all drug substances and products focused on providing active ingredients.

J. The agency that categorizes controlled substances into five schedules (I, II, III, IV, and V) based on their potential for abuse.

EXERCISE 29.3 MATCHING #2: DRUGS AND THEIR PRIMARY INDICATIONS

Instructions: Match each drug class or group in column A with its corresponding primary indication in column B by writing the appropriate letter in the space provided.

Column A

1. _____ Chemotherapy drugs
2. _____ Mitotane or trilostane
3. _____ Immunosuppressive drugs
4. _____ ACE inhibitors
5. _____ Antibiotics
6. _____ Glucocorticoids and mineralocorticoids
7. _____ Methimazole or radioactive iodide
8. _____ Anticoagulants
9. _____ Antitussives
10. _____ Insulin
11. _____ Antihypertensive
12. _____ Anticonvulsants
13. _____ Antiparasitics
14. _____ NSAIDs
15. _____ Diuretics
16. _____ L-thyroxine
17. _____ Antifungal drugs
18. _____ Inotropic agents
19. _____ Anticonvulsants
20. _____ Antiarrhythmics

Column B

A. Diabetes mellitus
B. Hyperadrenocorticism
C. Prevent life-threatening thrombi
D. Immune-mediated diseases
E. Dermatophyte infections
F. Hypoadrenocorticism
G. Neoplastic diseases (cancers)
H. Hyperthyroidism
I. High blood pressure
J. Respiratory conditions
K. Seizure disorders
L. Inflammation
M. Edema
N. GI nematode and arthropod infestations
O. Hypothyroidism
P. Vasodilation
Q. Improved contractility of cardiac muscle
R. Control heart rhythm abnormalities
S. Epilepsy
T. Bacterial infections

EXERCISE 29.4 MATCHING #3: ADVERSE DRUG REACTIONS

Instructions: Column A is a list of characteristics that apply to drug reactions. Indicate whether each characteristic applies to dose-dependent reactions, idiosyncratic reactions, or both by writing an "A," "B," or "C" in the space provided.

Column A

1. _____ Associated with an immune-system response.

2. _____ Occur at standard and inappropriate doses.

3. _____ Unpredictable.

4. _____ Treatment requires drug avoidance.

5. _____ May be prevented by therapeutic drug monitoring.

6. _____ Affect all members of a species.

7. _____ Not dose dependent.

8. _____ Not related to the action of the drug.

9. _____ Predictable.

10. _____ Often affect more than one species.

11. _____ Therapeutic drug monitoring will not prevent them.

12. _____ May or may not be related to the action of the drug.

13. _____ Occur after several days of treatment.

14. _____ May or may not affect multiple species.

15. _____ More severe at higher doses.

16. _____ Often respond to dose reduction.

17. _____ Affect a small portion of treated animals.

Column B

A. Dose-dependent drug reactions

B. Idiosyncratic drug reactions

C. Both dose-dependent and idiosyncratic drug reactions

EXERCISE 29.5 MATCHING #4: ANTIBACTERIAL DRUGS

Instructions: Match each antibacterial drug in column A with the corresponding class to which it belongs in column B by writing the appropriate letter in the space provided. (Note that responses may be used more than once.)

Column A

1. _____ Cephalexin
2. _____ Marbofloxacin
3. _____ Oxytetracycline
4. _____ Amikacin
5. _____ Sulfamethoxazole
6. _____ Ampicillin
7. _____ Metronidazole
8. _____ Tilmicosin
9. _____ Florfenicol
10. _____ Gentamicin
11. _____ Amoxicillin
12. _____ Cefpodoxime
13. _____ Tylosin
14. _____ Enrofloxacin
15. _____ Erythromycin
16. _____ Trimethoprim
17. _____ Azithromycin
18. _____ Lincomycin
19. _____ Clindamycin
20. _____ Doxycycline

Column B

A. Cephalosporins
B. Aminoglycosides
C. Sulfonamides
D. Potentiated sulfonamides
E. Fluoroquinolones
F. Amphenicols
G. Macrolides
H. Lincosamides
I. Tetracyclines
J. Nitroimidazoles
K. Penicillins

Chapter **29** Pharmacology and Pharmacy

EXERCISE 29.6 MATCHING #5: MECHANISM OF ACTION

Instructions: Match each commonly used drug in column A with its mechanism of action in column B by writing the appropriate letter in the space provided. (Note that responses may be used more than once.)

Column A

1. _____ Benazepril

2. _____ NSAIDs

3. _____ Digitoxin

4. _____ Organophosphate

5. _____ Apomorphine

6. _____ Trimethoprim

7. _____ Furosemide

8. _____ Pyrethirins

9. _____ Famotidine

10. _____ Hemparin

11. _____ Aspirin

12. _____ Enalapril

13. _____ Omeprazole

14. _____ Sulfamethoxazole

15. _____ Diphenhydramine

16. _____ Lidocaine

Column B

A. Histamine antagonist.

B. Prevents synthesis of folate.

C. Suppresses prostaglandin synthesis by inhibiting cyclooxygenase.

D. Functions as a vasodilator by inhibiting angiotensin-converting enzyme.

E. Binds to histamine receptors.

F. Prevents metabolism of acetylcholine by inhibiting acetylcholinesterase.

G. Blockade of fast sodium channels (slow action potential conduction).

H. Produces sedation as a dopamine receptor agonist.

I. Prevents sodium and water reabsorption by inhibiting the $Na^+/K^+/2Cl^-$ transporter in the loop of Henle.

J. Increases the strength of heart muscle contraction by inhibiting $Na^+/K^+/$ATPase.

K. Inhibits bacterial production of folic acid.

L. Proton pump inhibitor.

M. Interferes with clot formation by inhibiting the conversion of prothrombin to thrombin.

EXERCISE 29.7 MATCHING #6: DRUGS USED TO TREAT GASTROINTESTINAL DISEASE

Instructions: Match each drug or group of drugs used to treat gastrointestinal disease in column A with the corresponding class to which it belongs in column B by writing the appropriate letter in the space provided. (Note that responses may be used more than once.)

Column A

1. _____ Dolasetron and ondansetron

2. _____ Cisapride

3. _____ Cyprobeptadine

4. _____ Famotidine and ranitidine

5. _____ Sucralfate

6. _____ Docusate potassium

7. _____ Maropitant

8. _____ Prochlorperazine and chlorpromazine

9. _____ Loperamide

10. _____ Pancrealipase

11. _____ Metoclopramide

12. _____ Omeprazole

13. _____ Xylazine

Column B

A. Prokinetic

B. Antacid/ulcer therapy

C. Antiemetic

D. Antiemetic/prokinetic

E. Emetic

F. Laxative/emollient

G. Appetite stimulant

H. Digestive enzyme supplement

EXERCISE 29.8 MATCHING #7: DRUGS USED TO TREAT CARDIOVASCULAR DISEASE

Instructions: Match each drug or group of drugs used to treat cardiovascular disease in column A with the corresponding class to which it belongs in column B by writing the appropriate letter in the space provided.

Column A

1. _____ Atenolol and propranolol

2. _____ Pimobendan

3. _____ Diltiazem

4. _____ Furosemide and spironolactone

5. _____ Lidocaine and quinidine

6. _____ Benazepril and enalapril

7. _____ Hydralazine

8. _____ Amlodipine

9. _____ Digoxin

10. _____ Sotalol

11. _____ Sildenafil

Column B

A. Diuretic

B. ACE inhibitor (antihypertensive)

C. Positive inotrope

D. Calcium-channel blocker (class IV antiarrhythmic)

E. β-Adrenergic blocker (class II antiarrhythmic)

F. Phosphodiesterase V inhibitor (antihypertensive)

G. Fast sodium channel blocker (class I antiarrhythmic)

H. Arteriolar dilator (antihypertensive)

I. Calcium-channel blocker (antihypertensive)

J. Phosphodiesterase III inhibitor (balanced vasodilator/positive inotrope)

K. β-adrenergic blocker (class III antiarrhythmic)

EXERCISE 29.9 MATCHING #8: DRUGS PROHIBITED FOR USE IN FOOD-PRODUCING ANIMALS

Instructions: Match each drug or drug class in column A with the reason that it is banned in food-producing animals in column B by writing the appropriate letter in the space provided. (Note that responses may be used more than once.)

Column A

1. _____ Fluoroquinolones

2. _____ Clenbuterol

3. _____ Chloramphenicol

4. _____ Glycopeptides (vancomycin)

5. _____ Diethylstilbestrol (DES)

6. _____ Nitrofurans

7. _____ Sulfonamides

8. _____ Nitroimidazoles

Column B

A. Microbial drug resistance in humans

B. Vaginal cancer in humans exposed in utero

C. Carcinogenicity

D. Toxicity and death of exposed humans

E. Carcinogenicity and mutagenicity

F. Idiosyncratic bone marrow toxicosis in humans

EXERCISE 29.10 TRUE OR FALSE: COMPREHENSIVE

Instructions: Read the following statements and write "T" for true or "F" for false in the blanks provided. If a statement is false, correct the statement to make it true.

1. _____ To achieve therapeutic blood levels, hydrophilic drugs must be administered by injection.

2. _____ Drugs leave the vascular space by the process of adsorption.

3. _____ Biotransformation tends to make most drugs more hydrophilic prior to elimination in the urine or bile.

4. _____ Drug metabolism most often occurs in the kidney.

5. _____ Drug side effects are commonly related to the drug's mechanism of action.

6. _____ Glucocorticoids are classified according to the receptor they bind to.

7. _____ The term *antibiotic* is equivalent to the term *antibacterial*.

8. _____ The most common side effects of antimicrobial drugs are vomiting and diarrhea.

9. _____ When treating disseminated fungal infections, most systemic antifungal drugs are given for approximately 10 days to 2 weeks.

10. _____ Treatment of feline hyperthyroidism with radioactive iodine is generally curative.

11. _____ Mitotane kills the cells in the adrenal gland that produce cortisol, whereas trilostane does not.

12. _____ The molecular structure of insulin varies widely among the common domestic species.

13. _____ Because insulin is usually given in very small doses, a tuberculin syringe should be used to administer it.

14. _____ Glargine insulin has a bioactivity of 40 U/mL.

15. _____ Therapeutic strategies used in the treatment of gastrointestinal (GI) disease include nonspecific supportive therapies and targeted therapies based on the primary underlying disease process.

Chapter **29 Pharmacology and Pharmacy**

16. _____ Treatment of congestive heart failure is one of the main indications for diuretics such as furosemide.

17. _____ The class I antiarrhythmic lidocaine is administered orally to treat ventricular tachycardia.

18. _____ Potassium bromide may be used as an alternative to phenobarbital to control seizures in dogs with liver disease.

19. _____ Macrocyclic lactones, such as ivermectin and milbemycin oxime, have a prolonged effect because they are packaged in a slow-release form.

20. _____ Collies and related breeds have a genetic predisposition for CNS toxicity to milbemycins and avermectins.

21. _____ State laws cover drug distribution within the state, whereas federal laws cover manufacture of the drug.

22. _____ A new drug intended for use in animals other than humans must be approved by the FDA, but a new drug intended for use in animal feed does not require FDA approval.

23. _____ The use of a veterinary feed directive (VFD) drug requires a valid veterinarian-client-patient relationship.

24. _____ Dose-dependent drug reactions are unpredictable and do not respond to dose reduction or drug withdrawal.

25. _____ Drug compounding is a form of extralabel drug use.

26. _____ Vitamins, minerals, and herbs are considered to be dietary supplements, whereas nutraceuticals are classified as drugs.

27. _____ Internet companies are uniformly reliable sources of high-quality drugs and information about those drugs.

28. _____ A reverse distribution company (RDC) will dispose of expired drugs including controlled substances.

29. _____ The units used to express most drug dosages are gm/unit body weight (lb).

EXERCISE 29.11 MULTIPLE CHOICE: COMPREHENSIVE

Instructions: Circle the one correct answer to each of the following questions.

1. A drug's pharmacokinetics are not used to determine its
   a. Dose
   b. Withdrawal time
   c. Dosing regimen
   d. Action

2. A drug will be 100% bioavailable when it is given
   a. SC
   b. Orally
   c. IV
   d. IM

3. Because of a genetic mutation, Collies and a few other dog breeds have a nonfunctional p-glycoprotein pump. This abnormality makes these breeds more sensitive to the drug ivermectin because it
   a. Decreases protein binding of the drug
   b. Decreases action of the blood–brain barrier
   c. Increases its lipid solubility
   d. Increases tissue binding of the drug

4. One example of a drug that is metabolized by the body into a toxic metabolite is
   a. Acetaminophen
   b. Digoxin
   c. Enalapril
   d. Selamectin

5. Aspirin can be used in cats to prevent thrombus formation, but it must be used with caution because of
   a. The short half-life
   b. The slow metabolism in the cat
   c. The gastrointestinal side effects (bleeding)
   d. Secondary infection

6. The half-life of a drug is used to determine the
   a. Dose
   b. Prescription duration
   c. Dose interval
   d. Potency

7. A drug's pharmacokinetics are least likely to be affected by
   a. Kidney disease
   b. Liver disease
   c. Heart disease
   d. CNS disease

8. Blood flow to the kidneys is negatively impacted by
   a. NSAID-class drugs
   b. Penicillin-class drugs
   c. Benzodiazepine-class drugs
   d. Tetracycline-class drugs

9. Respiratory drugs include
   a. Bronchodilators and barbiturates
   b. Neuraminidase inhibitors
   c. Expectorants and mucolytics
   d. Nutraceuticals

10. "Dry eye" (a deficiency of the tear film) is a known dose-dependent adverse drug reaction to which class of antibacterial drugs?
    a. Potentiated sulfonamides
    b. Amphenicols
    c. Aminoglycosides
    d. Fluoroquinolones

11. Which of the following attributes is not associated with long-acting glucocorticoids?
    a. Doses cannot be effectively tapered.
    b. They stay in the body until they are naturally eliminated.
    c. They are available in oral, injectable, optical, otic, and ophthalmic forms.
    d. Their use increases the production of natural glucocorticoids.

12. The glucocorticoid _____ has a long duration of action.
    a. Prednisone
    b. Betamethasone
    c. Hydrocortisone
    d. Triamcinolone

13. Which of the following immunosuppressive drugs causes a wide variety of adverse effects, including polyphagia, polydipsia, polyuria, and delayed wound healing?
    a. Azathioprine
    b. Cyclosporine A
    c. Prednisolone
    d. Chlorambucil

14. The penicillin-class drug or combination that has activity against beta-lactamase is
    a. Ampicillin
    b. Penicillin G
    c. Amoxicillin
    d. Amoxicillin and clavulanate

15. Which class of antibacterial drugs is known for causing kidney toxicity?
    a. β-Lactams
    b. Fluoroquinolones
    c. Tetracyclines
    d. Aminoglycosides

16. The cephalosporin-class antibacterials are classified according to
    a. The duration of action
    b. The subclass
    c. Generation (first, second, third, etc.)
    d. Strength

17. Which two classes of antibacterial drugs have efficacy against protozoa?
    a. Sulfonamides and nitroimidazoles
    b. Penicillins and cephalosporins
    c. Tetracyclines and amphenicols
    d. Aminoglycosides and lincosamides

18. Which class of antibacterials is known to damage cartilage in young animals and cause blindness in cats as a part of its adverse effect profile?
    a. Amphenicols
    b. Macrolides
    c. Fluoroquinolones
    d. Sulfonamides

19. Which two antibacterial drugs and/or drug classes are banned in food-producing animals?
    a. β-Lactams and enrofloxacin
    b. Tetracycline and the macrolides
    c. Chloramphenicol and nitroimidazoles
    d. Aminoglycosides and lincosamides

20. Which of the following drugs is an imidazole-class antifungal that is used to treat dermatophytes in addition to disseminated fungal infections?
    a. Fluconazole
    b. Amphotericin B
    c. Clotrimazole
    d. Ketoconazole

21. Which antifungal agent does not adversely affect the liver as a part of its adverse effect profile?
    a. Amphotericin B
    b. Itraconazole
    c. Ketoconazole
    d. Fluconazole

22. Hyperthyroidism is a condition that is seen most frequently in
    a. Cats
    b. Horses
    c. Dogs
    d. Cattle

327

23. Insulin is a hormone produced in the beta cells of the pancreas and is responsible for cellular uptake of
    a. glucose.
    b. phosphate.
    c. potassium.
    d. Red blood cells

24. Which of the following types of insulin can be given intravenously?
    a. NPH
    b. PZIR
    c. Glargine
    d. Regular

25. NPH insulin is an example of
    a. Intermediate-acting insulin
    b. Long-acting insulin
    c. Peakless insulin
    d. Short-acting insulin

26. The phrase "first pass effect" refers to which organ?
    a. Heart
    b. Kidney
    c. Liver
    d. Brain

27. Which diuretic produces an effect on the basis of its physical characteristic alone?
    a. Hydrochlorothiazide
    b. Spironolactone
    c. Mannitol
    d. Furosemide

28. Amlodipine is most commonly used to treat
    a. Canine pulmonary hypertension
    b. Hypertension in cats and dogs
    c. Congestive heart failure
    d. CHF secondary to mitral insufficiency

29. Which of the following antiarrhythmics is a β-adrenergic blocker?
    a. Lidocaine
    b. Sotalol
    c. Diltiazem
    d. Quinidine

30. The abbreviation a.c. on written prescription means
    a. Before meals
    b. Right ear
    c. Two times a day
    d. Left eye

31. Which of the following antiparasitics is effective against cestodes?
    a. Pyrantel
    b. Fenbendazole
    c. Netobimin
    d. Praziquantel

32. Ectoparasite agents are most commonly given
    a. Subcutaneously
    b. Orally
    c. Topically
    d. Intramuscularly

33. Which of the following ectoparasiticides targets the parasite's growth and development by inhibiting development of the parasite's exoskeleton?
    a. Imidacloprid
    b. Lufenuron
    c. Fipronil
    d. Carbamate

34. Which agency regulates the manufacture and distribution of veterinary drugs and food additives?
    a. Environmental Protection Agency (EPA)
    b. Drug Enforcement Agency (DEA)
    c. U.S. Department of Agriculture (USDA)
    d. FDA's Center for Veterinary Medicine

35. The Drug Enforcement Agency (DEA) categorizes controlled drugs
    a. As Schedule I, II, III, IV, or V
    b. As Rx or non-Rx
    c. Based on their chemical structure
    d. Based on the severity of their side effects

36. Schedule II controlled substances have a high abuse potential and require completion of a special form when ordering them. Which of the following controlled substances is classified as a Schedule II substance?
    a. Codeine
    b. Phenobarbital
    c. Fentanyl
    d. Ketamine

37. Nutraceuticals
    a. Are subject to safety evaluations by the FDA
    b. Are made using a standardized manufacturing process
    c. Are classified as over-the-counter drugs
    d. May be administered without medical supervision

38. Which of the following abbreviations used in prescription writing is not universally understood by human medical professionals?
    a. s.i.d.
    b. p.r.n.
    c. t.i.d.
    d. q.o.d.

39. Which of the following medications is available in a transdermal form?
    a. Buprenorphine
    b. Methimazole
    c. Phenobarbital
    d. Furosemide

40. Which of the following is not true of the online pharmacy?
    a. Regulated by the FDA and the NABP
    b. Requires a valid hard copy provided directly from the prescriber
    c. Offers a toll-free phone number and street address
    d. Allows direct contact with its pharmacists for consultation

41. Percent solutions may be expressed as volume/volume ratio. For instance, a 5% solution contains
    a. 5 mL in 1 mL of solution
    b. 5 mL in 1 L of solution
    c. 5 mL in 100 mL of solution
    d. 5 mL in 100 L of solution

42. Which of the following metric system weight conversions is correct?
    a. 1 kg = 100 g
    b. 1 mcg = 1000 mg
    c. 10 ng = 1 mcg
    d. 1000 mg = 1 g

43. Which of the following metric system volume conversions is correct?
    a. 100 mL = 1 dL
    b. 100 mL = 1 L
    c. 1 mcL = 1000 mL
    d. 1000 mcL = 1 L

EXERCISE 29.12 FILL-IN-THE-BLANK: COMPREHENSIVE

Instructions: Fill in each of the spaces provided with the missing word or words that complete the sentence.

1. The study of drugs used in the diagnosis, treatment, or prevention of disease is known as _____.

2. The relationship between the amount of drug in the _____ and the concentration in the _____ is measured by the volume of distribution (Vd).

3. The protein that protects the brain from exposure to various drugs and substances by actively pumping them out of the cells is referred to as the _____.

4. Most drugs are eliminated from the body by the _____ into the _____.

5. It takes approximately _____ half-lives for a drug to reach steady state after it is first administered.

6. Whereas the antiseizure drug _____ is known to cause a dose-dependent adverse drug reaction involving the liver in dogs, the antiseizure drug _____ is known to cause an idiosyncratic adverse drug reaction involving the liver in cats.

7. Immunosuppressive drugs are used to treat _____ diseases.

8. The use of glucocorticoids concurrently with _____ _____ drugs (NSAIDs) is contraindicated because of the increased risk of gastrointestinal bleeding, _____, or perforation.

9. The method of choosing a specific antibacterial based on observation and experience is called _____ antibacterial therapy.

10. The two specific classes of drugs that are part of the larger β-lactam class are the _____ and _____.

11. The adverse effects of antifungal drugs result from targeting the _____ in the cell membranes of the treated patient.

12. _____ and _____ are two topical antifungal drugs used to treat yeast otitis.

13. Medical therapies for feline hyperthyroidism include the drug _____ and radioactive _____ therapy.

14. One cause of hyperadrenocorticism is overproduction of ACTH in the brain (called _____-dependent hyperadrenocorticism), and the other cause is overproduction of cortisol by an _____ tumor.

15. The concentration of insulin is expressed in _____ of activity per mL.

16. Congestive heart failure will result in an accumulation of fluid in the _____, _____ _____, and _____.

17. Drugs used to treat patients with heart failure include _____, _____, _____ and _____.

18. Diruetics eliminate fluid buildup by inhibiting the _____ of sodium at different parts of the _____.

19. The goal of therapy with lactulose in patients with hepatic encephalopathy is to make the stool _____, but not to produce _____.

20. Diuretic medications are intended to increase excretion of _____ and _____.

21. Digoxin has a narrow _____ _____ (a low ratio between the therapeutic plasma levels and toxic plasma levels).

22. The drugs enalapril and benazepril work by inhibiting _____ converting enzyme (ACE).

23. Whereas arrhythmias that originate from the atria are referred to as _____, arrhythmias that originate from the ventricles are referred to as _____.

24. The anticonvulsant of choice in cats is _____, because potassium bromide causes _____ symptoms in 40% of treated cats.

25. Endoparasites include three classes: (a) _____, (b) _____, and (c) _____.

26. Although used to control flies, ticks, mites, and mosquitoes, pyrethrins are not safe for use in _____.

27. The Animal Medicinal Drug Use Clarification Act (AMDUCA) enables veterinarians to use and prescribe animal and human drugs for _____ use under defined conditions.

28. The time interval between the last administered drug dose to a food-producing animal and the time that animal can be slaughtered or animal products such as eggs or milk can be used is known as the _____ _____.

29. The presence of a drug or its metabolite in cells, tissues, organs, or other edible products of an animal is referred to as a _____ _____.

30. An enteric coating is designed to prevent exposure of an oral medication to the acid environment of the _____ and delay absorption until it reaches the higher pH of the _____ _____.

31. Some injectable drugs are able to cross the oral mucous membranes of some species. An example of a drug that absorbs transmucosally in cats is the opioid analgesic _____.

32. No expiration date is required on the label of drugs regulated by the _____ *(an acronym).*

EXERCISE 29.13 DOSAGE CALCULATIONS: COMPREHENSIVE

Perform each of the following dosage calculations.

Specific instructions regarding this assignment:

A. *When performing calculations involving administration of oral tablets, express answers that are less than 1 tablet as a fraction (e.g., "½ tablet" instead of "0.5 tablet").*
B. *When performing calculations involving administration of injectable medications, express fractions of a milliliter (mL) as a decimal (e.g., "2.5 mL" instead of "2½ mL").*
C. *When writing instructions for the client, write it as you would on the label (e.g., "Give 1 tablet by mouth twice daily for 10 days" instead of "1 tab. P.O. BID × 10 d").*
D. *When writing instructions for the client, only limit the duration of administration (e.g., "Give 1 tablet once daily for 10 days" or "Give 1 tablet once daily until gone") if the medication is being given for a limited time. If the medication is ongoing, and the client will need to come in for a refill, do not include either of these phrases.*

1. **Order:** 22 mg/kg amoxicillin P.O. The patient weighs 25 lb. The tablet strength is 100 mg, and the tablets are scored. How many tablets will you give? (Note: You may round your answer down to the nearest ½ tablet.)

_____ **tablet(s)**

2. **Order:** 0.25 mg/lb butorphanol P.O. The patient weighs 30 lb. The tablet strength is 5 mg, and the tablets are scored. How many tablets will you give? (Note: You may round your answer down to the nearest ½ tablet.)

_____ **tablet(s)**

3. **Order:** 0.01 mg/lb fludrocortisone P.O. The patient weighs 60 lb. The tablet strength is 0.1 mg. How many tablets will you give?

_____ **tablet(s)**

4. **Order:** 0.5 mg/kg prednisolone. The patient weighs 66 lb. The tablet strength is 5 mg. How many tablets will you give?

_____ **tablet(s)**

5. **Order:** 62.5 mg sulfasalazine. The tablet strength is 500 mg. How many tablets will you give?

_____ **tablet(s)**

6. **Order:** 0.01 mg/lb soloxine SID. *(Note that this drug will be given for the remainder of the patient's life.)* The patient weighs 34 lb. The tablet strengths available are 0.1 mg, 0.2 mg, and 0.6 mg. The pills are scored. Determine the patient's total dose in mg, the most convenient pill size to dispense to achieve this dose (you may round down to the nearest size), how many tablets the owner will need to give each dose, the number of tablets you will dispense to supply this patient for 30 days, and instructions to the client.

This patient's total dose in mg (each time the drug is administered): _____

Pill size you would dispense: _____

Number of tablets the owner will give each dose: _____

The number of tablets to dispense: _____

Your instructions to the client: _____

_____

_____

_____

7. **Order:** 5 mg/kg amoxitabs BID for 10 days. *(This medication will not be ongoing.)* The patient weighs 25 lb. The tablet strengths available are 50 mg, 100 mg, 200 mg, and 400 mg. The pills are *not* scored. Determine the patient's total dose in mg, the most convenient pill size to dispense to achieve this dose (you may round down to the nearest size), how many tablets the owner will need to give each dose, the number of tablets you will dispense, and the instructions to the client.

This patient's total dose in mg (each time the drug is administered): _____

Pill size you would dispense: _____

Number of tablets the owner will give each dose: _____

The number of tablets to dispense: _____

Your instructions to the client: _____

_____

_____

_____

8. **Order:** 15 mg prednisolone BID for 2 weeks then 15 mg SID × 2 weeks; then 15 mg QOD for 2 weeks. *(This medication will not be ongoing.)* The tablet strength available is 5 mg only. The pills are scored. Determine how many tablets the owner will need to give each dose, the number of tablets you will dispense, and the instructions to the client.

Number of tablets the owner will give each dose: _____

The number of tablets to dispense: _____

Your instructions to the client: _____

_____

_____

_____

9. **Order:** 36 mg prednisolone injectable SQ. The prednisolone injection strength is 10 mg/mL. What volume will you administer expressed in mL?

_____ mL

10. **Order:** 14 mEq of potassium chloride is to be added to a 1 L bag of fluids. The KCl solution strength is 20 mEq/10 mL. How many mL will you add to the bag of fluids?

_____ mL

11. **Order:** 5 mg/kg sodium dexamethasone phosphate injectable IV. The patient weighs 35 lb. The solution strength is 4 mg/mL. Determine the total dose for this patient (mg) and how many mL you will give.

Total dose for the patient in mg: _____

How many mL you will give: _____

12. **Order:** 1 mg/lb lidocaine IV. The patient weighs 50 lb. The solution strength is 2%. How many mL do you give? Determine the total dose for this patient (mg) and how many mL you will give.

Total dose for the patient in mg: _____

How many mL you will give: _____

EXERCISE 29.14 CASE STUDY #1: SAFE USE OF CHEMOTHERAPY DRUGS

Allie, a 10-year-old, spayed female Golden Retriever is presented for treatment of lymphoma, a common cancer affecting the lymph nodes. With information gleaned from a complete workup including blood work, a needle biopsy, and radiographs, an appropriate chemotherapy protocol is devised that includes L-asparaginase, cyclophosphamide, prednisolone, vincristine, and doxorubicin. As most of these drugs are extremely toxic, precautions must always be taken when handling them to avoid personal exposure.

1. Discuss the nature of the precautions you would take to limit your exposure.

_____

_____

_____

_____

_____

_____

_____

_____

_____

2. It is very important that both doxorubicin and vincristine are given intravenously and that no amount of either drug, no matter how little, contacts the surrounding tissues. Why is this the case, and what precautions must be taken to ensure these drugs stay inside the vein?

_____

_____

_____

_____

_____

_____

334

EXERCISE 29.15 CASE STUDY #2: DISPENSING MEDICATIONS

Annie, a 4-year-old, spayed female black Labrador Retriever is presented for treatment of inhalant allergies. This is a recurrent problem in the fall, and allergy testing has indicated a sensitivity to several allergens, including ragweed pollen. At the height of the season, she often gets so itchy that she must be given both antihistamines and glucocorticoids to control it, or she will develop dermatitis with hair loss and a secondary pyoderma. At this point, Annie has no skin lesions but is very pruritic. The doctor wants to prescribe antihistamines and prednisolone now, so that the itching can be brought under control before she develops skin lesions.

1. Consider the following written prescription:

   Disp. #30, 5 mg, prednisolone; Sig: Give 1 tab PO q 12 h × 2d, then 1 tab q.o.d. until gone.

   a. Use your knowledge of abbreviations used in prescription writing to interpret this order by writing the prescription out in longhand.

   _____

   _____

   _____

   b. Now prepare a label to be affixed to the bottle with all the required information for a noncontrolled substance.

St. Francis Veterinary Associates
10000 Main Ave.
Anywhere, USA 98765
987-000-1234

---

30 Pain Management

LEARNING OBJECTIVES

When you have completed this chapter, you will be able to:

1. Pronounce, define, and spell all of the key terms in the chapter.
2. Explain how the technician can use effective communication, observation, and interpretation skills to advocate for the patient and to help provide effective and appropriate analgesia.
3. List common causes and physiologic and behavioral signs of pain in small animals, including the negative effects of untreated pain.
4. Describe the physiologic aspects of pain, including the phases of nociception in mammals; compare and contrast acute, chronic, inflammatory, neuropathic, somatic, and visceral pain; and explain the significance of the "wind-up phenomenon."
5. Do the following regarding treatment of pain in small animals:
   - Describe the basic principles of effective analgesia protocol design and pain management, including the concepts of preemptive and multimodal analgesia.
   - Compare and contrast agents used to treat pain in small animals, including nonsteroidal anti-inflammatory drugs (NSAIDs), local anesthetics, opioids, and alpha$_2$ agonists.
   - List the analgesics commonly given by constant rate infusion (CRI), and perform the calculations required to administer a drug by CRI.
   - List the "adjunctive analgesics" and nonpharmacologic treatment options for pain control; describe the uses and benefits of each.
6. Do the following regarding the treatment of pain in large animals:
   - List causes and signs of pain in large animals, and explain why large animals often are undertreated for pain.
   - Compare and contrast agents used to treat pain in large animals, including NSAIDs, opioids, alpha$_2$ agonists, and local anesthetics.
   - Discuss the role of joint supplements, chondroprotective agents, miscellaneous agents, alternative and complementary therapy, and good husbandry in the treatment of pain in large animals.
7. Describe analgesic agents and techniques commonly used in horses, cattle, sheep, goats, camelids, and pigs, and explain how economics and drug residues influence the decision to treat pain in food animals.

EXERCISE 30.1 MATCHING #1: TERMS AND DEFINITIONS

Instructions: Match each term in column A with its corresponding definition in column B by writing the appropriate letter in the space provided.

Column A

1. _____ Transduction
2. _____ Antagonist
3. _____ Agonist
4. _____ Nociception
5. _____ Breakthrough pain
6. _____ Transmission
7. _____ Agonist-antagonist
8. _____ Dysphoria
9. _____ Wind-up phenomenon
10. _____ Allodynia
11. _____ Neurotransmitters
12. _____ Hyperalgesia
13. _____ Multimodal analgesia
14. _____ Preemptive analgesia
15. _____ Partial agonist
16. _____ Modulation

Column B

A. A drug that blocks receptors.

B. Pain management administered before any trauma occurs to prevent expected pain.

C. Movement of a nerve impulse along peripheral nerves to the spinal cord.

D. A situation in which less and less stimulation is required to initiate pain.

E. A drug that stimulates some receptors and blocks others.

F. The combination of allodynia and hyperalgesia.

G. Transmission of pain impulses by fibers that normally carry pleasant or neutral impulses.

H. Conversion of mechanical, chemical, and thermal energy into electrical impulses.

I. Pain that occurs despite use of a usual protocol.

J. The process by which pain is detected by the nervous system.

K. Amplifying or dampening of a nerve impulse in the CNS.

L. The use of two or more analgesic drugs to alter more than one phase of the pain pathway.

M. An emotional state characterized by anxiety, depression, or unease.

N. A drug that causes overall decreased stimulation of receptors.

O. A drug that simulates receptors.

P. Chemicals that transmit nerve impulses between nerve cells.

EXERCISE 30.2 MATCHING #2: EXPECTED LEVEL OF PAIN ASSOCIATED WITH COMMON CONDITIONS AND PROCEDURES

Instructions: Match each condition or procedure in column A with its corresponding expected level of pain in column B by writing the appropriate letter in the space provided. (Note that responses may be used more than once.)

Column A

1. _____ Intervertebral disk herniation
2. _____ Laparotomy
3. _____ Castration
4. _____ Limb amputation
5. _____ Mass removal
6. _____ Declawing
7. _____ Fracture repair
8. _____ Dental procedures
9. _____ Ear canal ablation

Column B

A. Mild to moderate pain

B. Severe pain

EXERCISE 30.3 MATCHING #3: ANALGESICS AND ANALGESIC CLASSES

Instructions: Match each analgesic in column A with the corresponding class to which it belongs in column B by writing the appropriate letter in the space provided. (Note that responses may be used more than once.)

Column A

1. _____ Phenylbutazone
2. _____ Morphine
3. _____ Ketamine
4. _____ Naloxone hydrochloride
5. _____ Lidocaine
6. _____ Romifidine
7. _____ Buprenorphine
8. _____ Carprofen
9. _____ Xylazine
10. _____ Flunixin meglumine
11. _____ Butorphanol
12. _____ Mepivacaine
13. _____ Atipamezole
14. _____ Sodium hyaluronate
15. _____ Ketoprofen
16. _____ Dexmedetomidine
17. _____ Fentanyl
18. _____ Firocoxib
19. _____ Hydromorphone
20. _____ Tramadol
21. _____ Bupivacaine
22. _____ Detomidine
23. _____ Polysulfated GAGs
24. _____ Meloxicam

Column B

A. NSAID

B. α_2-Agonist

C. α_2-Antagonist

D. Local anesthetic

E. NMDA-receptor antagonist

F. Joint supplement and chondroprotective agent

G. Pure opioid agonist

H. Partial opioid agonist

I. Opioid agonist-antagonist

J. Opioid antagonist

K. Synthetic opioid

EXERCISE 30.4 TRUE OR FALSE: COMPREHENSIVE

Instructions: Read the following statements and write "T" for true or "F" for false in the blanks provided. If a statement is false, correct the statement to make it true.

1. _____ Like people, domestic animals tend to readily show that they are in pain.

2. _____ Pain tolerance varies widely between species and individuals within a species.

3. _____ In animals, pain is usually easy to differentiate from normal postoperative behaviors.

4. _____ Although pain has many negative physiologic effects, these effects are confined to the nervous system.

5. _____ Nociceptors are specialized nerve fibers that carry pain information, but not pleasant or neutral sensations.

6. _____ Allodynia is the phase of wind-up in which less and less stimulation is required to initiate pain.

7. _____ Administering analgesics after pain occurs is often just as effective as giving them before it occurs.

8. _____ Lower doses of individual analgesics can be used when an analgesic protocol includes agents from multiple classes that attack more than one phase of the pain pathway.

9. _____ Even though pain has many damaging consequences, it can also be beneficial by limiting activity.

10. _____ Even though multiple analgesics are often given concurrently, it is recommended that no more than one NSAID be given to a patient at a time.

11. _____ Lidocaine with epinephrine is helpful for feline declaw blocks because it reduces bleeding.

12. _____ Lidocaine, bupivacaine, or tetracaine can be used topically to reduce pain associated with minor procedures such as urethral catheterization.

13. _____ A bilateral infraorbital dental block is a technique that can be used to provide analgesia for dental extractions of the upper and lower dental arcades.

14. _____ Opioids classified as partial agonists have a decreased effect but very similar side effects to pure agonists.

15. _____ Giving butorphanol with a fentanyl patch will maximize the analgesic effects of the patch.

16. _____ Diazepam does not provide pain relief.

17. _____ Because it can cause heart toxicity, lidocaine is not recommended for use in cats.

18. _____ Analgesics are generally used more often in large animals than in small animals.

19. _____ Large animals do not experience pain in the same way as small domestic animals and people.

20. _____ GI ulceration is the primary side effect of NSAIDs in large animals.

EXERCISE 30.5 MULTIPLE CHOICE: COMPREHENSIVE

Instructions: Circle the one correct answer to each of the following questions.

1. Signs of pain can be classified as physiologic or behavioral. Examples of behavioral signs of pain are
   a. Tachycardia, dilated pupils, and howling
   b. Biting, hiding, and hypertension
   c. Tachypnea, reluctancy to move, and failure to groom
   d. Screaming, escaping, and tucking the abdomen

2. During which phase of nociception does the mechanical, chemical, or thermal energy that causes tissue damage get turned into electrical impulses by the nerve endings?
   a. Transduction
   b. Transmission
   c. Modulation
   d. Perception

3. The drug gabapentin has particular efficacy for
   a. Acute pain
   b. Deep pain
   c. Neuropathic pain
   d. Abdominal pain

4. NMDA-receptor antagonists such as ketamine have a particular place in preventing and treating
   a. Chronic pain
   b. Wind-up pain
   c. Neuropathic pain
   d. Preexisting pain

5. Drugs that provide analgesia by modifying inflammation are
   a. Opioids
   b. α_2-Agonists
   c. NSAIDs
   d. Local anesthetics

6. The analgesics of choice for treatment of osteoarthritis are
   a. NSAIDs
   b. Opioids
   c. Local anesthetics
   d. α_2-Agonists

7. Because of potential side effects of NSAIDs, patients should not receive them if they have
   a. Bleeding abnormalities
   b. Hypotension
   c. Stomach ulcers
   d. Any of the above

8. Dogs receiving NSAIDs are particularly prone to adverse effects relating to the GI system, whereas cats are particularly prone to adverse effects relating to the
   a. Liver
   b. CNS
   c. Kidneys
   d. Blood

9. Cats can be given NSAIDs when indicated but should never be given
   a. Meloxicam
   b. Carprofen
   c. Acetaminophen
   d. Aspirin

10. Local anesthetics work by
    a. Decreasing inflammation
    b. Blocking mu receptors
    c. Inhibiting norepinephrine release
    d. Disrupting neural transmission

11. A circumferential ring block for declawing requires an SQ injection of 0.5% bupivacaine at a dose of
    a. 1.0 mL/10 lb body weight
    b. 1.0 mL/10 kg body weight
    c. 1.0 mL per cat
    d. 0.1 mL/10 lb body weight

12. An epidural injection of lidocaine or morphine will provide analgesia to the
    a. Pelvis only
    b. Caudal abdomen only
    c. Tail only
    d. Caudal half of the body

13. The stinging sensation caused by injection of local anesthetics can be reduced by adding 0.1 mL of

    _____ to 10 mL of the local agent.
    a. Bupivacaine
    b. Epinephrine
    c. Sodium bicarbonate
    d. Saline

14. The class of opioids with the most severe side effects are the
    a. Pure agonists
    b. Partial agonists
    c. Mixed agonist-antagonists
    d. Antagonists

15. One of the following species is more sensitive to morphine and therefore requires lower doses of this pure agonist. Which one is it?
    a. Dog
    b. Cat
    c. Cow
    d. Horse

16. An opioid that has a significantly longer duration of action than most is
    a. Morphine
    b. Hydromorphone
    c. Butorphanol
    d. Buprenorphine

17. This synthetic drug is available in oral form and produces opioid-like stimulation of the mu receptor, but with fewer side effects.
    a. Fentanyl
    b. Dexmedetomidine
    c. Tramadol
    d. Hydromorphone

18. The drug romifidine is an α_2-agonist analgesic. Which of the drugs listed below is also in this class?
    a. Ketamine
    b. Acepromazine
    c. Dexmedetomidine
    d. Morphine

19. This class of analgesics works by inhibiting release of the neurotransmitter norepinephrine.
    a. NMDA inhibitors
    b. α_2-Agonists
    c. NSAIDs
    d. Anticonvulsants

20. Which of the following drug combinations is representative of the anesthetic protocol known as "kitty magic"?
    a. Morphine, acepromazine, and ketamine
    b. Fentanyl, ketoprofen, and ketamine
    c. Buprenorphine, meloxicam, and dexmedetomidine
    d. Buprenorphine, dexmedetomidine, and ketamine

21. As compared with morphine, the main advantages of fentanyl are
    a. Shorter half-life and faster onset of action
    b. Faster onset of action and longer half-life
    c. Longer half-life and slower onset of action
    d. Slower onset of action and shorter half-life

22. Which of the following drugs is safe for use in patients with GI disturbances and thus is a good choice for dogs with gastric dilation volvulus (GDV), unlike many analgesics.
    a. Carprofen
    b. Hydromorphone
    c. Lidocaine
    d. Dexmedetomidine

23. An NMDA receptor antagonist used to prevent wind-up phenomena is
    a. Gabapentin
    b. Xylazine
    c. Acepromazine
    d. Ketamine

24. In view of the efficacy gabapentin has in treating neuropathic pain, which of the following conditions would it be used to treat?
    a. Resistance to being touched at a location with no tissue damage
    b. Pain secondary to a severe infection
    c. Postsurgical incisional pain
    d. Limb pain resulting from trauma

25. The most commonly used NSAIDs in large animals are
    a. Flunixin meglumine and carprofen
    b. Carprofen and ketoprofen
    c. Ketoprofen and phenylbutazone
    d. Phenylbutazone and flunixin meglumine

26. The opioid most commonly used in large animals is
    a. Morphine
    b. Butorphanol
    c. Fentanyl
    d. Buprenorphine

27. Which of the following analgesic adjuncts is a nutraceutical and consequently is not regulated by the FDA?
    a. Gabapentin
    b. Tramadol
    c. Chondroitin sulfate
    d. Phenylbutazone

28. The analgesic class most commonly used in horses is
    a. Opioids
    b. α_2-Agonists
    c. NSAIDs
    d. Local anesthetics

29. The analgesic class most commonly used in ruminants is
    a. Opioids
    b. α_2-Agonists
    c. NSAIDs
    d. Local anesthetics

EXERCISE 30.6 FILL-IN-THE-BLANK: COMPREHENSIVE

Instructions: Fill in each of the spaces provided with the missing word or words that complete the sentence.

1. Signs of pain in animals can be categorized according to whether they are _____ (e.g., tachycardia or hypertension) or _____ (e.g., biting or guarding an incision).

2. Pain is now considered by some to be the fifth vital sign. The other four vital signs are _____, _____, _____, and _____.

3. Tissue damage results in inflammation. The classic signs of inflammation are localized _____, _____, and _____.

4. The phase of the pain pathway in which there is the awareness that something hurts is called _____.

5. Pain is subdivided into two categories based on the duration. The sensation experienced with each category differs. _____ pain is characterized by a sharp, stabbing sensation, whereas _____ pain is characterized by a dull, throbbing sensation.

6. An extreme form of pain sometimes occurs when the CNS is bombarded by persistent pain impulses. This extreme form is called "central sensitization" or _____ _____.

7. The four main categories of analgesic drugs are _____, _____, _____, and _____ _____.

8. To prevent adverse effects on kidney function, patients that are receiving NSAIDs should always have _____ _____ _____ monitored intraoperatively.

9. Adding the drug _____ to lidocaine at a 1:200,000 dilution will increase its duration of action.

10. Most cases of local anesthetic toxicity are a result of accidental _____ or _____ administration.

11. A correctly performed declaw block using bupivacaine will provide analgesia for up to _____ hours after surgery.

12. Morphine can be injected intra-articularly to provide analgesia of the joint. Use of this technique results in maintenance of a smooth plane of anesthesia when the joint capsule is incised. When this technique is not used, an increase in the _____ _____ is often observed as the joint capsule is entered.

13. Analgesia can be provided to patients following thoracotomy by injecting bupivacaine in the pleural space. When using this technique, the drug is thought to work by directly blocking the _____ nerves.

14. The specific effects that a particular opioid will have are dependent on the specific _____ in the CNS that it binds to.

15. Analgesia provided by opioids is primarily a result of binding of the drug to the _____ receptors in the CNS.

16. Hydromorphone has similar analgesic effects as morphine but is less likely to cause _____ or _____ (two adverse effects).

17. The injectable opioid _____ is readily absorbed across mucous membranes in cats as a result of the unique _____ _____ in this species and can consequently be given orally.

18. Analgesics in the class _____ work synergistically with opioids to _____ the intensity and duration of pain relief beyond what can be accounted for by the separate action of each drug.

19. The drug used to reverse the effects of the α_2-agonist dexmedetomidine is _____.

20. After being given any sedative, the patient should be placed in a quiet environment for _____ minutes to allow the drug(s) to take effect.

21. Different large animal species have different sensitivities to α_2-agonists. _____ are most resistant, _____ are moderately sensitive, and _____ are the most sensitive.

EXERCISE 30.7 CASE STUDY: ADMINISTERING ANALGESICS BY CONSTANT RATE INFUSION

Signalment: 4-year-old, 110-pound, neutered, male Bullmastiff.

History: This patient came up lame on the left rear limb while playing in the backyard 3 days ago. He has no history of previous medical problems.

Physical examination: The patient was three-legged lame on presentation, and physical findings were compatible with an anterior cruciate ligament rupture. All other findings were normal.

Preoperative workup: Results of routine preoperative blood work were normal.

Treatment plan: This patient was admitted to the hospital for surgical management of the anterior cruciate ligament rupture. The doctor has asked you to give this patient a 5 mcg/kg loading dose of fentanyl, followed by a 12 mcg/kg/hr (or 0.2 mcg/kg/min) CRI intraoperatively. The patient will be receiving lactated Ringer's solution in a 1 L bag at a rate of 10 mL/kg/hr. You are asked to calculate both the loading dose and the constant rate infusion for this patient.

1. Calculate the loading dose by following these steps:

   a. Calculate this patient's body weight in kg.

   Patient's body weight: _____ kg

   b. Calculate the loading dose of fentanyl in mL. The concentration of fentanyl is 0.05 mg/mL. Set this problem up by multiplying the body weight and the dose, and divide the product by the drug concentration.

   Loading dose of fentanyl: _____ mL

2. Now calculate the constant rate infusion by following the steps below.

   a. Calculate the fluid infusion rate for this patient in mL/hr. Set this problem up by multiplying the body weight and the prescribed fluid administration dosage.

   Fluid infusion rate during surgery: _____ mL/hr

   b. Calculate the number of hours the bag of lactated Ringer's solution will last. Set this problem up by converting the fluid bag size to mL and then dividing by the figure from the previous step.

   Number of hours the bag will last: _____ hours

   c. Calculate the number of minutes the bag of lactated Ringer's solution will last. Set this problem up by converting the figure from the previous step into minutes.

   Number of minutes the bag will last: _____ minutes

d. Calculate the total number of micrograms of fentanyl to add to the bag. Set this problem up by multiplying the patient weight by both the prescribed dose in mcg/kg/min and the figure from the previous step.

Number of micrograms to add to the bag: _____ **micrograms**

e. Convert this value to milligrams. Set this problem up by converting the figure from the previous step into milligrams.

Number of milligrams to add to the bag: _____ **milligrams**

f. Calculate the drug volume to add to the bag. Set this problem up by dividing the figure from the previous step by the drug concentration.

Drug volume to add to the bag: _____ **mL**

You will next add this volume of fentanyl to the bag after removing an equivalent volume of fluids from the bag. Then you will run the fluids for the duration of the surgery at the rate calculated in part 2a above using a controlled rate infusion pump.

31 Veterinary Anesthesia

LEARNING OBJECTIVES

When you have completed this chapter, you will be able to:

1. Pronounce, define, and spell all the key terms in this chapter.
2. Differentiate general anesthesia, sedation, tranquilization, neuroleptanalgesia, and local anesthesia; differentiate the periods of a general anesthetic event (premedication, induction, maintenance); and list the objectives of anesthesia and techniques used to achieve these objectives, including the concept of balanced anesthesia.
3. Discuss each aspect of patient preparation for an anesthetic procedure, including fasting, gathering historical information, physical assessment, stabilization, and physical status classification.
4. Do the following regarding injectable anesthetic agents:
   - Describe the ways anesthetic agents are classified, and differentiate agonists, partial agonists, agonist-antagonists, and antagonists.
   - Describe the effects, adverse effects, properties, and uses of anticholinergics, phenothiazine and benzodiazepine tranquilizers, alpha$_2$-adrenergic agents, opioids, propofol, alfaxalone, dissociatives, etomidate, and guaifenesin.
5. Explain how vapor pressure, blood-gas partition coefficient, and minimum alveolar concentration (MAC) influence the way inhalant anesthetics are used, and describe the effects, adverse effects, properties, and uses of halogenated inhalant anesthetics.
6. Do the following regarding the use of anesthetic equipment:
   - Discuss the characteristics, uses, and maintenance of endotracheal tubes, laryngoscopes, anesthetic masks, and anesthetic chambers.
   - Describe the characteristics of an anesthesia machine, including the four general machine systems.
   - Explain how to assemble an anesthetic machine, check for leaks, and set the pop-off valve before use.
   - Describe the structure, function, and use of each component of the carrier gas supply, including compressed gas cylinder, pressure gauge, pressure-reducing valve, flowmeter, and oxygen flush valve.
   - List and calculate the oxygen flow rates used for various species, systems, and periods of an anesthetic procedure.
   - Describe the structure, function, and uses of precision and nonprecision vaporizers.
   - Discuss rebreathing and nonrebreathing systems, and explain the criteria used to choose an appropriate breathing system for any given patient.
   - Describe the structure, function, and use of each component of the breathing system, including unidirectional flow valves, reservoir bag, pop-off valve, carbon dioxide absorber canister, pressure manometer, negative pressure relief valve, and breathing tubes.
   - Discuss the function and uses of passive and active scavenging systems.
   - Describe the procedures used to maintain anesthetic machines.
7. Do the following regarding endotracheal intubation:
   - Discuss the principles of endotracheal intubation, including the equipment needed to place an endotracheal tube and the criteria used to select and prepare an appropriate endotracheal tube for any given patient.
   - Describe placement of an endotracheal tube in a small animal, horse, adult ruminant, and small ruminant; how to check an endotracheal tube for proper placement; and how to inflate the cuff.
   - Discuss laryngospasm and other complications of intubation, including causes and methods of prevention.
   - Compare and contrast supraglottic airway devices and endotracheal tubes.
8. Do the following regarding anesthetic monitoring:
   - Explain the principles of anesthetic monitoring and how monitoring parameters can be used to identify the classic stages and planes of anesthesia.
   - Identify physical monitoring indicators of circulation, oxygenation, and ventilation.
   - Discuss the methods used to assess vital signs, including normal values, and common causes of abnormal values.
   - Describe methods used to assess reflexes and other monitoring indicators, and explain how they are used to determine anesthetic depth.
   - Discuss the function and setup of monitoring equipment used to assess circulation, oxygenation, and ventilation, and interpretation of data generated by these instruments.

345

9. Do the following regarding small animal anesthesia:
   - Describe the sequence of events required to take a small animal patient from consciousness to surgical anesthesia and back to consciousness.
   - Describe agents and methods commonly used to induce a small animal patient by IM or IV injection, mask, or chamber.
   - Describe agents and methods used to maintain anesthesia in a small animal patient and considerations for patient positioning, comfort, safety, and recovery.
10. Explain the sequence of events for an anesthetic event in a horse, including ways in which an equine anesthetic procedure differs from that of a small animal patient.
11. Explain the sequence of events for an anesthetic event in a ruminant, including ways in which a ruminant anesthetic procedure differs from that for a small animal patient.
12. List common problems and emergencies, associated causes, and interventions in relation to anesthesia.

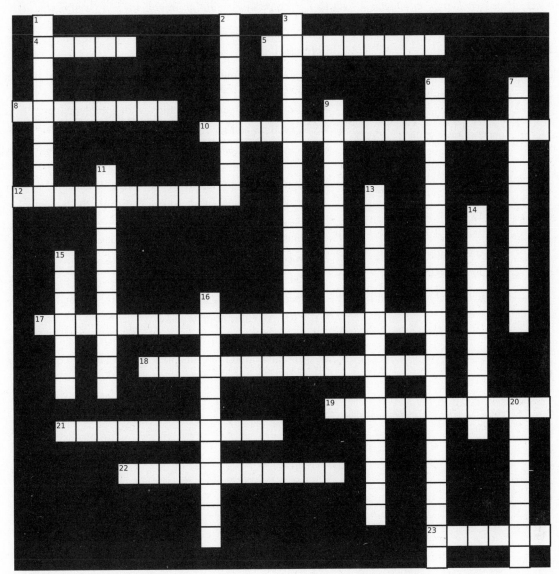

Across
4   A respiratory rate of 0 breaths/min.
5   The opposite of miosis.
8   A drug that induces sleep.
10 Also known as a circle system. (2 words)
12 Increased heart rate.
17 An anesthetic machine configuration used for patients weighing less than 2.5 kg. (2 words)
18 Decreased respiratory rate and/or tidal volume.
19 Mapleson E nonrebreathing circuit. (2 words)
21 The volume of air breathed in during each breath. (2 words)
22 A body temperature of 97° F in a cat.
23 Constricted pupils.

Down
1   Increased respiratory rate.
2   Lack of pain sensation.
3   Decreased RR and/or VT.
6   The product of respiratory rate and tidal volume. (3 words)
7   Air in the chest cavity.
9   Collapse of a portion of the lung.
11 Elevated blood CO2.
13 The percentage of binding sites on the hemoglobin molecules occupied by oxygen. (2 words)
14 Modified Mapleson D circuit. (2 words)
15 Reduced oxygen in the tissues.
16 A side effect of acepromazine that leads to hypotension.
20 A physical indicator of hypoxemia.

EXERCISE 31.2 MATCHING #1: TERMS AND DEFINITIONS

Instructions: Match each term in column A with its corresponding definition in column B by writing the appropriate letter in the space provided.

Column A

1. _____ Sedation
2. _____ Anesthetic induction
3. _____ Neuroleptanalgesia
4. _____ General anesthesia
5. _____ Balanced anesthesia
6. _____ Anesthesia
7. _____ Premedication
8. _____ Anesthetic protocol
9. _____ Ventilation
10. _____ Anesthetic maintenance
11. _____ Local anesthesia
12. _____ Tranquilization
13. _____ Narcosis

Column B

A. A state of profound sedation and analgesia produced by simultaneous administration of an opioid and tranquilizer.

B. Use of several anesthetic drugs with complementary effects.

C. Relaxation and reduced anxiety.

D. A list of the anesthetic drugs that will be given, including routes, amounts, and other details.

E. Going from a conscious state to Stage III anesthesia.

F. Artificial delivery of anesthetic gases into the patient's lungs.

G. A state of profound sedation, from which a patient can be aroused by loud noises or other stimulation.

H. Process used to keep a patient anesthetized.

I. The absence of sensation.

J. Unconsciousness and insensibility to feeling and pain.

K. A state of calm or drowsiness.

L. Loss of sensation in a small, isolated part or region of the body.

M. Administration of agents prior to the induction of anesthesia.

EXERCISE 31.3 MATCHING #2: ANESTHETIC MACHINE PARTS AND DESCRIPTIONS

Instructions: Match each anesthetic machine part in column A with its corresponding description in column B by writing the appropriate letter in the space provided.

Column A

1. _____ Pressure manometer
2. _____ Compressed gas cylinder
3. _____ Oxygen flush valve
4. _____ Line pressure gauge
5. _____ Pressure reducing valve
6. _____ Vaporizer
7. _____ Carbon dioxide absorber canister
8. _____ Reservoir bag
9. _____ Yoke
10. _____ Negative pressure valve
11. _____ Tank pressure gauge
12. _____ Flowmeter
13. _____ Pop-off valve
14. _____ Exhalation unidirectional valve

Column B

A. This part reduces the pressure of the gas from 40 to 50 psi to approximately 15 psi.

B. Carrier gas enters this part through the inlet port.

C. This part is most commonly used when preparing a patient for recovery or when a crisis has arisen.

D. This part provides the patient an adequate volume of anesthetic gases during inspiration to fill the lungs.

E. This part prevents rebreathing of carbon dioxide and allows the anesthetist to tell if the patient is breathing.

F. This part reduces the pressure of the gas in the system from tank pressure to 40 to 50 psi.

G. When this part reads 1000 psi, there is 300 L of oxygen left in an "E" size tank.

H. This part measures pressure of the gases in the patient's lungs.

I. This part should be emptied and refilled after 6 to 8 hours of machine use.

J. This part indicates pressure in the line entering the flowmeter.

K. This part should be closed while bagging or ventilating the patient.

L. When the oxygen pressure inside this part is 500 psi, it should be changed.

M. This part prevents asphyxiation if the bag is empty.

N. This part holds the oxygen tank on.

EXERCISE 31.4 MATCHING #3: COMPLICATIONS OF ENDOTRACHEAL INTUBATION AND CAUSES

Instructions: Match each complication of endotracheal intubation in column A with its corresponding cause in column B by writing the appropriate letter in the space provided. (Note that responses may be used more than once.)

Column A

1. _____ Aspiration of foreign material and fluid during dental cleaning.

2. _____ Dyspnea and hypoxia.

3. _____ Damage to the tube from chewing.

4. _____ Necrosis of the tracheal mucosa.

5. _____ Intubation of only one main stem bronchus, leading to hypoxia and difficulty in keeping the patient anesthetized.

6. _____ Changes in patient position may dislodge the tube from the glottis.

7. _____ Trauma or tracheal rupture resulting in pneumo-mediastinum and/or pneumothorax.

8. _____ Pollution of the workspace with anesthetic gas.

9. _____ Increased resistance to breathing with increased respiratory effort.

10. _____ Transmission of infectious agents leading to tracheitis, bronchitis, or pneumonia.

Column B

A. Tube too short.

B. Cuff overinflated/tube diameter too large.

C. Tube kinked or obstructed.

D. Tube not cleaned and disinfected.

E. Tube too long.

F. Cuff not inflated/underinflated or tube diameter too small.

G. Tube not removed before return to consciousness.

H. Overzealous intubation.

EXERCISE 31.5 MATCHING #4: MONITORING EQUIPMENT AND PARAMETERS

Instructions: Match each monitoring device in column A with the corresponding parameter or parameters it detects in column B by writing the appropriate letter in the space provided.

Column A

1. _____ Esophageal stethoscope

2. _____ Electrocardiograph

3. _____ Ultrasonic Doppler monitor

4. _____ Oscillometric monitor

5. _____ Pulse oximeter

6. _____ Apnea monitor

7. _____ Capnograph

Column B

A. Oxygen saturation and HR.

B. Relative HR and irregularity in heart sounds.

C. Carbon dioxide in inspired and expired air and RR.

D. Relative HR and systolic blood pressure.

E. Relative RR only.

F. Systolic, mean, and diastolic arterial blood pressure.

G. HR and rhythm.

EXERCISE 31.6 PHOTO QUIZ: ENDOTRACHEAL TUBE PARTS

Instructions: Match each endotracheal tube part with its corresponding name by writing the appropriate letter in the space provided.

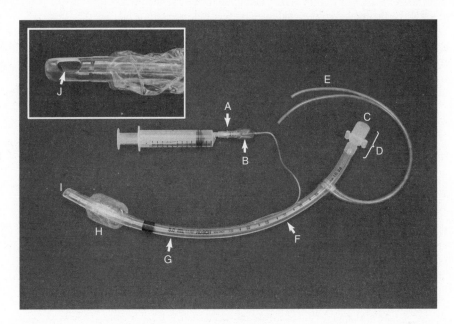

Part Names

1. _____ Connector
2. _____ Cuff
3. _____ Pilot balloon
4. _____ Valve
5. _____ Patient end
6. _____ Measurement of the internal diameter
7. _____ Murphy eye
8. _____ Machine end
9. _____ Tie
10. _____ Measurement of tube length

EXERCISE 31.7 TRUE OR FALSE: COMPREHENSIVE

Instructions: Read the following statements and write "T" for true or "F" for false in the blanks provided. If a statement is false, correct the statement to make it true.

1. _____ Anticholinergics are expected to increase tear and salivary secretions because of their parasympathetic nervous system blockade.

2. _____ Adverse effects of the phenothiazine tranquilizer acepromazine include vomiting and cardiac arrhythmias.

3. _____ The benzodiazepine diazepam should not be given IM because of pain when given by this route and erratic absorption from this site.

4. _____ As a result of significant adverse cardiovascular effects, the benzodiazepines should be given with caution in old, young, or ill patients.

5. _____ Ruminants are very sensitive to the drug xylazine, and therefore need only approximately one-tenth of the dose used for horses.

6. _____ An advantage of using the antagonist yohimbine to reverse the effects of xylazine is that dangerous adverse effects will be reversed, but the analgesic effects will persist.

7. _____ In addition to providing analgesia, opioid agonists produce cough suppression, respiratory depression, bradycardia, and hypotension.

8. _____ Most opioid agonists have a relatively long duration of action and must be administered only 2 to 3 times a day.

9. _____ Rapid IV administration of the ultra-short-acting anesthetic propofol can cause apnea, which may be severe.

10. _____ The barbiturate anesthetics are classified based on the receptors they affect.

11. _____ The intravenous, injectable anesthetic etomidate is not commonly used, in part because it has more significant adverse effects than other commonly used agents.

12. _____ Drugs that are milky in appearance should, as a rule, not be administered intravenously. The drug propofol is no exception to this rule.

13. _____ An inhalant anesthetic with a high blood-gas partition coefficient produces faster inductions than one with a low blood-gas partition coefficient.

14. _____ The halogenated inhalant anesthetic sevoflurane induces a more significant dose-dependent hypotension than isoflurane and so must be used with caution.

15. _____ Anesthetic masks may be used to induce but not to maintain general anesthesia.

16. _____ Oxygen is the carrier gas used during all anesthetic procedures.

17. _____ Oxygen flowmeters have an indicator that either is shaped like a ball or like a "rotor" (a bobbin-like shape). When setting oxygen flow, read the top of the ball or center of the rotor indicator.

18. _____ Precision vaporizers are located in the breathing circuit so that the patient's respiratory drive is able to move the carrier gas through the vaporizer as the patient breathes.

19. _____ A semiclosed rebreathing system is a safe, practical system to use with all patients greater than or equal to 2.5 kg in body weight.

20. _____ Closed rebreathing systems are a practical and economical alternative for both small and large animal patients.

21. _____ When in use, a reservoir bag should be approximately one-quarter full at peak expiration.

22. _____ When using a semiclosed rebreathing system, the pop-off valve should be kept partially open except when providing manual ventilation.

23. _____ An endotracheal tube should extend from the tip of the nose to the larynx.

24. _____ Under the traditional system of stages and planes of anesthesia, there are four stages, and stage IV is divided into four planes.

25. _____ Physical status class ASA I patients should be monitored every 5 minutes at a minimum.

26. _____ In general, vital signs are only loosely correlated with depth of anesthesia.

27. _____ Cyanotic mucous membranes are an early indicator of hypoxemia.

28. _____ Abdominal breathing is a breathing pattern in which there is a long pause after inhalation and a short pause after exhalation.

29. _____ The corneal reflex is not reliable in small animals but is useful to determine if a large animal patient is too deep.

30. _____ The electrocardiogram is an accurate indicator concerning whether or not the heart is beating.

31. _____ When administering injectable anesthetics by the intramuscular route, generally they are given "to effect."

32. _____ When turning a patient from side to side, the endotracheal tube should be temporarily disconnected from the breathing circuit.

33. _____ As soon as the patient is in the recovery area, most of the danger has passed and the frequency of anesthetic monitoring can be decreased.

34. _____ Horses naturally can breathe only through their noses and will become distressed and compromised if they are unable to.

35. _____ Many ruminants are difficult to handle and require heavy sedation, along with physical restraint prior to and during anesthetic induction.

36. _____ During surgery, all ruminants should have the head positioned higher than the body.

37. _____ During anesthetic recovery, once a ruminant is in sternal recumbency, does not require support, and is in no danger of bloating, it can be left unattended.

38. _____ Hypoventilation is an uncommon complication during equine and ruminant anesthetic procedures.

EXERCISE 31.8 MULTIPLE CHOICE: COMPREHENSIVE

Instructions: Circle the one correct answer to each of the following questions.

1. Which of the following general fasting recommendations is incorrect?
   a. Dogs: No food × 8 to 12 hours
   b. Adult cattle: No food × 24 to 48 hours
   c. Adult equine: No food × 8 to 12 hours
   d. Pediatric patients: No food × 2 to 4 hours

2. A patient that has a life-threatening disease such as a ruptured bladder should be put in which of the following ASA physical status classifications?
   a. ASA I
   b. ASA II
   c. ASA III
   d. ASA IV
   e. ASA V

3. Anticholinergics are expected to
   a. Decrease the heart rate in dogs
   b. Thicken the airway mucous in cats
   c. Constrict the bronchi in any species
   d. Protect against cardiac arrhythmias in cats

4. Which of the following drugs is commonly given in doses that are significantly lower than the doses listed on the label?
   a. Diazepam
   b. Dexmedetomidine
   c. Acepromazine
   d. Glycopyrrolate

5. Young, healthy dogs are resistant to the tranquilizing effects of
   a. Diazepam
   b. Acepromazine
   c. Xylazine
   d. Butorphanol

6. Which of the following agents often causes vomiting in cats?
   a. Acepromazine
   b. Xylazine
   c. Atropine
   d. Midazolam

7. α_2-Agonists have significant cardiovascular system effects. These drugs cause all of the following effects with the exception of
   a. High heart rate
   b. Decreased cardiac output
   c. Decreased blood pressure
   d. Heart block

8. All of the following are examples of pure opioid agonists except
   a. Fentanyl
   b. Hydromorphone
   c. Morphine
   d. Buprenorphine

9. This mixed opioid agonist-antagonist is used to treat mild to moderate pain, and as an antitussive.
   a. Hydromorphone
   b. Buprenorphine
   c. Butorphanol
   d. Fentanyl

10. The antagonist used to reverse the effects of opioid agonists such as morphine is
    a. Yohimbine
    b. Naloxone
    c. Tolazoline
    d. Flumazenil

11. Which of the following injectable drugs is *not* a controlled substance?
    a. Propofol
    b. Thiopental sodium
    c. Diazepam
    d. Methohexital

12. Which of the following drugs does not provide significant analgesia?
    a. Morphine
    b. Dexmedetomidine
    c. Fentanyl
    d. Propofol

13. Dissociatives should not be given to patients with seizure disorders for which of the following reasons?
    a. Increases salivation
    b. May induce seizure-like activity during recovery
    c. Causes thickened mucous production and choking
    d. Creates corneal dryness

14. The use of barbiturates as anesthetics has gradually declined over the past several decades due to the availability of ultra-short-acting injectable drugs such as
    a. Methohexital and pentobarbital
    b. Phenobarbital and methohexital
    c. Thiopental sodium
    d. Alfaxalone and propofol

15. Which of the following barbiturate drugs is still regularly used for induction of general anesthesia in laboratory animals by intraperitoneal injection?
    a. Methohexital
    b. Pentobarbital
    c. Phenobarbital
    d. Thiopental sodium

16. Which of the following injectable anesthetics is most appropriate to use as an induction agent in patients with severe heart disease because it has little effect on cardiovascular function?
    a. Methohexital
    b. Propofol
    c. Thiopental sodium
    d. Etomidate

17. Which of the following properties of inhalant anesthetics reveals information regarding the type of vaporizer used to administer it?
    a. Minimum alveolar concentration (MAC)
    b. Vapor pressure
    c. Blood-gas partition coefficient
    d. Boiling point

18. Oxygen administration is necessary throughout anesthesia because it
    a. Carries the anesthetic
    b. Compensates for diminished RR
    c. Compensates for diminished VT
    d. All of the above

19. What specific type of endotracheal tube is designed specifically for birds and other animals that do not have an expandable trachea?
    a. Murphy tube
    b. Silicone tube
    c. Cuffed tube
    d. Cole tube

20. Laryngoscopes are most often used in
    a. Dogs, cats, and horses
    b. Pigs, small ruminants, and camelids
    c. Horses, pigs, and adult ruminants
    d. Cats, adult ruminants, and camelids

21. The force that moves the gases around a rebreathing circuit is
    a. The pressure in the oxygen tank
    b. The unidirectional valves
    c. The patient's lungs
    d. The flowmeter

22. Which of the following is not the name of a nonrebreathing circuit?
    a. Lack
    b. Bain
    c. Murphy
    d. Jackson-Rees

23. Carbon dioxide absorbent granules should be changed at all of the following times except
    a. When they are soft and can be crushed with the fingers
    b. When they have turned violet or blue
    c. When they turn from white to off-white
    d. After 6 to 8 hours of use

24. An activated charcoal cartridge removes halogenated anesthetic from waste gases. It should be changed
    a. After 6 to 8 hours of use
    b. When it gains 50 g of weight
    c. When it changes color
    d. After 6 to 8 uses

25. Using the guidelines listed in the text, a _____ mm endotracheal tube should be prepared for a 30-kg dog.
    a. 9.5 to 10
    b. 10.5 to 11
    c. 11.5 to 12
    d. 12.5 to 13

26. Which of the following is an indicator that the endotracheal tube is in the esophagus instead of the trachea?
    a. Only one firm tube-like structure is palpable in the neck
    b. The patient whines or cries following placement
    c. The reservoir bag expands and contracts with respiratory movements
    d. The patient coughs during placement

27. Laryngospasm is most commonly encountered in
    a. Dogs, cats, and horses
    b. Horses, pigs, and adult ruminants
    c. Cats, adult ruminants, and dogs
    d. Pigs, small ruminants, and cats

28. The stage of anesthesia during which the patient loses voluntary control but has involuntary reactions such as vocalizing, reflex struggling, and paddling, and during which reflexes are present and muscle tone is marked, is
    a. Stage I
    b. Stage II
    c. Stage III
    d. Stage IV

29. Pedal and palpebral reflexes absent, corneal reflex present, midrange pupils, no voluntary movement, and normal heart and respiratory rates that increase in response to surgical stimulation indicate which of the following stages of anesthesia in a canine patient?
    a. Stage III, Plane 1
    b. Stage III, Plane 2
    c. Stage III, Plane 3
    d. Stage III, Plane 4

30. During anesthesia, a variety of heart rhythms may be seen, depending on the species. Sinus arrhythmia is normal in
    a. Dogs, cats, and horses
    b. Horses, cats, and adult ruminants
    c. Cats, adult ruminants, and dogs
    d. Dogs, horses, and adult ruminants

31. Which equipment can be used to monitor blood pressure indirectly?
    a. Pulse oximeter and Doppler monitor
    b. Oscillometric monitor and capnograph
    c. Doppler monitor and oscillometric monitor
    d. Capnograph and pulse oximeter

32. Malignant hyperthermia is a complication of general anesthesia that is most commonly seen in
    a. Pigs
    b. Dogs
    c. Cats
    d. Horses

33. Which of the following is not a typical location for placement of an ultrasonic Doppler probe?
    a. The ventral surface of the forepaw proximal to the metacarpal pad
    b. The lateral surface of the tail
    c. The dorsomedial surface of the hock
    d. The ventral surface of the hind paw proximal to the metatarsal pad

34. Which of the following is not a usual location for placement of a blood pressure cuff?
    a. Around the foreleg
    b. Around the metatarsus
    c. Around the tail base
    d. Around the upper front limb (humerus)

35. Sensors from which of the following monitoring equipment increase mechanical dead space?
    a. Pulse oximeter and apnea monitor
    b. Apnea monitor and capnograph
    c. Capnograph and Doppler monitor
    d. Doppler monitor and pulse oximeter

36. Which of the following drugs or combinations is not commonly used for anesthetic induction in small animal patients?
   a. Isoflurane
   b. Propofol
   c. Ketamine and diazepam
   d. Etomidate

37. All of the drugs listed below must be given intravenous (IV) except one, which can be given either IV or intramuscular (IM). Which drug can be given IM?
   a. Ketamine
   b. Etomidate
   c. Propofol
   d. Methohexital

38. During anesthetic recovery, the oxygen flow rate should be turned to
   a. 5 to 10 mL/kg/min
   b. 20 to 40 mL/kg/min
   c. 50 to 100 mL/kg/min
   d. 200 to 300 mL/kg/min

39. Which of the following is not a sign of normal recovery?
   a. Vocalization
   b. Excitement
   c. Hyperventilation
   d. Seizures

40. In contrast to most other domestic animals, many surgical procedures can be done using local or regional anesthetic techniques in this species.
   a. Feline
   b. Canine
   c. Bovine
   d. Equine

41. During general anesthesia, ruminants are less prone than other domestic species to
   a. Hypotension
   b. Hypoventilation
   c. Regurgitation
   d. Bloating

42. Animals of which species often breathe rapidly and shallowly, somewhat like a panting dog, during general anesthesia?
   a. Horse
   b. Cow
   c. Pig
   d. Cat

43. To prevent atelectasis during general anesthesia, healthy small animal patients should be bagged approximately every
   a. 1 to 2 minutes
   b. 2 to 5 minutes
   c. 5 to 10 minutes
   d. 20 to 30 minutes

44. When anesthetizing a dog, to prevent regurgitation of stomach contents, you should
   a. Position the head level with or slightly higher than the body
   b. Position the head lower than the body
   c. Pack gauze into the throat
   d. Position the patient in lateral recumbency

EXERCISE 31.9 FILL-IN-THE-BLANK: COMPREHENSIVE

Instructions: Fill in each of the spaces provided with the missing word or words that complete the sentence.

1. Neuroleptanalgesia is a state of profound sedation and analgesia produced by simultaneous administration of an

   _____ and a _____.

2. The focus of a preanesthetic physical assessment should be the _____, _____,

   and _____ systems.

3. Drugs classified as agonists bind to receptors and exert one or more effects. Drugs classified as _____

   _____ exert a decreased effect at the receptors, those classified as mixed _____

   partially reverse the effects of pure agonists, and those classified as _____ completely block the action of the corresponding agonist.

4. The preanesthetic medications used to counteract bradycardia and excess salivation are called _____. The drugs _____ and _____ are examples of these agents.

5. The main adverse effect on the cardiovascular system caused by acepromazine is _____.

6. The two drugs contained in the combination telazol are the benzodiazepine _____ and the dissociative _____.

7. The reversal agent can be given after either formulation of dexdomitor to awaken patients undergoing minor procedures.

8. Opioid drugs work by stimulating specific receptors in the brain and spinal cord. The effect of each opioid depends on its affinity for the various receptors. For instance, opioid agonists primarily stimulate the _____ receptors.

9. The dissociative anesthetics most commonly used in veterinary patients are _____ and _____.

10. Dissociative anesthetics cause a unique state called _____, in which the patient appears to be awake but is immobile and does not respond to its surroundings.

11. A combination of diazepam and ketamine is often used to induce general anesthesia in small animals. To do this, these drugs are mixed in a _____:_____ ratio by volume, and given at a dosage of about 1 mL of the mixture for every _____ pounds of body weight. So a 50-pound dog would need about _____ mL of this mixture for induction.

12. The drug combination "TKX" contains the drugs _____, _____, and _____.

13. _____, a drug used as an induction agent in healthy dogs and cats, may cause hyperthermia, especially in dogs.

14. A drug used as a muscle relaxant and sedative in large animals is _____ (also known as "GG" or glyceryl guaiacolate).

15. The anesthetic combination of xylazine, ketamine, and guaifenesin, used to maintain general anesthesia in horses, is commonly called "_____ _____."

16. To produce surgical anesthesia in the average patient, you must select a vaporizer dial setting of approximately _____ times the minimum alveolar concentration (MAC).

17. The inhalant anesthetic _____ induces more rapid inductions and recoveries than any other halogenated agent.

18. When checking a nonrebreathing system for leaks, the inflated reservoir bag should remain inflated for at least _____ seconds if no leaks are present.

19. When checking a rebreathing system for leaks, the reservoir bag should be inflated to a pressure of _____ cm of water. No leaks are present if the pressure decreases to no less than _____ cm of water over 10 seconds, or if an oxygen flow of no more than _____ mL/min is necessary to maintain pressure.

20. When setting the pop-off valve of a rebreathing system, the oxygen should be turned on to the maximum rate you anticipate will be needed for the procedure. The pop-off valve should then be opened until the pressure manometer indicates a pressure of _____ to _____ cm of water.

21. When turning on any dial or valve on an anesthetic machine, the dial or valve should be turned in a _____ direction.

22. An E-size oxygen cylinder with a pressure of 500 psi contains approximately _____ L of oxygen. At a flow rate of 2 L/min, the oxygen will last approximately _____ minutes.

23. An H-size oxygen cylinder with a pressure of 500 psi contains approximately _____ L of oxygen, which will last approximately _____ hours at a flow rate of 2 L/min.

24. To avoid confusion, an isoflurane vaporizer is identified by the color _____, and a sevoflurane vaporizer is identified by the color _____.

25. A nonrebreathing circuit is recommended for patients weighing less than _____ kg of body weight, but is mandatory for patients weighing less than _____ kg of body weight.

26. If a rebreathing system is used for a 5-kg patient, it should be fitted with _____ breathing tubes.

27. A 45-pound patient requires use of a _____ L rebreathing bag.

28. The pressure manometer should read no more than _____ cm of water when providing manual or mechanical ventilation to small animals, and should read no more than _____ cm of water when providing manual or mechanical ventilation to large animals, unless the chest cavity is open.

29. The primary benefit of pediatric breathing tubes is that they decrease mechanical _____ _____.

30. The anesthetic machine should be professionally serviced at least _____.

31. When inflating the cuff of the endotracheal tube, compress the reservoir bag and inflate the cuff until the leak just ceases at a pressure of _____ cm of water.

32. Anesthetized patients often experience decreased respiratory rate, and approximately a _____% decrease in VT. These patients often require periodic manual ventilation about every _____ to _____ minutes during anesthesia to prevent this complication.

33. Eye position is _____ during light anesthesia, gradually shifts to _____ position, and finally shifts back to _____.

34. The width of a blood pressure cuff should be _____% to _____% of the circumference of the extremity.

35. Oxygen saturation of hemoglobin greater than _____% is normal; between _____% and _____% indicates desaturation; less than _____% indicates hypoxemia; and less than _____% for longer than 30 seconds is a medical emergency.

36. In a normal anesthetized patient, the carbon dioxide level as measured with a capnograph should be _____ mm Hg during inspiration, and _____ to _____ mm Hg at the end of expiration.

37. When giving an injectable anesthetic IM, the onset of action will be _____ and the duration of action will be _____ than if the same drug were given IV.

38. When inducing a patient by chamber, use an oxygen flow rate of _____ L/min, and _____% to _____% isoflurane or _____% to _____% sevoflurane.

39. Hypotension in a horse is defined as a mean arterial blood pressure of less than _____ mm Hg.

40. Ruminants normally _____ gas to expel it from the rumen. Because this does not happen during anesthesia, _____ can occur.

41. Regurgitation of stomach contents is very common in ruminants during anesthesia, especially when the anesthetic depth is _____ or _____.

EXERCISE 31.10 CASE STUDY: COMPREHENSIVE

You are serving as an anesthetist for a 6-month-old, 48-pound female mixed-breed dog scheduled for an ovariohysterectomy. The doctor has prescribed the following anesthetic protocol:

Preanesthetic medications:	Hydromorphone 0.1 mg/kg IM
	Dexmedetomidine 0.005 mg/kg IM
Anesthetic induction:	Propofol 4 mg/kg IV to effect
Anesthetic maintenance:	Isoflurane 1.5% to 2.5% via endotracheal tube

You are expected to premedicate, induce, and maintain this patient, and to monitor her throughout the anesthetic event until fully recovered. Answer the following questions regarding anesthetic management of this case.

1. First you must prepare and administer the prescribed preanesthetic medications for this patient.

   a. Calculate the volume of each preanesthetic medication you will administer to this patient. (The concentration of hydromorphone is 2 mg/mL. The concentration of dexmedetomidine is 0.5 mg/mL.)

   Volume of hydromorphone you will administer (mL): _____

   Volume of dexmedetomidine you will administer (mL): _____

   b. What general effects would be expected from these premedications?

   Hydromorphone: _____

   _____

   Dexmedetomidine: _____

   _____

c. The patient should be placed in a quiet location while the preanesthetic medications take effect. Why is this necessary?

_____

_____

d. How much time should you allow for the medications to take effect before proceeding?

_____

2. Next, you must prepare the anesthetic machine and associated equipment including the equipment required for endotracheal intubation.

a. Using the rules-of-thumb regarding selection of an endotracheal tube, what tube size (internal diameter in mm) would you prepare for this patient? _____ **mm**

b. What other equipment would you prepare for endotracheal intubation?

_____

_____

_____

c. Would you select a rebreathing or a nonrebreathing circuit for this patient? Why?

_____

_____

_____

d. What size rebreathing bag would you prepare for this patient? _____ **L bag**

e. When using a semiclosed rebreathing system, what are the steps for setting the pop-off valve?

_____

_____

_____

f. Calculate the oxygen flow rate for this patient following IV induction, during any change in anesthetic depth, or during recovery in L/min.

_____ **L/min**

g. Now calculate the oxygen flow rate for this patient during anesthetic maintenance.

_____ **L/min**

h. You are using a machine with size E oxygen tanks. The tank pressure gauge shows 1200 psi. Approximately how many liters of oxygen are left in the tank?

_____ **L**

i. At an oxygen flow rate of 2 L/min, approximately how long (in hours) would this oxygen supply last?

_____ hours

3. Now you must induce this patient with propofol.

a. Calculate the volume (in mL) of propofol you will draw up for this patient. The concentration of propofol is 10 mg/mL.

_____ mL

b. Will you administer the entire calculated dose to this patient? Why or why not?

_____

_____

_____

c. Describe the specific technique you will use to administer the propofol.

_____

_____

_____

_____

_____

_____

d. What general effects do you expect from this agent?

_____

_____

_____

_____

_____

e. What adverse effects may occur if the propofol is injected too rapidly?

_____

_____

4. During anesthetic maintenance, you will be monitoring this patient to be sure that it is safe, and to determine anesthetic depth.

a. Summarize the findings regarding vital signs and machine parameters you would expect to see during Stage III, Plane 2 general anesthesia (medium surgical anesthesia).

Vital Signs:

Heart rate/rhythm	
Respiratory rate	
Respiratory character	
Body temperature	
Mucous membrane color	
Capillary refill time	
Pulse quality	

Machine Monitoring Parameters

Oxygen saturation	
Systolic arterial blood pressure	
Diastolic arterial blood pressure	
Mean arterial blood pressure	
Minimally acceptable mean during anesthesia	

b. Which of these vital signs and machine parameters are indicators of circulation, which are indicators of oxygenation, and which are indicators of ventilation?

Indicators of circulation: _____

_____

Indicators of oxygenation: _____

_____

Indicators of ventilation: _____

_____

c. Now summarize the findings regarding reflexes, ocular signs, and other indicators that would indicate that your patient is in Stage III, Plane 2 general anesthesia (medium surgical anesthesia).

Reflexes, Ocular Signs, and Other Indicators

Palpebral reflex	
Pedal reflex	
Swallowing reflex	
Corneal reflex	
Pupillary light reflex	
Pupil size	
Eyeball position	
Muscle tone	
Lacrimation	
Response to surgical stimulation	

5. The surgery was completed without incident, and the patient is ready for recovery.

   a. Indicate how you would prepare your patient for recovery, including the appropriate oxygen flow rate for this patient.

   _____

   _____

   _____

   _____

   _____

   _____

   _____

_____

_____

b. Discuss steps you would take to hasten recovery.

_____

_____

_____

c. What signs would tell you that the recovery is progressing normally?

_____

_____

_____

d. How do you know when you can remove the endotracheal tube?

_____

32 Surgical Instruments and Aseptic Technique

LEARNING OBJECTIVES

1. Pronounce, define, and spell all the key terms in this chapter.
2. Do the following regarding general surgery instruments and stapling equipment:
   - Name and describe commonly used surgical instruments.
   - Know the basic operation and properties of carbon dioxide and diode lasers, and develop a basic knowledge of laser safety protocol.
   - State advantages of surgical stapling, and list common surgical stapling devices.
3. Discuss vascular sealing devices and list commonly used instruments and equipment for ophthalmic, orthopedic, arthroscopic, and laparoscopic procedures.
4. Do the following regarding surgical instrument packs, instrument care, and the use of surgical drapes and gowns:
   - List surgical instruments and supplies routinely included in general and emergency surgical packs for small and large animals.
   - Describe procedures for cleaning, packing, and sterilizing instruments.
   - Describe procedures for folding and packing cloth surgical drapes and gowns.
5. Do the following regarding the processes of sterilization and disinfection as part of aseptic technique:
   - Differentiate between sterilization and disinfection.
   - List and describe physical and chemical methods of sterilization and methods of quality control of sterilization methods.
   - Know the appropriate sterilization processes for sensitive equipment.
   - State safe storage times and conditions for sterile packs.
   - List and describe common antiseptic and disinfectant agents.
   - Describe requirements for preparation of the operating room and maintenance of operating room sterility.
6. Describe preparation requirements for patients, including skin preparation, patient positioning, and draping.
7. Describe preparation requirements for the surgical team, and explain the procedures that may be used for hand scrubbing before surgery, the procedure for donning surgical attire, and the procedures for opening sterile items.

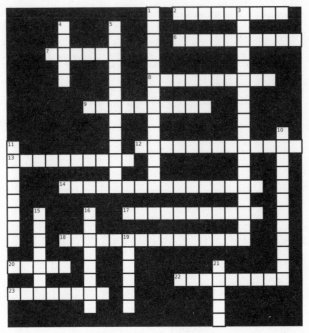

Across

2 One of the two self-retaining retractors commonly used to retract muscle during orthopedic and neurologic surgical procedures.

6 A group of surgical instruments named _____ forceps are used to crush blood vessels and tissues in order to stop the source of bleeding.

7 The common name for the frequently used disinfectant, sodium hypochlorite.

8 The general name for instruments, the primary function of which is to improve visualization in the surgical field during soft-tissue and orthopedic procedures.

9 Partially or fully threaded bone screws that comprise wider threads designed to increase gripping in soft bone.

12 An antiseptic agent that has effective antimicrobial properties as well as a rapid onset and long-lasting residual activity.

13 The type of cleaning unit designed to remove debris that is tightly bound to instruments and clean areas on the instruments that cannot be reached by scrub brushes.

14 Large hemostatic forceps with longitudinal grooves in the jaws and cross-grooves at the tip.

17 The type of cloth drape that comes premade with an opening in the center for easy placement over the predetermined incision site.

18 The jaws of needle holders that are of high quality often contain replaceable _____ _____ inserts that help grip needles and prevent wear. (2 words)

20 Another name for emergency sterilization.

22 The smooth, stainless steel bone pins that can range in diameter from 1/16 to 1/4 inch.

23 The iodine solution for skin that is not commonly used in veterinary medicine, and is comprised of 50% alcohol and 2% iodine.

Down

1 A disinfectant solution that is used for cold sterilization. Can cause chemical synovitis and chondrocyte damage if not rinsed off.

3 A cannula-type instrument into which the obturator is placed for arthroscopic procedures. (2 words)

4 One of the two self-retaining retractors commonly used to retract muscle during orthopedic and neurologic surgical procedures.

5 The chemical gas that is capable of killing all microorganisms. (2 words)

10 The process that allows one to create and maintain a desired level of abdominal distention during laparoscopic procedures.

11 Instruments designed with small cup-like formations on one or both ends used to scrape dense tissues like cartilage or bone.

15 The retractor that comprises one single blade and a handle; used to lever tissues out of the line of view.

16 The hand-held instrument characterized by sharp tips that appear cupped; used for cutting small pieces of dense tissues like cartilage, bone, or fibrous tissues.

19 The sharp pointed instrument inserted inside an arthroscope sleeve.

21 Surgical wire with T-shaped handles used in orthopedic procedures for cutting bone in a saw-like motion.

EXERCISE 32.2 DEFINITIONS: KEY TERMS

Instructions: Define each term in your own words.

1. Coherent light: _____

   _____

2. Latent thermal damage: _____

   _____

3. Collateral thermal damage: _____

   _____

4. External fixation: _____

   _____

5. Asepsis: _____

   _____

6. Aseptic technique: _____

   _____

7. Exogenous route: _____

   _____

8. Endogenous route: _____

   _____

9. Sterilization: _____

   _____

10. Filtration: _____

    _____

11. Disinfectant: _____

    _____

12. Antisepsis: _____

    _____

13. Antiseptic agents: _____

    _____

14. Cold trays: _____

_____

15. Quarter drapes: _____

_____

16. Towel clamps: _____

_____

EXERCISE 32.3 MATCHING: SURGICAL INSTRUMENTS

Instructions: Match each definition in column A with its corresponding word in column B by writing the appropriate letter in the space provided.

Column A

1. _____ "Heavy-duty" operating scissors commonly used for cutting dense tissues.

2. _____ Instruments used to grasp needles and pass suture material through tissues in addition to aiding with suture tying.

3. _____ Thumb forceps with delicate intermeshing teeth, which make them good for grasping delicate tissues atraumatically.

4. _____ The needle holder that is equipped with scissors built into the instrument.

5. _____ Thumb forceps that are relatively atraumatic with multiple sets of delicate teeth and long narrow jaws that are often used for vascular surgeries.

6. _____ A traumatic type of thumb forceps with a broad curved surface that is good for handling needles.

7. _____ The classification of instruments with a locking mechanism that are used to clamp tissues.

8. _____ The self-retaining retractor that facilitates retraction of the ribs for surgical site exposure within the thoracic cavity.

9. _____ Traumatic tissue forceps that are used to securely grasp tissues but that leave the tissues "crushed." Therefore, these forceps should only be used on tissues that are to be removed during the procedure.

10. _____ The hemostatic forceps designed with large transverse grooves used to clamp bundles of tissues and large vessels.

11. _____ Thumb forceps with jaws composed of large interdigitating teeth that are primarily used for fascia or skin.

12. _____ One of the two types of hemostatic forceps that are similar in design to Halsted mosquito forceps but that differ from one another slightly in jaw-tooth pattern. Used to perform the function of crushing medium vessels and tissues.

13. _____ Intestinal tissue forceps designed with atraumatic flexible jaws, which allows for safe clamping of viable portions of the bowel in addition to other delicate tissues.

14. _____ Hemostatic forceps that are relatively small in size and designed to occlude small vessels.

15. _____ The general type of forceps used for tissue manipulation that is designed with a "spring action." Used by compressing the two metal handles together to make the jaws meet.

16. _____ Hemostatic forceps that are similar to the Rochester-Pean but have interdigitating teeth at the tips used for grasping tissues. They are commonly utilized in orthopedic or large animal surgery.

Column B

A. Kirschner wire

B. Rochester-Ochsner

C. Allis

D. Adson

E. Babcock

F. Halsted mosquito

G. Jamshidi

H. DeBakey

I. Kelly

J. Russian

K. Rochester-Carmalt

L. Mayo dissecting scissors

M. Rochester-Pean

N. Conical

O. Olsen-Hegar

P. Army-Navy

Q. Needle holders

R. Malleable

S. Finochietto

T. Rat-tooth

U. Kerrison

V. Doyen

W. Trephine

X. Tissue forceps

Y. Thumb forceps

17. _____ The tissue forceps that are similar to Allis tissue forceps but provide less tissue security as a result of having a less traumatic effect on tissues.

18. _____ Hemostatic forceps that are large in size with longitudinal grooves and cross-grooves at the tip of the jaws which aid in traction for crushing and clamping across vessels. They are commonly used in spay procedures.

19. _____ A hand-held surgical retractor that is designed with smooth blades and used to retract skin, fat, or muscles.

20. _____ A specific type of rongeurs used for spinal surgeries with a "gun-shaped" appearance.

21. _____ A T-shaped stainless steel instrument that has a cutting cylindrical blade. Similar to the appearance of a general biopsy punch.

22. _____ The type of bone pin that is similar to an intramedullary pin but is smaller in size and may be used to pin small fragments of bone.

23. _____ The type of needle that shares similarities with a trephine but is often disposable, making it only good for a single use.

24. _____ An atraumatic hand-held surgical retractor composed of specialized metal that allows the retractor to be bent into a desired shape, making it especially useful for retracting thoracic and abdominal organs.

25. _____ The type of obturator used to penetrate the synovial membrane of the joint capsule to allow further advancement of the arthroscope sleeve into the joint space. Provides a reduced risk of causing articular cartilage damage.

EXERCISE 32.4 PHOTO QUIZ #1: SURGICAL INSTRUMENT PARTS

Instructions: Name each surgical instrument part (indicated by the arrows).

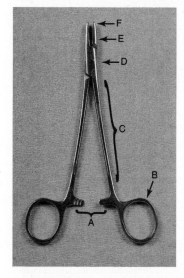

Part Names

A._____

B._____

C._____

D._____

E._____

F._____

EXERCISE 32.5 PHOTO QUIZ #2: SURGICAL INSTRUMENTS

Instructions: Match each general class of surgical instruments with its corresponding photo by writing its name in the space provided. Then respond to each of the follow-up queries.

General Classes of Surgical Instruments

A. Suction tips

B. Scissors

C. Self-retaining retractors

D. Thumb forceps

E. Scalpel handles and blades

F. Tissue forceps

G. Hemostatic forceps

H. Needle holders

I. Hand-held retractors

1. General class of instruments: _____

Name each instrument and then indicate how you can differentiate each by its size and jaw pattern.

Name: **Criteria used to differentiate:**

A. _____   _____

B. _____   _____

C. _____   _____

D. _____   _____

E. _____   _____

F. _____   _____

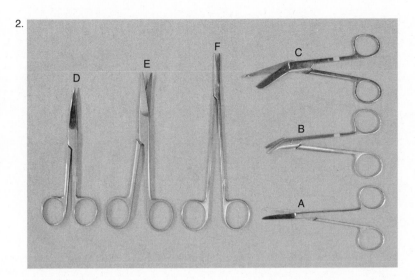

2. General class of instruments: _____

Name each instrument and then indicate whether it is primarily used to cut wire suture, delicate tissue, bandage material, suture, or fascia and other dense tissue or if it is used for general-purpose cutting.

Name: **Primary use:**

A. _____   _____

B. _____   _____

C. _____   _____

D. _____   _____

E. _____   _____

F. _____   _____

3.

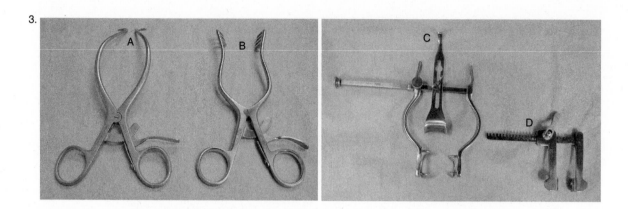

3. General class of instruments: _____

Name each instrument and then indicate whether it is primarily used to expose the abdominal cavity, expose the thoracic cavity, or retract muscle for orthopedic and neurologic surgeries.

Name: **Primary use:**

A. _____   _____

B. _____   _____

C. _____   _____

D. _____   _____

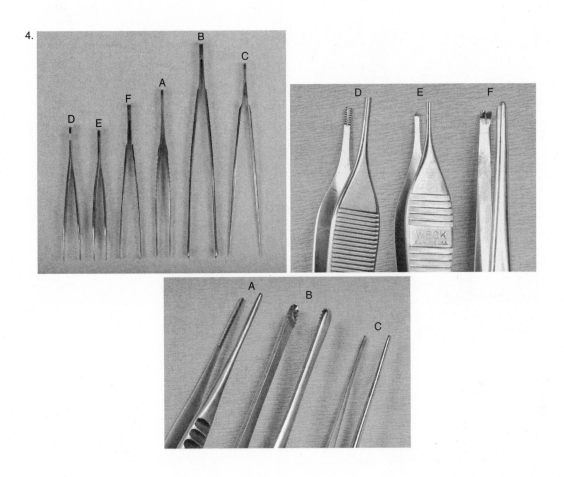

4. General class of instruments: _____

Name each instrument and then indicate whether it is primarily used to hold tissue and needles, skin and fascia, delicate tissue, vessels, needles only (because of tissue trauma), or wound dressing.

Name: **Primary use:**

A. _____   _____

B. _____   _____

C. _____   _____

D. _____   _____

E. _____   _____

F. _____   _____

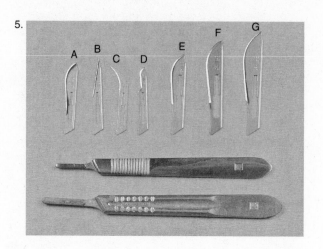

5. General class of instruments: _____

Indicate the number of each blade.

A. _____ B. _____ C. _____ D. _____

E. _____ F. _____ G. _____

Indicate the number of the scalpel handle on the bottom: _____

   Which blades will fit on this handle? _____

Indicate the number of the scalpel handle on the top: _____

   Which blades will fit on this handle? _____

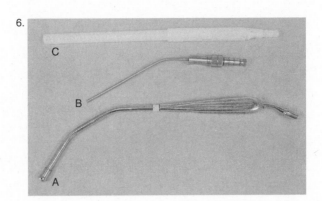

6. General class of instruments: _____

Name each instrument and then indicate whether it is primarily used to suction fluid from a body cavity or a joint or for general-purpose suctioning.

Name: **Primary use:**

A. _____   _____

B. _____   _____

C. _____   _____

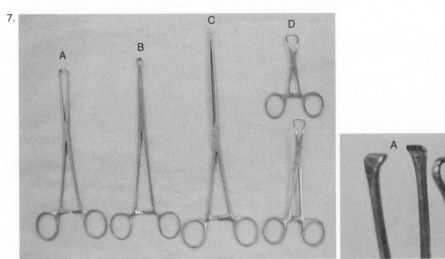

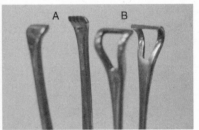

7. General class of instruments: _____

Name each instrument and then indicate whether it is primarily used to hold tissue that will be removed, bowel and other delicate tissues, tissue that will not be removed, or surgical drapes.

Name: **Primary use:**

A. _____   _____

B. _____   _____

C. _____   _____

D. _____   _____

Chapter **32** Surgical Instruments and Aseptic Technique

8.

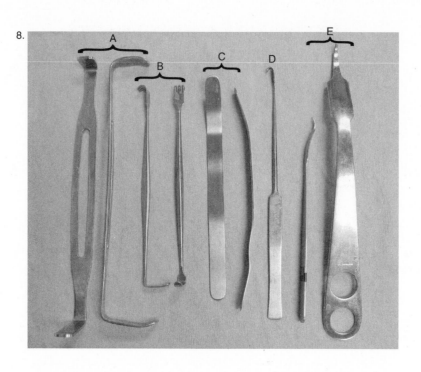

8. General class of instruments: _____

Name each instrument and then indicate whether it is primarily used to retract skin, fat and muscle, abdominal and thoracic organs, the horn of the uterus, or tissues during orthopedic surgery.

Name: **Primary use:**

A. _____   _____

B. _____   _____

C. _____   _____

D. _____   _____

E. _____   _____

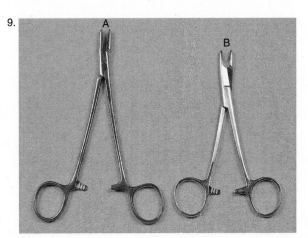

9. General class of instruments: _____

What is the specific name of each instrument?

Name:

A. _____

B. _____

What is the difference between these two instruments?

_____

EXERCISE 32.6 TRUE OR FALSE: COMPREHENSIVE

Instructions: Read the following statements and write "T" for true or "F" for false in the blanks provided. If a statement is false, correct the statement to make it true.

1. _____ It is necessary to shave between the patient and the ground plate when using electrocautery technology in order to prevent the occurrence of burns.

2. _____ The use of a ground plate is required for bipolar electrosurgery.

3. _____ The wavelength and frequency of light emitted by a laser are uniform.

4. _____ When using a laser, adipose (fat) tissue is more likely to cause scatter radiation than bone.

5. _____ CO_2 laser beams are produced from a liquid medium.

6. _____ CO_2 lasers emit a "free" laser beam.

7. _____ The diode laser and YAG laser have similar wavelengths.

8. _____ The beam of the YAG or diode laser is transmitted by fibers.

9. _____ CO_2 lasers create greater collateral and latent thermal damage compared to Nd:YAG and diode lasers.

10. _____ The majority of lasers used in the medical field are class IV and are capable of causing damage to the skin and eyes.

Chapter **32** Surgical Instruments and Aseptic Technique

11. _____ Certain laser types can penetrate through clear glass.

12. _____ Lasers generate a potentially toxic substance called "plume" when used on tissues.

13. _____ Brown-Adson thumb forceps are not commonly used in the veterinary field.

14. _____ Surgeons commonly hold thumb forceps in their dominant hand to grasp tissues for dissection or suturing.

15. _____ Kelly forceps are characterized by transverse grooves that extend along the entire length of the jaw, whereas the jaws of Crile forceps only contain grooves on the distal aspect.

16. _____ Another name for the "spay hook" is the Snook ovariohysterectomy hook.

17. _____ Most bone-holding forceps are self-retaining.

18. _____ Chisels and osteotomes are produced from a hard metal and therefore can be used to cut other materials besides bone.

19. _____ The threads of bone pins are located only on the end of the pin.

20. _____ External fixators are used to hold bone pins in position and can be made of metal or acrylic material.

21. _____ Bone screws should never be used in conjunction with a bone plate or interlocking nail.

22. _____ Large bone screws commonly have a slotted head.

23. _____ Arthroscopes are used to examine joint structures of large and small animals.

24. _____ The majority of arthroscopic equipment is designed specifically for veterinary use.

25. _____ Once a fibrous joint capsule has been penetrated by a sharp trocar, the trocar is replaced with the arthroscope.

26. _____ Gas insufflation with the use of CO_2 or nitrous oxide is an acceptable method of joint distention.

27. _____ Pressurized bag systems are used to deliver fluid into the joint.

28. _____ Arthroscopy may be performed on horses with the use of local anesthetics and sedatives.

29. _____ Nitrous oxide gas is used to insufflate the abdomen when performing laparoscopy.

30. _____ Stainless steel surgical instruments with a polished finish are preferred over those with a satin finish.

31. _____ Only surgical instruments made from the same material should be ultrasonically cleaned at the same time.

32. _____ Oil is used to lubricate and maintain proper function of surgical instruments.

33. _____ Cloth drapes and gowns are designed for repeated use.

34. _____ Radiation is a safe alternative for sterilizing certain materials that would otherwise be damaged by other methods of sterilization.

35. _____ As compared with dry heat, wet heat requires a greater period of time to achieve sterilization and is also more difficult to control.

36. _____ Wet heat sterilization with boiling water at ambient pressures is a reliable method to achieve sterilization.

37. _____ After the sterilization process is finished, the pack should be allowed to self-cool prior to handling by fully opening the autoclave door for at least 20 minutes.

38. _____ It is common among veterinary practices to use a combination of autoclave tape on the outside of a surgical pack as well as a chemical indicator strip in the center of the pack to assure proper sterilization was achieved.

39. _____ Liquid chemicals should not be used for instrument sterilization.

40. _____ Ethylene oxide is a toxic, colorless, and explosive gas used for instrument sterilization.

41. _____ Ethylene oxide gas is capable of penetrating through paper and plastic packaging materials.

42. _____ Proper placement of surgical packs and materials in the sterilization chamber is extremely important in order for effective sterilization to take place with the use of ethylene oxide gas.

43. _____ Disinfectants are capable of killing vegetative bacteria as well as effective at destroying spores.

44. _____ Iodine compounds are antimicrobial agents that are extremely effective against bacterial spores.

45. _____ Aqueous iodine solutions contain a lower level of free iodine than iodophors, resulting in less bactericidal activity.

46. _____ By diluting iodophor stock solutions, the bactericidal activity will increase and the cytotoxicity will decrease.

47. _____ Povidone-iodine is commonly used in the veterinary field as a surgical scrub and is effective in reducing bacteria.

48. _____ The residual bactericidal effect of povidone-iodine is greatly reduced by the presence of organic matter.

49. _____ Chlorhexidine is an antiseptic agent that provides effective antimicrobial activity without causing significant skin irritation or complications, as seen with povidone-iodine solutions.

50. _____ Methyl alcohol is more effective than ethyl and isopropyl alcohol when used as a disinfectant.

51. _____ Glutaraldehyde is an effective antimicrobial agent that can be used on living tissues.

52. _____ Arthroscope and laparoscope components (light cable and camera) should be cleaned only by gas or cold sterilization.

53. _____ A presurgical scrub is performed on the patient either in the surgical preparation room or inside the operating room to maintain asepsis.

54. _____ The final sterile scrub should be performed on the patient just before entering the operating room.

55. _____ "One-step prep" skin preparation solutions may be used in place of traditional scrubs for preparing surgery sites, as they have comparative antimicrobial killing capabilities.

56. _____ Feline castration surgical prep involves shaving the scrotum.

57. _____ Lateral recumbency is the most desirable position for most abdominal surgeries.

58. _____ The sleeves, the front of the gown, and the neckline are considered to be sterile on a "scrubbed-in" person.

59. _____ "Scrubbed-in" assistants are responsible for opening all sterile items for the surgeons.

Instructions: Circle the one correct answer to each of the following questions.

1. The laser energy applied to tissue is measured in
   a. Volts
   b. Watts
   c. Joules
   d. Amperes

2. Which of the following laser types is not commonly used in the veterinary field?
   a. CO_2
   b. Nd:YAG
   c. Argon
   d. Diode

3. CO_2 lasers are primarily used for
   a. Vaporization of tissues
   b. Precise cutting and vaporization of tissues
   c. Transendoscopic surgery
   d. Deep-tissue penetration

4. Which of the following is most susceptible to damage from laser injury?
   a. Thyroid glands
   b. Eyes
   c. Reproductive organs
   d. Hands

5. The surgical scissors most commonly utilized for soft-tissue dissection are
   a. Metzenbaum scissors
   b. Mayo dissecting scissors
   c. Iris scissors
   d. Operating scissors

6. The type of surgical instrument sometimes used to secure surgical drapes and instrument cords (such as those used for cautery) is
   a. Allis tissue forceps
   b. Babcock forceps
   c. Doyen forceps
   d. Russian thumb forceps

7. Tissue forceps are used for
   a. Cutting and clamping tissues
   b. Occluding and grasping vessels
   c. Crushing and cutting tissues
   d. Clamping and holding tissues

8. Which of the hemostatic forceps listed are most commonly used for large animal surgery or orthopedic procedures?
   a. Rochester-Ochsner forceps
   b. Rochester-Pean forceps
   c. Crile forceps
   d. Kelly forceps

9. The Poole suction tip is primarily used in the
   a. Abdominal cavity
   b. Thoracic cavity
   c. Joints
   d. Both A and B

10. Which of the following is not a recognized material used for orthopedic implants?
    a. Cobalt-chromium alloys
    b. Titanium
    c. Stainless steel alloy
    d. Aluminum alloys

11. The most commonly used arthroscope for canine arthroscopy is
    a. 4-mm outer diameter, and a 25-degree angled lens
    b. 4-mm outer diameter, and a 32-degree angled lens
    c. 5-mm outer diameter, and a 10-degree angled lens
    d. 2.7-mm outer diameter, and a 32-degree angled lens

12. The inner pressure of an insufflated abdominal cavity should not exceed
    a. 10 to 15 mm Hg
    b. 15 to 20 mm Hg
    c. 20 to 25 mm Hg
    d. 25 to 32 mm Hg

13. Which of the following is not classified as an exogenous source of contamination?
    a. Air
    b. Surgical instruments
    c. Patient skin
    d. Oral cavity bacteria

14. Which of the following is not a surgical wound classification used to determine the degree of vigilance required regarding aseptic technique?
    a. Sterile
    b. Clean
    c. Clean-contaminated
    d. Contaminated

15. Which of the following is not classified as a general type of physical sterilization?
    a. Filtration
    b. Radiation
    c. Heat
    d. Ethylene oxide

16. Which of the following statements is true regarding radiation sterilization?
    a. Materials that are easily damaged should not be sterilized by radiation.
    b. Radiation destroys microorganisms.
    c. Radiation produces high temperatures during the sterilization process.
    d. Radiation is not used for sterilization of medical supplies.

17. The most common sterilization method is
    a. Wet heat
    b. Filtration
    c. Radiation
    d. Hydrogen peroxide gas plasma

18. Which of the following products is most effectively sterilized by dry heat?
    a. Rubber
    b. Fabrics
    c. Metals
    d. Oils

19. Reliable methods of heat sterilization for fabrics and metals include
    a. Saturated steam under pressure
    b. Boiling water
    c. Dry heat
    d. Both A and B

20. Which of the following products is most effectively sterilized by moist heat?
    a. Powders
    b. Petroleum products
    c. Oils
    d. Rubber

21. The adequate amount of spacing between each pack in an autoclave chamber to ensure proper steam penetration is
    a. 2.5 to 7.5 cm
    b. 3.5 to 8.5 cm
    c. 5.0 to 10 cm
    d. 7.5 to 12 cm

22. The recommended exposure time and temperature for flash-sterilization is
    a. 2 minutes at 250° F
    b. 3 minutes at 131° C
    c. 4 minutes at 270° F
    d. 5 minutes at 131° F

23. To prevent rapid cooling of packs after a sterilization cycle has finished, the autoclave door should be slightly cracked open for a minimum of
    a. 5 minutes
    b. 10 minutes
    c. 15 minutes
    d. 20 minutes

24. Fusible pellet glass indicators provide evidence that a(n)
    a. Pressure of 27 psi was reached
    b. Adequate level of steam saturation was achieved
    c. Time of 15 minutes passed
    d. Temperature of 118° C was reached

25. Which of the following statements is false in regard to culture test indicators?
    a. They use spores of a particular strain of bacteria.
    b. They yield rapid results.
    c. They are the only type of indicator that provides evidence that microorganisms were destroyed.
    d. They do not indicate if proper steam penetration has been achieved.

26. Which of the following events would render a sterile surgical pack contaminated?
    a. The pack was stored in an open cabinet.
    b. The pack was stored in an upside-down position.
    c. The outside of the pack came in contact with a nonsterile instrument.
    d. The pack was dropped but the tape sealing the pack remained intact.

27. The general operating temperature for ethylene oxide is between
    a. 21° C and 140° C
    b. 15° C and 60° C
    c. 21° C and 60° C
    d. 21° F and 70° F

28. The minimal humidity requirement for effective sterilization to occur by the use of ethylene oxide is
    a. 20%
    b. 25%
    c. 32%
    d. 35%

29. Which of the following statements is not true of hydrogen peroxide gas plasma sterilization?
    a. Gas plasma is capable of inactivating mycobacteria and bacterial spores
    b. Gas plasma is capable of inactivating viruses and fungi
    c. Gas plasma is considered to be safer for the environment when compared with ethylene oxide
    d. Gas plasma sterilization is considered to be a more hazardous form of chemical sterilization when compared with ethylene oxide

30. The residual bactericidal activity of povidone-iodine when left on the skin is
    a. 2 to 4 hours
    b. 4 to 6 hours
    c. 6 to 8 hours
    d. 8 to 10 hours

31. Skin irritation or acute dermatitis related to the use of povidone-iodine iodophors in veterinary practice can affect up to
    a. 10% of canine patients
    b. 25% of canine patients
    c. 50% of canine patients
    d. 75% of canine patients

32. The proper dilution for chlorhexidine antiseptic agents in order to produce a 0.05% lavage solution for open wound treatment is
    a. 1:40 with sterile water
    b. 1:40 with saline
    c. 1:20 with sterile water
    d. Both a and b

33. The required exposure time when soaking instruments to achieve cold sterilization should exceed
    a. 32 minutes
    b. 1 hour
    c. 2 hours
    d. 3 hours

34. For which of the following procedures is it not acceptable to use cold-sterilized instruments?
    a. Dental surgery
    b. Superficial laceration
    c. Abscess debridement
    d. Lumpectomy

35. The general rule of thumb for clipping the perimeter around the incision site is
    a. 2 to 5 cm
    b. 3 to 10 cm
    c. 5 to 15 cm
    d. 10 to 20 cm

36. The general recommendation for initial skin preparation of a surgical site consists of scrubbing and rinsing
    a. 2 times
    b. 3 times
    c. 4 times
    d. 5 times

37. Which of the following statements is not true regarding the surgical hand scrub?
    a. The two basic methods include "counted brush strokes" and "timed"
    b. The "counted brush stroke" method is more commonly used
    c. 10 to 25 brush strokes are performed on all surfaces prior to rinsing
    d. The initial scrub of the day should be at least 5 minutes

38. Which of the following is not acceptable for scrubbed-in personnel?
    a. Resting gloved hands on a sterile drape
    b. Clasping gloved hands in front of the body between shoulders and waist
    c. Crossing arms at chest height
    d. Touching the gown within the sterile zone while wearing gloves

39. Which of the following is a false statement regarding towel clamps?
    a. The Roeder towel clamp has a metal ball stop on the jaws
    b. The Backhaus towel clamp prevents deep tissue penetration
    c. Towel clamps are designed to secure drapes to the patient
    d. Towel clamps have tips that join together like "tongs"

EXERCISE 32.8 FILL-IN-THE-BLANK: COMPREHENSIVE

Instructions: Fill in each of the spaces provided with the missing word or words that complete the sentence.

1. Lasers emit energized light produced from a crystal, a _____, or a _____.

2. A laser's _____ within the light spectrum determines the effect it will have on tissue.

3. The result of laser-tissue interaction is dependent on the tissue's _____ and _____.

4. In addition to the expected effect of a laser on the surgery site, lasers also cause thermal tissue damage that is classified either as _____ or _____.

5. The two most commonly used needle holders in the veterinary field are _____ and _____.

6. Adson thumb forceps are commonly used for the dissection of delicate _____ tissue and _____.

7. _____ and _____ hemostatic forceps share similarities in appearance but differ in their jaw tooth pattern, which covers the entire jaw in one and only the distal aspect of the jaw in the other.

8. The _____ _____ is a specialized surgical instrument designed to act as a hand-held retractor that is used to grasp uterine horns during ovariohysterectomy procedures.

9. The suction tip designed for general purpose use is referred to as a _____ tip.

10. The periosteal elevator most commonly utilized in small animal orthopedics is known as the _____ elevator.

11. The type of bone-holding forceps equipped with a ratcheted handle for secure bone clamping is known as the _____ bone-holding forceps.

12. Two surgical devices made from soft metals that are used for bone cutting are the _____ and _____.

13. The points of bone pins come in varieties, like the _____, trocar, or _____ trocar.

14. The most commonly used sizes of stainless steel cerclage wire for small animal surgery are _____ gauge, _____ gauge, and _____ gauge.

15. The two basic types of bone screws are the _____ and the _____.

16. When using a laparoscope, the abdominal cavity is accessed through the _____ _____ in horses or through the _____ _____ in both dogs and horses.

17. The use of a sharp _____ and a cannula is needed to penetrate subcutaneous tissues and the lining of the peritoneum in order to create a portal for a laparoscope.

18. The most commonly used gas for insufflation is _____ because it is noncombustible, making it relatively safe.

19. The box lock of instruments should remain in the _____ position when going through the ultrasonic cleaner.

20. Instruments with a _____ finish are less resistant to discoloration and spotting caused by cleaning.

21. After instruments are cleaned, they should be rinsed thoroughly with _____ water and allowed to completely dry prior to autoclaving to prevent _____ formation.

22. _____ and _____ heat are the two general types of heat sterilization.

23. The two primary methods of sterilization used by manufacturers for packaging and the production of certain surgical supplies are _____ and _____.

24. Downward displacement or _____ displacement sterilizers use steam introduced into the top of the autoclave chamber to push air to the bottom.

25. Rapid and even penetration of steam by use of a _____ sterilizer is achieved by a vacuum pump that evacuates air before steam is allowed to enter the chamber.

26. Ethylene oxide and _____ _____ are the two most commonly used agents for gas sterilization.

27. Ethylene oxide sterilization is slowly being overtaken by _____ _____ sterilization because it is safer for personnel and the environment.

28. _____ indicators are used to evaluate exposure to saturated steam for an adequate period of time, whereas _____ indicators are used to test for sterility.

29. The quaternary ammonium compound most commonly used as a disinfectant is _____ chloride.

30. The two most commonly used aldehydes in veterinary medicine are _____ and _____.

31. The _____ skin preparation is performed in the patient preparation room to remove gross contamination.

32. _____ recumbency means the animal is placed on its back.

33. _____ recumbency means the animal is laying on either the right or left side of the body.

34. _____ recumbency means the animal is lying on its belly.

35. The two methods for donning surgical gloves are _____ gloving and _____ gloving.

EXERCISE 32.9 CASE STUDY: INSTRUMENT CLEANING AND PACKING

Signalment: Mary, a 1-year-old female domestic shorthair tabby.

Chief complaint: Mary is being admitted to the hospital for a routine spay.

Minimum database: Mary's database is normal, including physical examination findings and basic lab work. There is no history of previous medical problems.

Disposition of the case: Mary's surgery went well with no complications. Now you are responsible for cleaning, maintaining, repacking, and sterilizing the instruments used for this case. Your goals are to ensure efficient operation of the surgery suite, prevent instrument damage, and ultimately prepare the instruments in such a way that makes them safe for use on the next surgical case.

Please answer the following questions related to this case.

1. Describe the protocol that should be followed to prevent instrument corrosion.

_____

_____

_____

2. Explain the process of cleaning instruments, listing each step in the proper order. Include information regarding both hand cleaning and ultrasonic cleaning, including the agents and equipment used.

_____

_____

_____

_____

_____

_____

3. How should instruments be rinsed, dried, and lubricated?

_____

_____

_____

4. Instruments should always be inspected before repacking them. During this inspection, what will you look for?

_____

_____

_____

5. What are the principles of packing the instruments in preparation for sterilization? What instruments would be in a typical pack?

_____

_____

_____

_____

_____

6. Explain the principles of using an autoclave to sterilize the pack, including preparation, loading the autoclave, maintenance, and ensuring safety.

_____

_____

_____

_____

_____

Find the words listed below. The words may be located horizontally, vertically, or diagonally, and may be reversed.

```
G E S T E I N M A N N P I N U H A D A O A S
R B A A N I A O A R T H R O S C O P E L I Y
H S R N I O S O E L E C L Q L E N T C A C E
E B N Q D P S S R O N G E U R S H O L P D L
L R O R I O L T E R S D E A I Y H O E A C N
E D R N X P R P E O P G H T L O H H E R S T
E I O P E R I O S T E A L E L E V A T O R B
R S E G H C Q G E A C N N R T T Y C S S E L
O I O C R C U L S N R E L N S D A G S C I I
R N L C O O A T R U O F L A B T L E S O R P
R F L N L D I I T X F I T R A U I T E P H C
N E I I H I U I I I G O T Y T A L Y L E O L
S C R A C U I D F O N A V A S O P I N A C D
N T D F E I E I I N I G R M L O R O I C A S
A A R R L I H C E A D A F M O U L E A C E Y
G N I N I A T E R F L E S O O S G A T O P O
E T A S R O H P O D O I G N R G S N S R P H
Y L L O I I O T E T H R F I I C A E A D O A
A R L E T I H H F O E O O U R A E O N I E F
E N A T R N Y O L F N O E M P U R P S O R S
L C H H N D E T I R O L H C O P Y H S N O T
L E O N E L L Y N O B S R U D H I D P P C B
```

SelfRetaining
Phenols
Balfour
Hypochlorite
PeriostealElevator
Alcohol
BonecuttingForceps
QuaternaryAmmonium
BoneholdingForceps
HallAirDrill
SteinmannPin
Arthroscope
Triangulation
Rongeurs
Laparoscope
StainlessSteel
Accordion
Glutaraldehyde
EthyleneOxide
Disinfectant
Iodophors
Chlorhexidine

33 Surgical Assistance and Suture Material

LEARNING OBJECTIVES

When you have completed this chapter, you will be able to:
1. Pronounce, define, and spell all the key terms in this chapter.
2. Describe the role of the veterinary technician in surgical assistance for large and small animal patients.
3. Explain preoperative preparation as it applies to the small animal surgical patient, including review of clipping and surgical scrub techniques with respect to patient positioning. Discuss considerations for operating room sterility and instrument table organization.
4. Discuss intraoperative duties of the surgical assistant, including surgical lighting, instruments, hemostasis, suture cutting, lavage and suction, camera manipulation, tissue manipulation, retraction, and organ positioning.
5. Describe the most common permanent and temporary forms of surgical implants and their uses.
6. Discuss the considerations involved in choosing a type of suture material, and list and describe commonly used suture materials and needles and their application.
7. Describe the role of the surgical assistant in the postoperative management of patients.
8. Discuss surgical assisting in equine patients, including draping techniques, instrument setup, tissue handling, and common types of suture materials.

EXERCISE 33.1 MATCHING #1: TERMS AND DEFINITIONS

Instructions: Match each term in column A with its corresponding definition in column B by writing the appropriate letter in the space provided.

Column A	Column B
1. _____ Fenestrated	A. Does not allow water to penetrate.
2. _____ Impervious	B. Surgical incision into the abdominal cavity.
3. _____ Ingesta	C. Relating to surgery on the skeleton.
4. _____ Laparotomy	D. Having a window or one created in a surgical drape.
5. _____ Orthopedic	E. "Squeezed on," as with a suture needle onto suture.
6. _____ Swaged	F. Food material in the intestinal tract.

EXERCISE 33.2 MATCHING #2: CHARACTERISTICS OF SUTURE MATERIAL

Instructions: Match each characteristic of suture material in column A with its corresponding classification in column B by writing the appropriate letter in the space provided.

Column A

1. _____ Passes more easily through tissue.
2. _____ Better knot security.
3. _____ Greater capillary action.
4. _____ More susceptible to bacterial colonization.
5. _____ Made of a single strand.

Column B

A. Monofilament

B. Multifilament

EXERCISE 33.3 MATCHING #3: TRADE AND GENERIC NAMES OF SUTURE MATERIAL

Instructions: Match each trade name in column A with its corresponding generic name in column B by writing the appropriate letter in the space provided.

Column A

1. _____ Vicryl
2. _____ Dexon
3. _____ Monocryl
4. _____ PDS
5. _____ Maxon
6. _____ Nylon
7. _____ Prolene
8. _____ Novafil
9. _____ Mersilene

Column B

A. Polydioxanone

B. Polybutester

C. Polyglyconate

D. Polyglactin 910

E. Polypropylene

F. Polyester

G. Poliglecaprone 25

H. Polyamide

I. Polyglycolic acid

EXERCISE 33.4 MATCHING #4: CLASSIFICATION OF SUTURE MATERIAL

Instructions: Match each suture material in column A with its corresponding classification in column B by writing the appropriate letter in the space provided. (Note that responses may be used more than once.)

Column A

1. _____ Polyglyconate
2. _____ Stainless steel
3. _____ Polybutester
4. _____ Silk
5. _____ Polypropylene
6. _____ Polydioxanone
7. _____ Polyglycolic acid
8. _____ Poliglecaprone 25
9. _____ Polyglactin 910
10. _____ Polyamide
11. _____ Polyester

Column B

A. Monofilament, absorbable

B. Monofilament, nonabsorbable

C. Multifilament, absorbable

D. Multifilament, nonabsorbable

E. Monofilament or multifilament, absorbable

F. Monofilament or multifilament, nonabsorbable

Instructions: Respond to the queries associated with each photo in the spaces provided.

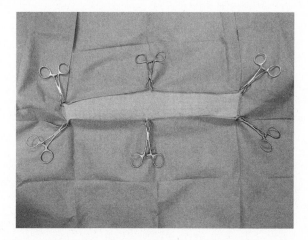

1a. Identify the instruments in this image.

_____

1b. What are the principles that must be followed when placing these clamps?

_____

_____

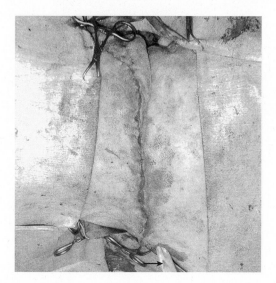

2a. Identify the type of drain used in this image.

_____

2b. What is the purpose for this drain in this case?

_____

2c. Is this drain passive or active? What does this mean regarding the way that it works?

_____

_____

2d. What are some of the principles of caring for this drain?

_____

_____

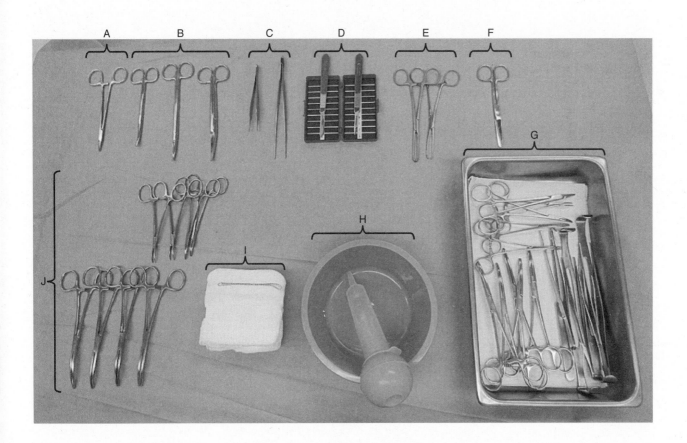

3. Examine this sterile field, identify the labeled instruments and supplies according to general type, and describe the primary purpose for each. *(For instance, the needle holders on the upper left [A] are used to handle suture needles and material while suturing tissue.)*

A. _____

   Primary purpose: _____

B. _____

   Primary purpose: _____

C. _____

   Primary purpose: _____

D. _____

    Primary purpose: _____

E. _____

    Primary purpose: _____

F. _____

    Primary purpose: _____

G. _____

    Primary purpose: _____

H. _____

    Primary purpose: _____

I. _____

    Primary purpose: _____

J. _____

    Primary purpose: _____

EXERCISE 33.6 TRUE OR FALSE: COMPREHENSIVE

Instructions: Read the following statements and write "T" for true or "F" for false in the blanks provided. If a statement is false, correct the statement to make it true.

1. _____ The main purpose for drapes is to cover the hair, which is not sterile.

2. _____ Once a towel clamp is removed from the patient, it is considered contaminated and must be removed from the surgery site and instrument table.

3. _____ Sterile stockinettes can be used as an additional drape material to allow the surgeon and surgical assistant to maneuver a leg without continually touching the skin.

4. _____ When a surgery is performed on an extremity, it is often desirable for the limb to be prepped using the hanging-limb technique.

5. _____ Oral surgeries are considered sterile procedures.

6. _____ Between uses, instruments should be placed back on the surgical table in the same location from which they came in order to have them readily accessible for both surgeon and surgical assistant.

7. _____ The handles used to adjust operating room lights should be placed before the patient is draped.

8. _____ Utilizing a surgical assistant to pass instruments is convenient for the surgeon but increases surgery time.

9. _____ Any portion of the scissors may be used for cutting suture as long as you are not in the surgeon's way.

10. _____ Bipolar (as opposed to unipolar) electrocautery is used when extreme precision is necessary.

11. _____ Iso-osmotic fluids are used for lavage of wounds and surgical sites.

12. _____ Once prepped, the skin is considered sterile.

13. _____ The urinary bladder is located in the cranial part of the abdomen.

14. _____ USP 2-0 suture is smaller in diameter than USP 2 suture.

15. _____ Suture with high memory holds knots better than suture with low memory.

16. _____ Suture material classified as absorbable loses the majority of its breaking strength in 21 days.

17. _____ Catgut absorbs in an unpredictable fashion.

18. _____ Polypropylene suture has the greatest tensile strength of all suture materials.

19. _____ Swaged needles are more traumatic to tissue.

20. _____ A taper-point needle would be the most appropriate choice for subcutaneous tissue.

21. _____ Formation of a watertight seal is an advantage of continuous suture patterns.

22. _____ The surgical nurse is vital to decreasing surgery and anesthesia time in the large animal patient.

23. _____ Irrigation during bone drilling is helpful in removing debris but is not required.

24. _____ Self-retaining retractors are critical to adequate organ exposure in equine abdominal surgery.

25. _____ Gauze sponges are an essential tool for providing hemostasis in both large and small animal patients.

EXERCISE 33.7 MULTIPLE CHOICE: COMPREHENSIVE

Instructions: Circle the one correct answer to each of the following questions.

1. When placing quarter drapes, the drape should be placed
   a. A few cm from the incision and pulled closer to the incision if needed to adjust it
   b. A few cm from the incision and pulled farther away from the incision if needed to adjust it
   c. Five to 10 cm from the incision and pulled closer to the incision if needed to adjust it
   d. Five to 10 cm from the incision and pulled farther away from the incision if needed to adjust it

2. If a surgical glove becomes contaminated during surgery, it should be
   a. Removed and replaced
   b. Covered
   c. Flushed with sterile saline
   d. Wiped clean

3. Quarter drapes are held in place by
   a. Allis tissue forceps
   b. Babcock forceps
   c. Rochester forceps
   d. Backhaus towel clamps

4. When preparing for an abdominal exploration, the patient should be placed in
   a. Right lateral recumbency
   b. Dorsal recumbency
   c. Sternal recumbency
   d. Left lateral recumbency

5. The proper patient position for a right lateral intercostal thoracotomy is
   a. Dorsal recumbency
   b. Left lateral recumbency
   c. Right lateral recumbency
   d. Sternal recumbency

6. A break in aseptic technique is most likely to occur
   a. As the patient is being prepped
   b. Interoperatively
   c. As the patient is being draped
   d. During suturing and as the drapes are being removed

7. Surgical instruments that are most commonly used should be placed in a location that the surgeon can easily access. These instruments most commonly include
   a. Retractors, scalpel, and hemostats
   b. Hemostats, needle holders, and retractors
   c. Scalpel, tissue forceps, and scissors
   d. Scissors, needle holders, and thumb forceps

8. The portions of the surgery gown that are considered sterile are
   a. Front from waist to shoulders
   b. Front and sides from waist to shoulders
   c. Front and sides from midchest to waist
   d. Front from midchest to waist

9. Scalpel blades are placed on the scalpel handle using
   a. Halstead mosquito forceps
   b. Allis tissue forceps
   c. Your fingers
   d. A needle holder

10. The suction tip that is best for suctioning large volumes of fluid out of body cavities is called the
   a. Yankauer tip
   b. Hohmann tip
   c. Poole tip
   d. Frazier tip

11. Which organ can be lifted out of the abdomen during an exploratory laparotomy, because it is very mobile?
   a. Liver
   b. Spleen
   c. Kidney
   d. Stomach

12. A dog's left kidney can be best viewed by retracting the
   a. Duodenum ventrally and to the left
   b. Descending colon and spleen to the right
   c. Ascending colon to ventrally and caudally
   d. Spleen cranially

13. Which retractors are the most appropriate choice for retracting lungs when performing a thoracotomy?
   a. Gelpi
   b. Army-Navy
   c. Malleable
   d. Senn

14. Which of the following tissues heals more slowly and therefore requires the use of nonabsorbable suture?
   a. Tendon
   b. Stomach
   c. Bladder
   d. Uterus

15. Which of the following sutures is available with an antibacterial coating?
   a. Silk
   b. Polydioxanone
   c. Catgut
   d. Polyglactin 910

16. Which suture has the best handling characteristics but stimulates inflammation?
   a. Catgut
   b. Polyglycolic acid
   c. Silk
   d. Polydioxanone

17. The most commonly used curved needles are
   a. 1/4-circle and 5/8-circle
   b. 3/8-circle and 1/2-circle
   c. 5/8-circle and 1/2-circle
   d. 3/8-circle and 1/4-circle

18. A cutting needle would be the most appropriate choice for
   a. Skin
   b. Intestine
   c. Fascia
   d. Bladder wall

19. The suture needle point recommended for suturing organs like the liver and kidney is
   a. Cutting
   b. Reverse cutting
   c. Taper
   d. Blunt

20. The closure of the equine abdominal wall usually requires
   a. USP 4-0 or 5-0 suture
   b. USP 2-0 or 3-0 suture
   c. USP 0 or 1 suture
   d. USP 2 or 3 suture

EXERCISE 33.8 CASE STUDY: SUTURE NEEDLES

You are working at a busy multiple-doctor practice as the head surgery technician. A new veterinary assistant has come to talk to you because she is confused about the different suture needles. When the doctor asked her to get one earlier in the day, she had no idea what to do. She asks you to give her some information about needles so she will have a better understanding of them and can get the proper one when asked. Explain the structure and function of suture needles, including the general shapes they come in, the different types of points, and the methods of suture attachment. In each case, discuss the circumstances under which each type is used.

a. Shapes: _____

_____

_____

_____

_____

_____

b. Needle points: _____

_____

_____

_____

_____

_____

c. Suture attachment: _____

_____

_____

_____

_____

_____

34 Small Animal Surgical Nursing

LEARNING OBJECTIVES

1. Pronounce, define, and spell all the key terms in this chapter.
2. Do the following regarding surgical preparation and animal positioning:
   - Describe the perioperative responsibilities of the veterinary technician.
   - Describe indications and use of prophylactic antibiotics.
   - Describe signs of blood loss in the postoperative patient.
   - Discuss concerns related to hypothermia in perioperative patients and be able to manage it.
   - Evaluate surgical incisions for complications and be able to removal skin sutures or staples.
3. Understand restraint of the anesthetized patient for surgical procedures.
4. Differentiate between elective and non-elective surgery.
5. List and describe perioperative considerations for commonly listed surgical procedures.
6. List considerations related to client education for discharged surgical patients.

EXERCISE 34.1 CROSSWORD PUZZLE: TERMS AND DEFINITIONS

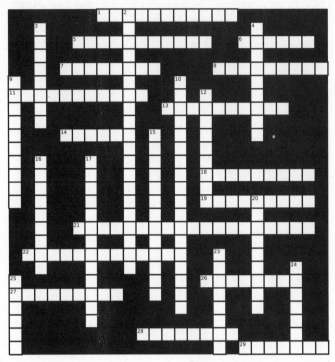

Across
1 The term used to describe low blood pressure.
5 Male cats with urologic syndrome may experience urethral _____.
6 A dog should be placed in _____ recumbency for a simple orchidectomy procedure.
7 The name of the hernia found more commonly in female dogs.
8 A common symptom of cats with urologic syndrome.
11 A specific type of collar used to prevent animals from licking and/or chewing at an affected area.
13 A term that means surgical removal of the testicles.
14 The term cesarean delivery was derived from the name of _____, who was thought to be the first person to be born by this surgical technique.
18 A specific type of hernia in which omentum and intraabdominal fat protrudes through a defect in the abdominal wall.
19 A syndrome associated with a loss of stamina in working breeds that is a complication of ovariohysterectomy.
21 A surgical procedure performed in male dogs with penile scar tissue to establish normal urine flow. (2 words)
22 The name of the hernia where a classic visual sign is a "tucked-up" abdomen.
26 Cesarean delivery is usually performed on animals experiencing _____.
27 The most critical anesthetic period for an animal with a diaphragmatic hernia.
28 _____ radiographs should be taken to confirm the diagnosis of a diaphragmatic hernia.
29 During an ovariohysterectomy procedure, before closing the abdominal wall, the _____ stump must be visualized to check for hemorrhage.

Down
2 A surgical procedure performed in male cats that experience urethral obstruction secondary to feline urologic syndrome. (2 words)
3 The removal of the scrotum at the same time as removing the testicles is called scrotal _____.
4 Some animals experiencing urologic syndrome may need lifesaving measures to protect their heart if this electrolyte value is too high.
9 A term used to describe general bleeding.
10 The surgical treatment recommended for an animal with a pyometra.
12 The term used to describe narrowing of the opening of the urethra because of excessive formation of scar tissue.
15 A complication of an umbilical hernia in which there is a loss of intestinal blood supply.
16 A term used to describe bloody urine.
17 A term used for intestinal entrapment.
20 A surgical procedure performed to remove bladder stones.
23 The drug used to increase uterine muscular contractions.
24 An alternative name for bladder stones.
25 The medical term for an internal organ.

EXERCISE 34.2 DEFINITIONS: KEY TERMS

Instructions: Define each term in your own words.

1. Abdominocentesis: _____

_____

2. Capillary refill time: _____

_____

3. Anastomosis: _____

_____

4. Arthrodesis: _____

_____

5. Enterotomy: _____

_____

6. Onychectomy: _____

_____

7. Strangulation: _____

_____

8. Thoracocentesis: _____

_____

9. Urethrostomy: _____

_____

EXERCISE 34.3 MATCHING: TERMS AND DEFINITIONS

Instructions: Match each term in column A with its corresponding definition in column B by writing the appropriate letter in the space provided.

Column A

1. _____ Evisceration
2. _____ Gastrotomy
3. _____ Intussusception
4. _____ Ileus
5. _____ Osteochondrosis
6. _____ Ostectomy
7. _____ Celiotomy
8. _____ Orchidectomy
9. _____ Dehiscence

Column B

A. The telescoping of one portion of an animal's bowel into another.

B. The surgical removal of part of a bone.

C. The surgical removal of an animal's testicles.

D. Surgical incision into the abdominal cavity.

E. The uncontrolled exposure of abdominal organs through a surgical incision as a result of trauma or dehiscence.

F. Temporary loss of intestinal motility.

G. A surgical incision made into the stomach.

H. Abnormally thickened portion of the articular cartilage.

I. Separation of the sutured layers of an incision.

Chapter **34 Small Animal Surgical Nursing**

Instructions: Read the following statements and write "T" for true or "F" for false in the blanks provided. If a statement is false, correct the statement to make it true.

1. _____ It is acceptable for surgical patients to have access to water prior to surgery.

2. _____ It is best to vaccinate a puppy or kitten the day of surgery rather than before.

3. _____ Prophylactic antibiotics should be given to all animals undergoing surgery.

4. _____ To achieve therapeutic drug levels in a surgical wound, antibiotics should be administered no less than 20 minutes prior to the first incision.

5. _____ It is not unusual for a patient's PCV and TP to drop to 10% as a result of anesthesia and surgery.

6. _____ The size of the surgical incision can affect the patient's body temperature during a surgical procedure.

7. _____ Heat lamps are a safe alternative to heating blankets to maintain adequate body temperature in an anesthetized patient.

8. _____ For small dogs and cats, it is acceptable to use a warm water bath postoperatively to raise their body temperature quickly.

9. _____ During an anesthetic procedure, the combination of an increased heart rate and low blood pressure is a direct indicator of pain, which should be managed by increasing the anesthetic levels.

10. _____ It is best to assess how much pain an animal is in postoperatively prior to administering pain medication.

11. _____ Topical antibiotic ointments can delay the healing process when applied directly to incision sites.

12. _____ Noxious-tasting agents should be placed directly on an incision to prevent licking and chewing.

13. _____ Tail docking is most commonly performed for aesthetic reasons to conform to breed standards.

14. _____ Tail docking should always be performed under anesthesia.

15. _____ Ideally, dewclaws should be removed during the first week of the animal's life.

16. _____ The medical term for surgical removal of the claw and the third phalanx associated with it is "onychectomy."

17. _____ Gastric dilation-volvulus is a condition commonly seen in toy dog breeds.

18. _____ Spaying a dog or cat during estrus does not affect the potential risks of the surgical procedure.

19. _____ Remaining ovarian tissue left from a spay procedure may result in recurrent heat cycles and stump pyometra.

20. _____ Animals that have been spayed may have an increase in body weight after the surgery.

21. _____ In preparation for canine castration, the scrotum is normally shaved and draped into the surgical field.

22. _____ Alcohol should not be used when preparing the scrotum for castration in male dogs and cats.

23. _____ Shaving scrotal hairs is an acceptable alternative to plucking scrotal hairs when prepping for feline castration.

Instructions: Circle the one correct answer to each of the following questions.

1. The surgical procedure that is most likely to require the veterinary technician to act as a surgical assistant is a(n)
   a. Orthopedic procedure
   b. Hernia repair
   c. Feline ovariohysterectomy
   d. Laceration or abscess repair

2. At what body temperature is it safe to stop using heat sources to warm the patient postoperatively?
   a. 103° F
   b. 102° F
   c. 101° F
   d. 100° F

3. Which of the following procedures would be considered least painful?
   a. Fracture repair
   b. Amputation
   c. Declaw
   d. Mass removal

4. What is the earliest that it is safe to remove sutures after a surgical procedure?
   a. 6 to 8 days
   b. 10 to 14 days
   c. 20 to 24 days
   d. 25 to 30 days

5. Which surgery would be considered a nonelective procedure?
   a. Declaw
   b. Splenectomy
   c. Castration
   d. Ovariohysterectomy

6. What is the ideal age to perform tail docking on puppies?
   a. 2 to 3 days
   b. 3 to 5 days
   c. 6 to 10 days
   d. 10 to 12 days

7. What are three known techniques used for feline claw removal?
   a. Rescoe nail trimmers, #12 scalpel blade, CO2 laser
   b. Surgical scissors, #15 scalpel blade, CO2 laser
   c. #12 scalpel blade, surgical scissors, Rescoe nail trimmers
   d. Rescoe nail trimmers, #15 scalpel blade, CO_2 laser

8. Postoperative bandages placed after an onychectomy should be removed how many hours after surgery?
   a. 12 hours
   b. 24 hours
   c. 6 hours
   d. 8 hours

9. What is not a typical early complication of an onychectomy procedure?
   a. Loose bandage
   b. Removal of the bandage by the patient
   c. Skin sloughing
   d. Hemorrhage

10. What is the proper name for surgical incision into the abdominal cavity?
    a. Celiotomy
    b. Gastrotomy
    c. Pyometra
    d. Orchidectomy

11. The most common approach to the abdominal cavity is
    a. Ventral midline
    b. Paramedian
    c. Paracostal
    d. Flank

12. What is the standard clipping for ventral midline celiotomy surgery?
    a. 2 cm cranial to xiphoid to 2 cm caudal to pubis, and to the nipples laterally
    b. 2 cm cranial to umbilicus to 2 cm caudal to pubis, and 2 to 4 cm lateral to the nipples
    c. 2 cm cranial to xiphoid to 2 cm caudal to pubis, and 2 to 4 cm lateral to the nipples
    d. 2 cm cranial to umbilicus to 2 cm caudal to pubis, and to the nipples laterally

13. What is the proper term used to describe an incision that is made into the stomach?
    a. Enterotomy
    b. Cystotomy
    c. Perineal urethrostomy
    d. Gastrotomy

14. What color should a normal gastrointestinal track be when viewed in an open abdominal surgery?
    a. Pale tan
    b. Brown
    c. Gray
    d. Pink

15. A devitalized intestinal track can be recognized by
    a. Bleeding of the cut surface
    b. Decreased motility
    c. Red discoloration
    d. Lack of fluorescein dye uptake

16. Which of the following is not a classic clinical sign of gastric dilation-volvulus?
    a. Vomiting
    b. Retching
    c. Increased appetite
    d. Distention of stomach

17. Which radiographic view of the abdomen is most beneficial when evaluating stomach rotation or bloat on a dog?
    a. Left lateral
    b. Right lateral
    c. VD
    d. DV

18. Which of the following is not a good indication for castrating a dog or cat?
    a. Decreasing population growth
    b. Treatment of perineal hernias
    c. Elimination and/or correction of aggression
    d. Prevention of reproductive system tumors

19. Which of the following is removed during a spay?
    a. Broad ligament and the ovaries
    b. Ovaries and uterus
    c. Suspensory ligament and uterine horn
    d. Oviducts and ovaries

20. A spay hook is a surgical instrument that is specifically used to
    a. Exteriorize the uterine horns
    b. Elevate the ovaries to the level of the incision
    c. Immobilize the uterine vessels
    d. Ligate the uterine body

21. When performing a spay after parturition, it should be done when the puppies or kittens are weaned and lactation ceases, or approximately
    a. 2 to 4 weeks later
    b. 4 to 6 weeks later
    c. 6 to 8 weeks later
    d. 8 to 10 weeks later

22. A condition of the uterus involving endometrial hyperplasia, increased uterine secretions, and accumulation of fluid in the uterus with secondary infection is known as
    a. Pyometra
    b. Uterine prolapse
    c. Mucometra
    d. Hydrometra

23. Which is not a major indication for feline castration?
    a. Prevent fighting
    b. Decrease urine odor
    c. Prevent roaming
    d. Decrease vocalization

24. What is the most common indication for cystotomy in small animals?
    a. Remove tumors
    b. Correct congenital defects
    c. Remove cystic calculi
    d. Repair traumatic rupture in bladder

25. The name for a hernia in which abdominal contents protrude into the thoracic cavity is
    a. Umbilical hernia
    b. Diaphragmatic hernia
    c. Inguinal hernia
    d. Abdominal hernia

26. Approximately what percentage of mammary tumors in cats are malignant?
    a. 10% to 15%
    b. 25% to 50%
    c. 50% to 60%
    d. 80% to 90%

27. The most common neurologic disorder involving the spine in dogs is
    a. Atlantoaxial subluxation
    b. Spinal trauma
    c. Lumbosacral stenosis
    d. Spontaneous intervertebral disk rupture

28. What are the first three steps that should always be performed when encountering an animal with a long-bone fracture?
    a. (1) Stabilize the animal, (2) check for open wounds associated with the fracture, and (3) immobilize the fracture.
    b. (1) Administer pain medication, (2) assess the fracture, and (3) immobilize the fracture.
    c. (1) Anesthetize the animal for emergency surgery, (2) administer pain medication, and (3) immobilize the fracture.
    d. (1) Manipulate the bones back into place, (2) administer pain medication, and (3) immobilize the fracture.

29. After long bone or joint surgery, what level of activity is most appropriate for optimal recovery?
    a. Leash walking
    b. Playing with other dogs
    c. Cage confinement
    d. Off-leash activities

Instructions: Fill in each of the spaces provided with the missing word or words that complete the sentence.

1. Evisceration is the uncontrolled exposure of organs through a surgical incision because of _____ of the wound.

2. Ileus is the term used to describe temporary loss of _____ motility.

3. _____ is an infection along tissue planes.

4. The _____ _____ _____ is the required time it takes for blood to refill small capillary beds of mucus membranes after digital blanching has occurred.

5. _____ is the term used to describe accumulation of blood serum beneath an incision site after surgery.

6. Onychectomy is the removal of the claw and the associated _____ phalanx.

7. Celiotomy (laparotomy) is a surgical incision into the _____ cavity.

8. Vomiting, retching, and severe distention of the stomach are classic signs of _____ _____.

9. Animals suffering from GVD are usually in _____, and if left untreated, the animals will die as a result of cardiovascular collapse.

10. A gastropexy is performed on the _____ ventrolateral aspect of the body wall near the last rib.

11. The primary indication for ovariohysterectomy is the prevention of _____ and subsequent production of unwanted puppies and kittens.

12. Ovariohysterectomy performed before the animal's first estrus cycle will greatly decrease the risk of _____ neoplasia in dogs.

13. Another name for false pregnancy is _____.

14. There is not an optimal age for canine castration, but it is often performed around _____ months of age.

15. _____ is the term used to describe a bacterial infection in the uterus with purulent fluid accumulation.

16. The accumulation of sterile fluid within the uterus causing a mild to moderate distention is known as _____ or _____.

17. In addition to preventing unwanted pregnancies, major indications for feline castration are to decrease urine odor and to prevent fighting, roaming, and _____ _____.

18. _____ delivery is when an incision is made into the abdominal cavity and then into the uterus to deliver a neonate.

19. Cesarean delivery is usually performed on animals that are experiencing _____.

20. _____ is the incision into the urinary bladder to expose the interior contents or lumen of the urinary bladder.

21. Perineal urethrostomy in male cats is often recommended to manage multiple episodes of _____ associated with feline urologic syndrome.

EXERCISE 34.7 CASE STUDY #1: DELIVERY OF PUPPIES BY CESAREAN SECTION

A 3-year-old pregnant female Mastiff is scheduled for a planned cesarean section tomorrow at the practice where you were recently hired. You are going to be a part of a small team that will receive and care for the newborn puppies. Wanting to provide competent care, you study your notes the night before to be sure you are prepared to assist. Also, because time is of the essence when reviving puppies delivered by cesarean, you want to prepare the necessary equipment well beforehand.

1. Besides the equipment necessary to clamp and tie off the umbilical cords, what other equipment would you prepare?

_____

_____

_____

2. What exactly will you do when you are handed the first neonate?

_____

_____

_____

_____

_____

_____

_____

_____

_____

EXERCISE 34.8 CASE STUDY #2: MONITORING FOR POSTOPERATIVE BLEEDING

You have just completed an ovariohysterectomy on a 1-year-old female bearded Collie mix named Mandy. This patient was in heat at the time of the surgery, and there was more bleeding than usual during the procedure. Although the surgery went well, the doctor has asked you to monitor this patient for intraabdominal hemorrhage postoperatively. Answer the following questions regarding management of this case.

1. What changes in this patient's vital signs and general physical findings would alert you that this serious postoperative complication was occurring?

_____

_____

_____

_____

_____

2. What general diagnostic tests could be done to help determine if intraabdominal bleeding was occurring?

_____

_____

_____

_____

_____

3. If signs of hemorrhage were observed, what general types of treatment strategies may be used for Mandy?

_____

_____

_____

_____

_____

_____

_____

_____

4. Mandy recovered uneventfully and was ready for discharge the following day. Discuss in detail the appearance of a normal incision postoperatively between the time of surgery and suture removal. Then discuss the signs that an incision is not healing normally.

a. Appearance of a normal incision postoperatively:

_____

_____

_____

_____

_____

b. Signs that an incision is not healing normally:

_____

_____

_____

_____

_____

_____

_____

_____

_____

_____

_____

_____

5. When Mandy's incision is healed, the sutures or staples will need to be removed.

   a. Typically, how many days after surgery are sutures or staples removed?

   _____

   b. Describe the procedure that will be used to remove her sutures or staples.

   _____

   _____

   _____

   _____

   _____

Find the words listed below. The words may be located horizontally, vertically, or diagonally, and may be reversed.

```
A E O E U Y P Z E T E E I R E G R A T U
I S A O T M R L N H V L A A M O R E S L
M E E N R O M D E E U D V N P S A L Y C
E A R C Z T T S O M I E G A S C L I B E
O P L S N C A L P A C I G L H T L S G A
A C T I V E T E L T S E I G A E O S E E
G M E C N R C T A O R N U E U X C E M O
C C T I T T I S S M E O Z S A D N A A O
C Y A N O S I S I A R I M I A T A E E E
Y R A M M A M N A H S T E C I L H E N P
D A Y V S G A L T A E T E S G S T M Y S
A I A A A L B E T U M D M F T M E D M R
R T E S L A K S Q R A A I O Y C B M E V
S G R A T I A I Y X E P O R T S A G R C
M H S I R T N I E O I E Y M L I Z R S I
I I N T E R V E R T E B R A L D I S C O
E L S M U A B G L A A S S L T O L U G I
L N D O Q P A S S I V E O I G V E E I A
A Z T V R E M D A A R S I N T C A B O O
E U L L E A R R D R A A O G O M R R L A
```

Seroma
GDV
Hematoma
Nose
Dehiscence
Mammary
Drain
Neoplasia
ElizabethanCollar
Lumpectomy
Active
Metastasize
Passive
Analgesics
Strikethrough
IntervertebralDisc
Formalin
Tourniquet
Radial
Germinal
Laser
Cyanosis
Ileus
LineaAlba
Gastropexy
PartialGastrectomy

35 Large Animal Surgical Nursing

LEARNING OBJECTIVES

When you have completed this chapter, you will be able to:

1. Pronounce, spell, and define all key terms in this chapter.
2. Describe the preoperative preparation needed for equine patients, as well as the responsibilities of the veterinary technician before, during, and after equine surgery, including postoperative monitoring, medication administration, bandage care, and grooming.
3. List the surgical procedures commonly performed in equine patients and describe indications and preoperative, intraoperative, and postoperative considerations for common surgical procedures in equine patients, including gastrointestinal (GI) surgery, urogenital tract surgery, orthopedic surgery, and upper respiratory tract surgery.
4. List the surgical procedures commonly performed in bovine patients and describe indications and preoperative, intraoperative, and postoperative considerations for common surgical procedures in bovine patients, including surgical procedures related to conditions of the GI tract, musculoskeletal system, respiratory system, urogenital system, reproductive system, and ophthalmic system.
5. Discuss the surgical procedures of young stock, including dehorning, castration, and umbilical hernias and infections.
6. Do the following related to small ruminants:
   - Discuss selected conditions of small ruminants related to the urinary and ophthalmic systems.
   - Describe the surgical procedures commonly performed in small ruminants, including indications and preoperative, intraoperative, and postoperative considerations for common surgical procedures in small ruminants.

Instructions: Define each term in your own words.

1. Abomasopexy: _____

   _____

2. Colpotomy: _____

   _____

3. Laparotomy: _____

   _____

4. Omentopexy: _____

   _____

5. Rumenotomy: _____

   _____

6. Pyloropexy: _____

   _____

7. Rumenostomy: _____

   _____

8. Urachus: _____

   _____

Instructions: Read the following statements and write "T" for true or "F" for false in the blanks provided. If a statement is false, correct the statement to make it true.

1. _____ An organized system to keep track of instrument preferences and glove sizes used is especially important when multiple veterinarians and/or technicians serve in a single hospital.

2. _____ An Esmarch bandage is wrapped around the limb in a spiral fashion moving from proximal to distal to a point below the surgery site.

3. _____ When performing lower limb surgery in a horse, a tourniquet may be used to assist with hemostasis. To prevent any potentially serious side effects, a tourniquet should be applied for a maximum period of 2 hours.

4. _____ To help prevent myositis during general anesthesia in the equine patient, the down forelimb should be pulled forward to minimize the pressure on the triceps and radial nerve.

5. _____ Shoes are generally removed from an equine patient following surgery to prevent them from falling off and contaminating the surgery site.

6. _____ Postoperative myopathies are painful, whereas postoperative neuropathies are not as painful for the patient.

7. _____ When a bandage is placed on an equine limb, it needs to be monitored for swelling only below the bandage.

8. _____ Urinary calculi occur frequently in the equine patient.

9. _____ Urinary calculi in the mare can sometimes be removed following epidural anesthesia and manual dilation of the urethra.

10. _____ Equine castration requires extensive surgical facilities and specialized equipment.

11. _____ Dystocia is very common in horses when compared with cattle.

12. _____ The best way to repair major fractures of long bones in horses is with screws and bone plates.

13. _____ Treatment of flexural and angular deformities is dependent upon the severity of the deformity.

14. _____ Laminitis, a serious, often life-threatening disease in the horse, is defined as inflammation of the lamina in the spine.

15. _____ Equine upper airway diseases are often diagnosed using endoscopy. Sedation is used to make sure the expensive equipment is not damaged.

16. _____ Left laryngeal hemiplegia results in the paralysis of the left arytenoid cartilage, which prevents it from being adducted during inspiration.

17. _____ Following a surgical repair of a left arytenoid paralysis, the laryngotomy incision is left open to heal by second intention.

18. _____ Dorsal displacement of the soft palate in the equine patient is usually intermittent, appears during exercise, and dissipates when the horse swallows.

19. _____ The care of food animals requires appropriate chutes and stocks, unlike those in a non-food-animal clinic.

20. _____ When placing a jugular catheter in the bovine patient, it is advisable to make a stab incision in the skin to prevent burring of the catheter.

21. _____ Many anesthetic agents used in the bovine patient are used off-label.

22. _____ Drug withdrawal times are not important in both the food-animal and non-food-animal.

23. _____ Padding for the bovine patient undergoing general anesthesia is not as important as for the equine patient.

24. _____ With appropriate wound care, many oral lacerations in the bovine patient will resolve without much treatment because of the flushing effect of the saliva, which prevents oral bacterial accumulation.

25. _____ The majority of flank laparotomies in the bovine patient are performed while the patient is standing, using local anesthetic techniques.

26. _____ The majority of lameness in cattle is caused by foot problems.

27. _____ If a bovine patient has an acute lameness, septic arthritis is a common cause.

28. _____ A caudal epidural provides a loss of sensation to everything caudal to the tuber coxae and udder.

29. _____ After removal of an ovary in the bovine patient, you need to monitor for signs of hemorrhage, as this may be a serious postoperative complication.

30. _____ An advantage of performing a C-section in the left flank of the bovine patient is that the abomasum will obstruct other viscera and prevent them from eviscerating through the incision.

31. _____ Uterine prolapse commonly occurs in first-calf heifers and often recurs in subsequent calvings.

EXERCISE 35.3 MULTIPLE CHOICE: COMPREHENSIVE

Instructions: Circle the one correct answer to each of the following questions.

1. Which animal cannot regurgitate?
   a. Bovine
   b. Porcine
   c. Equine
   d. Caprine

2. The use of elastrator bands to perform castration of calves has been associated with the development of:
   a. tetanus.
   b. seromas.
   c. hematomas.
   d. sepsis.

3. Horses are administered NSAIDs postoperatively for which of the following reasons?
   a. Antifungal and analgesic properties
   b. Antibacterial and anti-inflammatory properties
   c. Antiemetic and analgesic properties
   d. Anti-inflammatory and analgesic properties

4. Which of the following statements is true of equine limb bandages?
   a. They are kept in place until skin sutures are removed.
   b. They are placed following recovery from anesthesia.
   c. They are removed at day 2 to 3 postoperatively to check wound healing and reapplied.
   d. A and C are correct.

5. The most common surgical approach to the equine abdominal cavity is through a
   a. Lateral flank incision
   b. Ventral midline incision
   c. Paramedian incision
   d. Paracostal incision

6. Which type of hernia is usually congenital?
   a. Umbilical
   b. Inguinal
   c. Incisional
   d. Hiatal

7. One of the most common intravenous drug combinations used for equine castration is
   a. Xylazine/lidocaine
   b. Lidocaine/ketamine
   c. Xylazine/ketamine
   d. Lidocaine/thiobarbiturate

8. The most common cause of equine ovarian disease necessitating removal of the ovary is
   a. Benign tumors
   b. Neoplasia
   c. Ovarian cysts
   d. Ectopic pregnancy

9. Mares with abnormal conformation can develop
   a. Pneumovagina and vaginal prolapse
   b. Pneumovagina and pneumouterus
   c. Pneumouterus and uterine prolapse
   d. Vaginal prolapse and uterine prolapse

10. Vesicovaginal reflux can lead to
    a. Endometrial inflammation
    b. Vaginal inflammation
    c. Bladder inflammation
    d. Kidney inflammation

11. Myositis is damage to or inflammation of:
    a. muscles.
    b. bones.
    c. nerves.
    d. lungs.

12. Laminitis rarely occurs in horses of less than _____ year(s) of age.
    a. 7
    b. 5
    c. 3
    d. 1

13. Prior to general anesthesia, feed should be withheld from an adult food-animal patient for
    a. 6 to 12 hours
    b. 12 to 24 hours
    c. 18 to 36 hours
    d. 36 to 48 hours

14. The NSAID that is licensed for use in the bovine patient is
    a. Flunixin
    b. Phenylbutazone
    c. Rimadyl
    d. Aspirin

15. Which regional analgesic technique involves injection of lidocaine cranial to transverse processes of L1, L2, and L3 in the bovine patient?
    a. Line block
    b. Inverted-L block
    c. Distal paravertebral block
    d. Proximal paravertebral block

16. Which regional analgesic technique involves injection of lidocaine vertically behind the last rib and horizontally below the transverse processes of the lumbar vertebrae?
    a. Line block
    b. Inverted-L block
    c. Distal paravertebral block
    d. Proximal paravertebral block

17. Which regional analgesic technique involves injection of lidocaine directly over the incision?
    a. Line block
    b. Inverted-L block
    c. Distal paravertebral block
    d. Proximal paravertebral block

18. Which regional analgesic technique involves injection of lidocaine parallel to transverse processes of the vertebrae L1, L2, and L4?
    a. Line block
    b. Inverted-L block
    c. Distal paravertebral block
    d. Proximal paravertebral block

19. What bovine disease may lead to peritonitis, liver or reticular abscesses, pericarditis, or vagal indigestion?
    a. Traumatic reticuloperitonitis
    b. Abomasal displacement
    c. Osteomyelitis
    d. Abomasal volvulus

20. A rumenotomy is performed by entering the patient's abdomen from an incision made in the
    a. Right flank
    b. Left flank
    c. Ventral midline
    d. Dorsal midline

21. For a patient with traumatic reticuloperitonitis, the surgery is performed by entering the patient's abdomen from an incision made in the
    a. Right flank
    b. Left flank
    c. Ventral midline
    d. Dorsal midline

22. Abomasal displacements are most likely to occur in the first _____ weeks after parturition.
    a. 6
    b. 8
    c. 12
    d. 16

23. In a bovine patient with foot problems, which claws are most likely involved because they are the weight-bearing claws?
    a. Front lateral and hind medial
    b. Front medial and hind medial
    c. Front lateral and hind lateral
    d. Front medial and hind lateral

24. In obstructive urolithiasis, the most common site of obstruction in cattle is the
    a. Tip of the prepuce
    b. Proximal sigmoid flexure
    c. Glans penis
    d. Distal sigmoid flexure

25. The procedure used as a salvage surgery in feedlot steers and bulls of low economic value with obstructive urolithiasis is the
    a. Ischial urethrostomy
    b. Perineal urethrostomy
    c. Ischial urethrectomy
    d. Perineal urethrectomy

26. Which specific retention suture is used in cows with vaginal or uterine prolapse?
    a. Buhner
    b. Mattress
    c. Inverted
    d. Everted

27. Cattle with pendulous sheaths, long prepuces, large preputial orifices, and the absence of retractor prepuce muscles are prone to
    a. Obstructive urolithiasis
    b. Preputial prolapse
    c. Paraphimosis
    d. Phimosis

28. The best time to dehorn a calf with a dehorning iron is at an age of
    a. 1 month
    b. 3 months
    c. 6 months
    d. 12 months

29. Which bovine castration method has been linked to the development of tetanus?
    a. Pulling the testicles until cord breaks
    b. Crushing the cord with an emasculotome
    c. Application of an elastrator band
    d. Transecting and breaking the cord

30. Entropion is the most common ocular disease of
    a. Neonatal calves
    b. Neonatal lambs
    c. Neonatal goats
    d. Neonatal foals

EXERCISE 35.4 CASE STUDY #1: EPIDURAL ANESTHESIA IN A MARE

A 3-year-old mare is presented with breeding problems. Upon examination, the veterinarian diagnoses urine pooling in her cranial vaginal cavity. After discussing the situation with the owner, the veterinarian elects to perform standing surgery on the mare the following day to repair the floor of the vagina, so that she can still potentially be used this breeding season. The veterinarian informs you that you will be administering the epidural anesthesia on the mare.

1. A veterinary assistant who is new to the practice asks you to explain what supplies you will need, what agent will you use, how you will do the epidural, what area will be numb, and if she needs to be aware of any side effects, as she will be holding the mare at the front of the stocks. How would you answer these questions?

    a. Supplies you will need: _____

    _____

    _____

    b. The agent you will use: _____

    _____

c. How you will do the procedure: _____

_____

_____

_____

_____

_____

d. The area that will be affected: _____

_____

e. Side effects: _____

_____

_____

EXERCISE 35.5 CASE STUDY #2: FORELIMB FRACTURE IN A HORSE

Your clinic receives a call that a 4-year-old thoroughbred stallion has injured his right forelimb. You and the DVM jump in the truck and drive to the track to evaluate the horse. Once radiographs are taken and processed, the DVM determines that the patient has a phalangeal fracture of his right forelimb and should be transported to the clinic for surgical repair. The owner agrees, and the DVM instructs you to place a splint on the horse for transport to the clinic.

1. Which type of splint will you use for this limb?

_____

2. You then discuss with the owner the safest way to trailer the horse for the ride to the clinic. What do you tell him?

_____

_____

_____

_____

_____

_____

EXERCISE 35.6 CASE STUDY #3: LEFT DISPLACED ABOMASUM (LDA) IN A COW

The clinic veterinarian is out on a farm call and calls to tell you she is sending a cow to the clinic that she suspects of having an LDA. The "ping" was not as definitive as she would have liked, and she wants to be sure of the diagnosis before surgery. She asks you to perform a Liptak test to confirm the diagnosis. She is sending the cow to the clinic for the test, as the farm she is from is all muddy from the recent heavy rain, and she is concerned about contamination. The cow will have surgery if the test confirms the diagnosis. She wants you to call her when you are done with the test so she is aware of the results. If the results are positive, she wants you to prepare the cow for surgery so that she can perform the surgery as soon as she arrives back at the clinic, before completing the rest of her appointments.

1. Explain how to do the Liptak test and what the test will show if the cow does indeed have an LDA.

    a. Liptak test procedure: _____

    _____

    _____

    _____

    b. What the test will show: _____

    _____

2. You call the veterinarian to tell her the results of the test, and she tells you to go ahead and get the cow ready for surgery. She will be using a left flank approach and wants you to use the distal paravertebral technique to anesthetize the area. She is confident in your ability to perform this block and that the cow will be properly prepared when she returns to perform the surgery.

    a. Describe the procedure for performing this block.

    _____

    _____

    _____

    _____

    _____

    _____

    _____

    _____

    b. What nerves are blocked using this technique?

    _____

    _____

    _____

413

36 Veterinary Dentistry

LEARNING OBJECTIVES

When you have completed this chapter, you will be able to:

1. Pronounce, define, and spell all of the key terms in this chapter.
2. Be familiar with terminology used in veterinary dentistry to designate location and direction; describe the modified Triadan system for numbering teeth; and describe normal occlusion in dogs and cats, common malocclusions, and orthodontic treatment in small animals.
3. Discuss aspects of the complete medical history as they relate to veterinary dentistry, and describe aspects of extra-oral and intraoral examinations in dogs and cats.
4. Describe equipment and supplies used for dental radiography, and compare paralleling, bisecting angle, and occlusal techniques in dental radiography.
5. Differentiate between the types of periodontal disease seen in dogs and cats, including stomatitis, gingivitis, and periodontitis. State the goal of periodontal debridement.
6. Describe equipment and procedures for professional dental cleaning using power and hand scalers, and explain methods for sharpening dental instruments.
7. Discuss the rationale and procedures for polishing teeth.
8. Compare and contrast regional nerve blocks for oral surgery for dogs and cats.
9. Explain the grading system for periodontal disease and the importance of home care in veterinary dentistry.
10. Discuss indications for restorative dentistry, endodontics, and exodontics.
11. Describe common dental conditions seen in small animals.
12. List and describe equine dental clinical practices, as well as common problems and treatments.

414

EXERCISE 36.1 CROSSWORD PUZZLE: TERMS AND DEFINITIONS

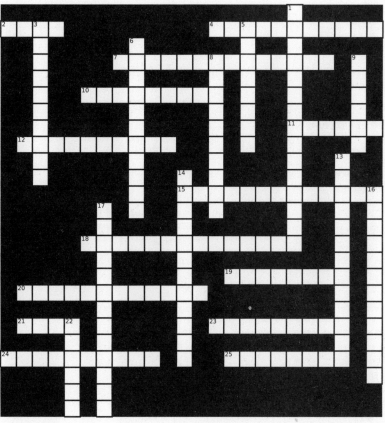

Across
2 The tip of the tooth root.
4 The study and treatment of the inside of the tooth and periapical tissues.
7 The condition in which the mandible is abnormally short in relation to the maxilla.
10 The area between the roots of a multirooted tooth.
11 Tooth decay that results from demineralization of hard tooth structures by acid-producing oral bacteria.
12 Term for mammals that have two sets of teeth (primary and deciduous).
15 The term used to indicate an upper jaw that is wider than the lower jaw (normal in most species).
18 Having a wide skull and a short maxilla.
19 Light brown or yellow, raised, mineralized deposit adherent to the tooth and root surfaces.
20 Anatomic term describing the attachment structures of the teeth.
21 Tooth structure that consists of nerves, blood vessels, lymphatics, and connective tissue.
23 Tooth type that has a large reserve crown and root structure that allows for continued growth over an animal's lifetime.
24 Diffuse inflammation of the entire oral cavity.
25 Hard layer covering the surface of the root of a tooth.

Down
1 Having a narrow skull and long maxilla.
3 The extraction of diseased teeth.
5 Gap between teeth seen normally in many species.
6 Tooth type in which the crown is relatively small compared with the size of the well-developed roots.
8 Inflammation of the gingiva.
9 Thin layer covering the crown that is the hardest tooth substance.
13 The most commonly used system of numbering teeth. (2 words)
14 Misalignment of the teeth or jaws.
16 Having a well-proportioned skull width and maxillary length.
17 Inflammation of the gingiva and other supporting tooth structures.
22 A white-tan film that collects on teeth and is composed of bacteria, exfoliated cells, food debris, and saliva.

Chapter **36** Veterinary Dentistry

Instructions: Match each description in column A with its corresponding anatomic or directional term that is used to describe the location of a structure or lesion in column B by writing the appropriate letter in the space provided.

Column A

1. _____ Portion of the tooth that is closest to the most caudal portion of the dental arch.

2. _____ Structure that is closer to the front of the head in comparison with another structure.

3. _____ A portion of the tooth closer to the tip of the root.

4. _____ The surface facing the lips that is visible from the front (in the case of incisors).

5. _____ The surface of the mandibular teeth adjacent to the tongue.

6. _____ Closer to the crown of the tooth in relation to another structure.

7. _____ The surface facing the lips or vestibule (also called buccal or labial).

8. _____ The surface of maxillary teeth adjacent to the palate.

9. _____ Toward the back of the head in comparison with another structure.

10. _____ Portion of the tooth in line with the dental arcade that is closest to the most rostral portion of the midline of the dental arch.

Column B

A. Rostral

B. Caudal

C. Vestibular

D. Facial

E. Lingual

F. Palatal

G. Mesial

H. Distal

I. Apical

J. Coronal

EXERCISE 36.3 MATCHING #2: TRIADAN NUMBERING SYSTEM

Instructions: Using the numeric Triadan system for tooth identification saves time when performing detailed dental charting. Match each canine or feline tooth listed with its corresponding Triadan number by writing the appropriate number in the space provided. (Refer to Figures 36-3 and 36-4 in the textbook for these numbers.) Recall that not all teeth are present in a normal adult cat and should be noted accordingly as "not present" if the tooth listed is not present in a normal adult cat.

1. _____ Canine left maxillary second incisor tooth.

2. _____ Feline right mandibular third premolar tooth.

3. _____ Canine left maxillary second molar tooth.

4. _____ Canine right maxillary canine tooth.

5. _____ Feline left mandibular second premolar tooth.

6. _____ Feline right mandibular third incisor tooth.

7. _____ Canine right maxillary fourth premolar tooth.

8. _____ Feline right maxillary first premolar tooth.

9. _____ Canine right mandibular third molar tooth.

10. _____ Feline left mandibular fourth premolar tooth.

11. _____ Canine deciduous right maxillary first incisor tooth.

12. _____ Feline deciduous left mandibular canine tooth.

416

EXERCISE 36.4 MATCHING #3: CLINICAL STAGES OF PERIODONTAL DISEASE

Instructions: Match each clinical description in column A with its corresponding grade of periodontal disease in column B by writing the appropriate letter in the space provided. (Note that responses may be used more than once.)

Column A

1. _____ Root débridement, gingival curettage, and periodontal surgery are often required.

2. _____ Inflammatory changes are confined to the gingiva (gingivitis).

3. _____ Root débridement or subgingival curettage *may* be required.

4. _____ Periodontitis where 50% or more of the attachment structures of the tooth have been lost.

5. _____ Early form of periodontitis.

6. _____ This grade is easily reversible with a routine dental cleaning.

7. _____ Periodontitis where 25% to 50% of attachment structures of the tooth have been lost.

8. _____ Epithelial attachment loss is present.

9. _____ Fair to guarded prognosis to save affected teeth.

10. _____ Frequently affected teeth cannot be saved.

Column B

A. Grade I periodontal disease

B. Grade II periodontal disease

C. Grade III periodontal disease

D. Grade IV periodontal disease

EXERCISE 36.5 MATCHING #4: HOME DENTAL CARE BRUSHING TECHNIQUES

Instructions: Match each description in column A with its corresponding brushing technique in column B by writing the appropriate letter in the space provided. (Note that responses may be used more than once.)

Column A

1. _____ Toothbrush bristles are placed along the gingival margin and the sulcus.

2. _____ A gentle sweeping motion of toothbrush bristles is directed apical to coronal.

3. _____ Toothbrush bristles do not enter the sulcus.

4. _____ The bristles are directed at a 45-degree angle toward the marginal gingiva.

5. _____ Toothbrush bristles are placed apical to the gingival margin.

6. _____ Toothbrush bristles enter the gingival sulcus.

7. _____ A mesial to distal motion of brushing is employed.

8. _____ Sometimes used in areas of periodontal surgery.

Column B

A. Bass brushing technique

B. Modified Stillman brushing technique

EXERCISE 36.6 MATCHING #5: LOCAL ANESTHETIC AGENTS

Instructions: Match each characteristic in column A with its corresponding local anesthetic agent in column B by writing the appropriate letter in the space provided. (Note that responses may be used more than once.)

Column A

1. _____ Onset of effect in 4 to 20 minutes.

2. _____ Onset of effect in 3 to 5 minutes.

3. _____ Duration of action 1.5 to 2 hours.

4. _____ Duration of action 4 to 10 hours.

5. _____ Most commonly used local anesthetic in veterinary dentistry

Column B

A. Bupivacaine 0.5%

B. Lidocaine 2%

EXERCISE 36.7 MATCHING #6: DENTAL NERVE BLOCKS

Instructions: Match each description in column A with its corresponding dental nerve block in column B by writing the appropriate letter in the space provided. (Note that responses may be used more than once.)

Column A

1. _____ For this block, the needle is placed 0.5 cm deep into the caudal hard palate of the cat and 1 cm deep into the caudal hard palate of the dog.

2. _____ The foramen for this block is located dorsal to the maxillary third premolar.

3. _____ This block affects sensation of the soft tissue and bone of the entire ipsilateral mandible.

4. _____ This block may cause numbness of the tongue and therefore self-inflicted trauma.

5. _____ The foramen for this block is located ventral to the mesial root of the mandibular second premolar.

6. _____ The foramen for this block is located caudal and ventral to the mandibular third molar in the dog and the mandibular first molar in the cat.

7. _____ This block requires a needle that is bent 1 cm from the tip.

8. _____ This block is placed just caudal to the maxillary second molar in the dog or the maxillary first molar in the cat.

9. _____ This block helps prevent sensation to the ipsilateral mandible rostral to the labial frenulum.

10. _____ Lidocaine may be the preferred local anesthetic for this block.

11. _____ This block causes a loss of sensation rostral only to the third premolar on the ipsilateral maxilla.

12. _____ This block prevents sensation of the entire maxillary quadrant on the buccal and palatal sides of the teeth.

13. _____ This block has an intraoral and extraoral approach described.

Column B

A. Infraorbital nerve block

B. Middle mental nerve block

C. Inferior alveolar nerve block

D. Maxillary nerve block

Instructions: Answer the questions for each picture.

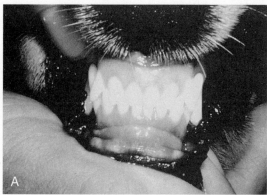

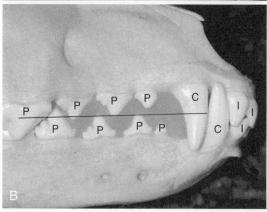

1. Identify this type of occlusion.

   _____

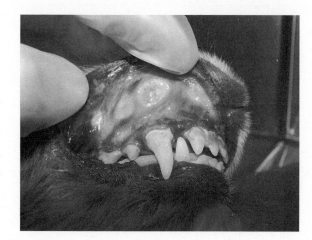

2. Identify this lesion in the dog.

   _____

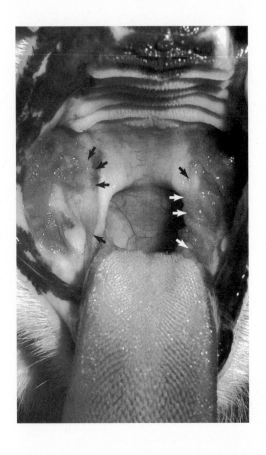

3. Identify this lesion in the cat that is lateral to the palatoglossal folds (see arrows).

_____

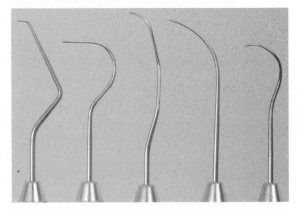

4. Identify these instruments and their uses.

_____

_____

_____

_____

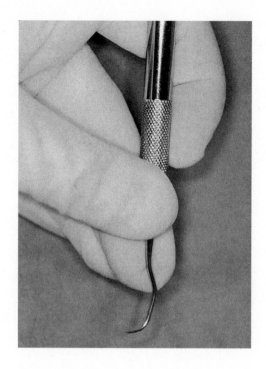

5. Identify this method of holding a dental instrument.

_____

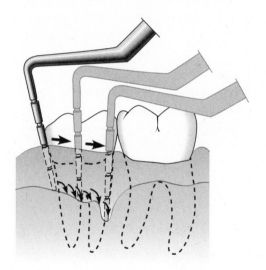

6. Identify this instrument and describe its proper use.

_____

_____

_____

_____

_____

_____

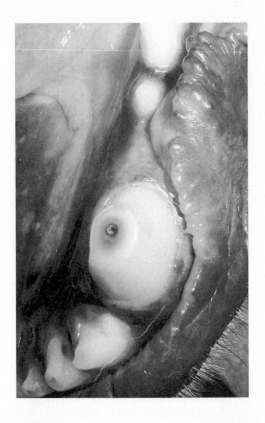

7. Identify this lesion. What instrument is used to confirm the diagnosis?

_____

_____

8. Identify this radiographic technique.

_____

_____

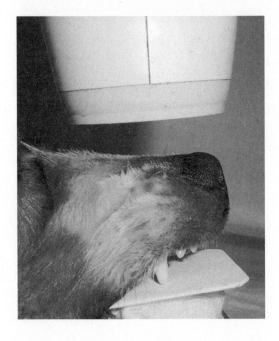

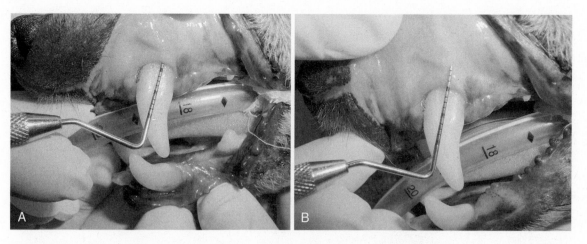

9. Based on this picture, what is the measurement of the gingival sulcus of this patient?

_____ mm

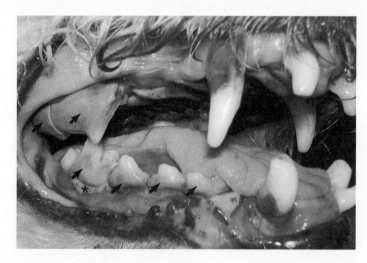

10. Based on this picture, what type of bone loss is occurring? How do you differentiate this from other types of bone loss?

_____

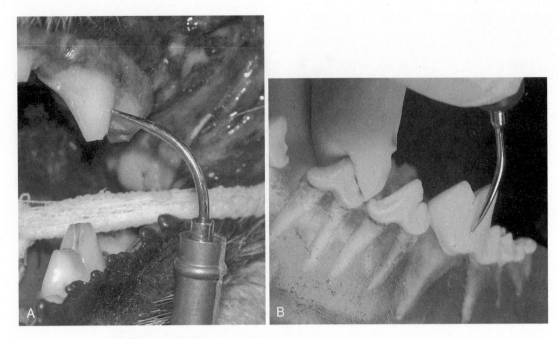

11. Which picture (A or B) depicts the correct angulation of the ultrasonic scaler tip?

_____

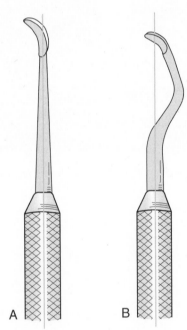

12. Which instrument (A or B) is better used for scaling the rostral portion of the mouth?

_____

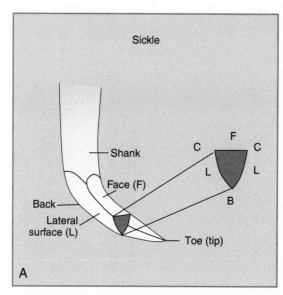

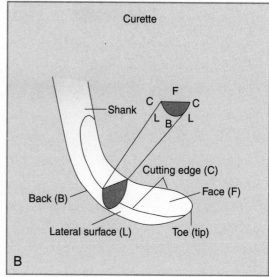

13. Identify where you would use each instrument (A and B) and the toe shape, back shape, and cross-sectional shape.

    a. Sickle scaler:

       i. Location of use _____

      ii. Toe shape _____

     iii. Back shape _____

     iv. Cross-sectional shape _____

    b. Curette:

       i. Location of use _____

      ii. Toe shape _____

     iii. Back shape _____

     iv. Cross-sectional shape _____

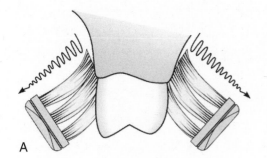

A

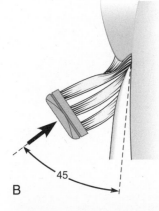

B

14. Identify the brushing techniques in A and B.

A. _____

B. _____

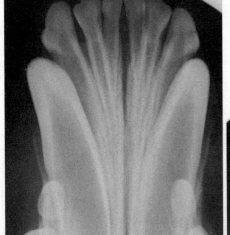

A

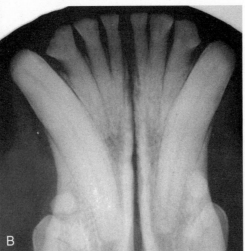

B

15. Which patient is older: A or B? How do you know this from looking at the radiographs?

_____

_____

_____

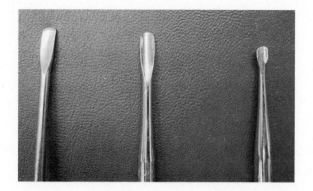

16. Identify each instrument form, left to right.

    Left: _____

    Middle: _____

    Right: _____

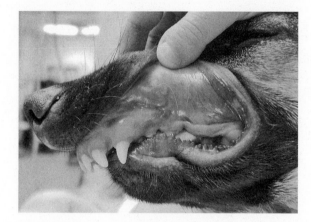

17. Identify this malocclusion by class.

    _____

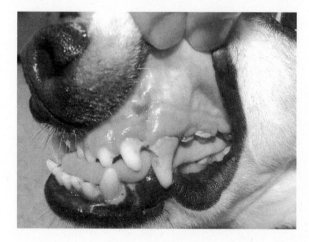

18. Identify this malocclusion by class.

    _____

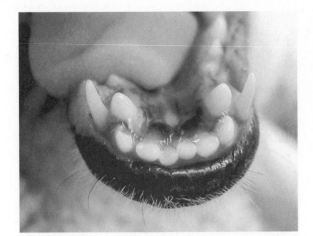

19. Identify the two disease states present in this patient.

    a. _____

    b. _____

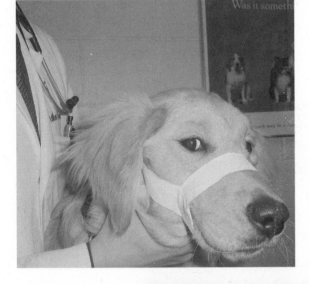

20. Describe this therapy and the most likely reason for its use.

    a. Therapy: _____

    b. Reason for its use: _____

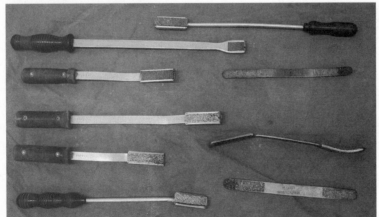

21. Identify these instruments, their use, and the species in which they are used.

    a. Instruments: _____

    b. What they are used for: _____

    c. Species: _____

Instructions: Read the following statements and write "T" for true or "F" for false in the blanks provided. If a statement is false, correct the statement to make it true.

1. _____ Each dental or oral surgical procedure should begin with a comprehensive extraoral and intraoral examination.

2. _____ Alveolar mucosa refers to the mucosa that begins at the mucocutaneous junction and lines the cheeks and lips.

3. _____ When performing an intraoral examination, missing teeth should be documented on the dental chart by placing an "X" through the missing tooth.

4. _____ The normal gingival sulcus depth is 0 to 3 mm in dogs and 0 to 1 mm in cats.

5. _____ Probing depths greater than normal should be documented on the dental chart as pockets.

6. _____ Abrasion refers to the normal wear associated with tooth-to-tooth contact of a patient over time with normal mastication.

7. _____ During periodontal examination of multirooted teeth, a bifurcation should be assessed from the buccal and lingual-palatal surfaces.

8. _____ Many dental x-ray units have an internally set level of kilovoltage and milliamperes, and only exposure time may be changed for a darker or lighter technique.

9. _____ Intraoral packaged film is the standard of the industry, used since the 1920s.

10. _____ To ensure good diagnostic quality, the dental sensor may be held in the patient's mouth, provided appropriate protective gear is worn by the handler.

11. _____ Direct method computed digital radiography involves the use of an electronic intraoral sensor, a computer, and the x-ray machine to capture the image and convert it to the digital format of pixels.

12. _____ The epithelial attachment to the tooth crown forms the bottom of the gingival sulcus, which is a moat-like structure surrounding the tooth.

13. _____ Early in the formation of plaque, the bacterial population consists mainly of endotoxin-producing Gram-positive anaerobic rods and spirochetes.

14. _____ When performing a dental cleaning, the most important patient safety precaution is to intubate the patient and check to ensure that the endotracheal tube cuff is fully inflated.

15. _____ Standard-size universal and broad-tip ultrasonic scalers are designed to provide better access to subgingival pockets and furcation areas.

16. _____ The ultrasonic scaler tip should be directed at a 90-degree angle toward the tooth surface to avoid damaging the enamel.

17. _____ A curette with a straight shank in relation to the long axis of the handle is best suited for use on rostral teeth.

18. _____ If the face of a curette is offset at an angle of 60 to 70 degrees, as in Gracey curettes, the instrument is considered to be area specific, and only one of the cutting edges may be adapted to the tooth.

19. _____ Sickle scalers are used to scale the crowns of the teeth and have a sharp tip that will cause lacerations if the instrument is used subgingivally.

20. _____ When sharpening hand instruments, the angle between the stone and the face should be no greater than 85 degrees.

21. _____ Sharpening stones typically used for dental instruments include Arkansas, India, ceramic, and a synthetic composition that differs in coarseness and the type of lubricant required to reduce heat friction.

22. _____ No restorative material is as strong as the original tooth structure.

23. _____ Pins and posts used in restorative dentistry add strength to the restoration.

24. _____ As an animal ages, the pulp chamber and root canal become narrower as a result of the continued production of secondary dentin.

25. _____ Dental radiographs are not needed when performing endodontics.

26. _____ Exodontics involves relatively straightforward and complication-free procedures.

27. _____ Complicated tooth fractures can lead to the formation of a periapical abscess, facial swelling, and draining tracts.

28. _____ Complicated tooth fractures should be monitored for a period of time before endodontic or exodontic therapy is performed.

29. _____ Tooth root abscesses in the horse have similar causes compared to those seen in the dog and cat.

30. _____ Horses do not get dental caries.

EXERCISE 36.10 MULTIPLE CHOICE: COMPREHENSIVE

Instructions: Circle the one correct answer to each of the following questions.

1. The radicular hypsodont type of dental morphology is found in which species?
   a. Rabbits
   b. Horses
   c. Cats
   d. Pigs

2. The canine and feline teeth used for shearing and grinding are the
   a. Canines
   b. Molars
   c. Premolars
   d. Both B and C

3. How many permanent teeth are there in the normal adult canine dentition?
   a. 32
   b. 36
   c. 42
   d. 44

4. At what age would a cat be expected to have all of its permanent teeth erupted?
   a. 6 months
   b. 8 months
   c. 10 months
   d. 12 months

5. Which of the clinical symptoms of oral disease may be manifested later in the disease process?
   a. Rubbing the face along furniture
   b. Anorexia
   c. Dropping food
   d. Pawing at the mouth

6. The only easily palpable major salivary gland of the dog and cat is the
   a. Sublingual
   b. Parotid
   c. Zygomatic
   d. Mandibular

7. Which tissue would not be considered part of the periodontium?
   a. Alveolar bone
   b. Gingival connective tissue
   c. Dentin
   d. Cementum

8. The instrument used to measure gingival sulcus depth is a periodontal
   a. Explorer
   b. Curette
   c. Probe
   d. Scaler

9. When performing dental radiographs, which technique is most useful for obtaining images of the mandibular teeth caudal to the second premolars?
   a. Bisecting angle technique
   b. Occlusal technique
   c. Paralleling technique
   d. Cone-cutting technique

10. Which anatomic structure would be the most radiopaque on a dental radiograph?
    a. Cementum
    b. Enamel
    c. Dentin
    d. Lamina dura

11. Once plaque has formed on a tooth, how long does it take to mineralize if left undisturbed?
    a. 1 day
    b. 3 days
    c. 7 days
    d. 2 weeks

12. For operator safety, what is the appropriate protective equipment that should be worn during a dental cleaning procedure?
    a. Gown, mask, gloves
    b. Cap, eye protection, gloves
    c. Mask, eye protection, gloves
    d. Gown, eye protection, gloves

13. Intrinsic staining of the teeth that is often seen on the occlusal surface of maxillary molars in dogs would not be caused by
    a. Trauma
    b. Tetracycline antibiotics during tooth development
    c. Food pigments
    d. Developmental defects

14. According to the Mobility Scoring Index, how would a patient's tooth be classified if mobility were increased in any direction other than axial over a distance of more than 0.5 mm and up to 1.0 mm?
    a. Stage 0 (M0)
    b. Stage 1 (M1)
    c. Stage 2 (M2)
    d. Stage 3 (M3)

15. Which form of local anesthetic delivery is most commonly used in veterinary dentistry?
    a. Splash block
    b. Local infiltration
    c. Regional anesthesia
    d. Both B and C

16. Which of the following is an example of regional anesthesia?
    a. Placing bupivacaine in an open wound to provide topical anesthesia
    b. Placing lidocaine at the foramen of the infraorbital nerve
    c. Placing bupivacaine into the periodontal ligament of the left maxillary fourth premolar
    d. Placing lidocaine into the periodontal ligament of the right mandibular first molar

17. Which of the following is/are reasons that bupivacaine 0.5% is commonly used in veterinary dentistry?
    a. Long duration of action
    b. Intraoperative pain management
    c. Postoperative pain relief
    d. All of the above

18. What is the maximum safe dose for bupivacaine 0.5% for the dog?
    a. 1 mg/kg
    b. 1.5 mg/kg
    c. 2 mg/kg
    d. 3 mg/kg

19. What is the maximum safe dose for bupivacaine 0.5% for the cat?
    a. 1 mg/kg
    b. 1.5 mg/kg
    c. 2 mg/kg
    d. 3 mg/kg

20. Which grade of periodontal disease often requires tooth extraction?
    a. I
    b. II
    c. III
    d. IV

21. What is the minimum depth of a periodontal pocket in which doxycycline can be placed?
    a. 3 mm
    b. 4 mm
    c. 6 mm
    d. 7 mm

22. Why is doxycycline gel a drug of choice for the treatment of periodontal pockets?
    a. It has good antimicrobial spectrum against periodontal pathogens.
    b. It has anti-inflammatory effects.
    c. It has a space-occupying effect, which prevents food and debris from filling the pocket.
    d. All of the above are reasons for using doxycycline gel.

23. What is recommended as an antibacterial oral rinse when treating periodontal disease?
   a. 0.12% chlorhexidine
   b. 1.2% chlorhexidine
   c. 0.2% chlorhexidine
   d. 2% chlorhexidine

24. Attempts to save teeth with advanced periodontal surgery should not be performed unless the client is able to
   a. Apply a 2% chlorhexidine rinse.
   b. Consent to doxycycline gel therapy.
   c. Perform daily tooth brushing.
   d. Provide a soft-food diet for the rest of the patient's life.

25. Why are human toothpastes not used for tooth brushing in veterinary patients?
   a. They cause gingival ulceration.
   b. The mint flavoring is toxic.
   c. They can cause stomach upset if swallowed.
   d. Both B and C

26. Which type of diet is best to help control plaque?
   a. A diet that has been manufactured and tested to reduce plaque accumulation
   b. Any diet of hard foods is appropriate.
   c. Soft diets are best in order to avoid gingival trauma from hard abrasive foods.
   d. All veterinary diets now provide plaque control.

27. Which organization has been established to recognize products that have been shown to meet predetermined standards of plaque and calculus retardation?
   a. The Veterinary Oral Health Council (VOHC)
   b. The American Veterinary Medical Association (AVMA)
   c. The American Veterinary Dental College (AVDC)
   d. The Food and Drug Administration (FDA)

28. How do mechanical cleansing diets help prevent plaque and tartar accumulation?
   a. Long fibers oriented in one direction within a large kibble are designed to scrape the side of the teeth as the teeth penetrate the kibble.
   b. Crisscrossed fibers oriented in a large kibble are designed to scrape the side of the teeth as the teeth penetrate the kibble.
   c. Small particles of digestible vegetable carbohydrate are placed in the large kibble designed to scrape the side of the teeth as the teeth penetrate the kibble.
   d. Microscopic particles of inert silica are placed in the large kibble designed to scrape the side of the teeth as the teeth penetrate the kibble.

29. What is the function of HMP in a chemical cleansing diet that helps prevent plaque and tartar accumulation?
   a. HMP decreases the production of saliva, which contains the minerals associated with tartar accumulation.
   b. HMP sequesters calcium in plaque fluids effectively preventing the mineralization of plaque.
   c. HMP binds with magnesium in order to decrease mineral deposition in plaque.
   d. HMP generates a thermal response in the oral cavity that effectively kills plaque-forming organisms.

30. Which of the following chew toys has no potential for harmful effects when used to help prevent plaque and tartar accumulation?
   a. Rawhide chews
   b. Cow hooves
   c. Hard nylon bones
   d. All of the choices listed above have some potential harmful effects.

31. Which of the following are indications for restorative dentistry?
   a. Dental caries
   b. Fractured teeth
   c. Endodontically treated teeth
   d. All of the above

32. Which type of dental crown has the greatest strength and requires less tooth removal?
   a. Porcelain
   b. Metal
   c. Zirconium
   d. Both A and C

33. On which teeth of the dog are crowns more commonly placed?
   a. Canines and mandibular first molars
   b. Maxillary fourth premolars and mandibular first molars
   c. Canines and maxillary fourth premolars
   d. Canines and maxillary first molars

34. What is the usual minimal age that conventional root canal therapy is usually performed on dogs and cats?
   a. 6 months of age
   b. 12 months of age
   c. 15 months of age
   d. 18 months of age

35. What does the term CUPS refer to?
   a. Chronic ulcerative papillary sepsis
   b. Chronic ulcerative paradental stomatitis
   c. Caustic ulcerative papillary stomatitis
   d. Canine upper premolar syndrome

36. Which of the following is/are indications for exodontics?
    a. A grave prognosis for saving a tooth
    b. Owner financial constraints that preclude use of salvage techniques
    c. Multiple anesthetic episodes are contraindicated
    d. All of the above are indications for exodontics

37. Once exodontia is performed, what is recommended as a lavage solution?
    a. Sodium hypochlorite
    b. Isotonic saline
    c. 0.12% chlorhexidine solution
    d. Both B and C

38. What is the suture type and pattern recommended to close an exodontic area?
    a. 4-0 or 5-0 absorbable braided in a simple interrupted pattern
    b. 4-0 or 5-0 absorbable monofilament in a simple interrupted pattern
    c. 4-0 or 5-0 nonabsorbable monofilament in a simple continuous pattern
    d. 4-0 or 5-0 nonabsorbable braided in a simple continuous pattern

39. In what location are feline resorptive lesions usually seen clinically?
    a. Cervical (neck) region
    b. Apex of the root
    c. Occlusal surface of the crown
    d. All locations are equally seen

40. What is the treatment of choice for cats with tooth resorption?
    a. Deep root planing followed by fluoride gel
    b. Root canal followed by crown restoration with glass ionomer
    c. Exodontics
    d. Nothing, because cats rarely have clinical signs with tooth resorption

41. Which of the following is *not* an example of a class I malocclusion (neutroclusion)?
    a. The mandible is relatively shorter than the maxilla.
    b. The mandibular canines are lingually displaced.
    c. The maxillary incisors are positioned lingual to the mandibular incisors.
    d. A maxillary premolar is positioned lingual to the opposing mandibular premolar.

42. Mandibular brachygnathism (mandibular distoclusion) belongs to which class of malocclusion?
    a. I
    b. II
    c. III
    d. IV

43. Mandibular prognathism (mandibular mesioclusion) belongs to which class of malocclusion?
    a. I
    b. II
    c. III
    d. IV

44. Dolichocephalic skull types are typical of
    a. Persian cats
    b. Labrador Retrievers
    c. Greyhounds
    d. Boxers

45. Which of the following is true for dental impressions?
    a. Dental impressions are important in the treatment plan for orthodontic disease.
    b. Alginate is the material used to fill the dental impression tray.
    c. Dental stone is used to fill the impression so as to create a positive image of the mouth.
    d. All of the above are true.

46. Which teeth in dogs are most commonly fractured?
    a. Maxillary fourth premolar
    b. Canine teeth
    c. Incisors
    d. Both A and B

47. Discolored teeth in the dog are most commonly a result of which disease or condition?
    a. Canine distemper
    b. Pulpitis (pulp necrosis)
    c. Periodontal disease
    d. Class IV malocclusion

48. Stomatitis, seen most commonly as lymphocytic-plasmacytic stomatitis in cats, has what cause?
    a. Immune-mediated
    b. Uremia
    c. Viral disease
    d. Foreign-body reaction

49. What therapy provides resolution to stomatitis in approximately 80% of cases in cats?
    a. Doxycycline at 2 mg/kg for 14 days
    b. Dental cleanings every 3 months
    c. Full mouth or nearly full mouth extractions
    d. Crown restorations

50. What is the cause of masticatory myositis?
    a. Viral infection of the muscle of mastication
    b. Antibody formation toward a specific component of myosin found only in the muscles of mastication
    c. A caustic reaction to a 2% chlorhexidine oral rinse
    d. Periapical abscess formation from an untreated complicated fracture of the maxillary fourth premolar

51. What is the definitive method of diagnosis for masticatory myositis?
    a. Serum and muscle tissue antibody analysis
    b. Viral isolation with electron microscopy
    c. History of inappropriate use of chlorhexidine with cytology of oral mucosa
    d. Internal oral examination and dental radiography of the maxillary fourth premolar

52. What is the usual treatment of choice for masticatory myositis?
    a. Saline rinses of the oral cavity twice daily for 2 weeks
    b. Acyclovir orally once daily for 1 month
    c. Endodontic or exodontic treatment of the maxillary fourth premolar fracture
    d. An immunosuppressive dose of steroids tapered to a maintenance dose

53. What is the most common type of jaw fracture in the dog and cat?
    a. Temporomandibular disarticulation
    b. Ramus fracture
    c. Symphyseal separation of the mandible
    d. Fracture of the angle of the mandible

54. Attrition refers to wear:
    a. due to chewing inappropriately.
    b. from teeth contacting teeth.
    c. from chewing at hair.
    d. from chewing on metal.

55. What is the purpose of the varied grooves and ridges on the occlusal surfaces of the premolars and molars in the horse?
    a. Determination of age
    b. Grinding of food
    c. Defense against predators
    d. Prehension of food

56. Which of the following are clinical signs of severe dental disease in the horse?
    a. Ocular, nasal, or oral discharge
    b. Weight loss
    c. Head shaking or tilting
    d. All of the above

57. To perform a thorough oral examination in the horse, which of the following procedures is necessary?
    a. General anesthesia
    b. Local anesthesia
    c. Sedation
    d. Both B and C

58. What is the term used to describe the process of mechanically adjusting the occlusal surface of horse teeth by removing raised areas?
    a. Floating
    b. Bishoping
    c. Curettage
    d. Sailing

59. What is one of the clinical signs associated with wry nose in the horse?
    a. Difficulty suckling
    b. Difficulty prehending food
    c. Severe dyspnea
    d. All of the above

60. What is the mechanism by which horses, teeth are kept clean?
    a. Daily brushing
    b. Placement of HMP in drinking water
    c. Normal mastication of abrasive substances
    d. All of the above

EXERCISE 36.11 FILL-IN-THE-BLANK: COMPREHENSIVE

Instructions: Fill in each of the spaces provided with the missing word or words that complete the sentence.

1. Because of the variation in severity of disease at the time of treatment, the term *dental prophylaxis* is largely being replaced with the term _____ _____ _____.

2. Members of the _____ of _____ _____ technicians have completed a credentialing process and passed a specialty examination to verify an advanced level of dental knowledge.

3. The root apices of _____ teeth are open for a limited time during tooth eruption and development, and therefore do not continually grow or erupt.

4. The smooth, convex bulge located on the palatal side of the gingival third of incisor teeth is called the _____.

5. The adjective _____ is used to describe the maxillary fourth premolar and mandibular first molar of dogs and cats, which play a significant role in shearing food during mastication.

6. A history of sneezing after drinking water may indicate the presence of a(n) _____ _____, which is a common problem in small-breed dogs with advanced periodontal disease.

7. An important component of the extraoral examination is a technique called _____ _____, which involves gently pushing on the closed eyelids with your thumbs to assess ability of the globes to move caudally in the orbit.

8. The _____ _____ is a raised structure located on the midline behind the maxillary incisors of dogs and cats.

9. The rostral two-thirds of the hard palate are covered by palatal mucosa that has hard ridges or _____, ranging from 8 to 10 in number.

10. Radiographic evaluation of areas that have missing teeth is imperative because _____ _____ can develop as a result of an unerupted tooth.

11. Dental instruments are held with a(n) _____ _____ _____, in which the first three fingers are in a triangular position on the instrument and the ring finger is used as a rest on an adjacent oral structure.

12. The _____ _____ is a cribriform plate of bone lining the tooth socket and appears radiographically as a white line adjacent to the periodontal space.

13. The term _____ _____ more truly describes the periodontal health of a tooth because it accounts for both pocket depth and gingival recession.

14. _____ _____ occurs when the dental x-ray beam misses portions of the sensor, plate, or film, resulting in areas with no image.

15. Inaccurate vertical angulation of the x-ray beam causes the resultant image to appear shortened, which is termed _____, or lengthened, which is termed _____.

16. The _____ _____ is composed of strong fibers that connect the tooth to alveolar bone.

17. A normal anatomic structure called the _____ _____ _____ is located apical to the mandibular second premolar in dogs and can be misinterpreted as periapical pathology when superimposed over a tooth root.

18. The term _____ _____ refers to the use of nonsurgical instrumentation to remove hard and soft deposits from all tooth surfaces along with the disruption of nonadherent bacteria within the gingival sulcus.

19. In today's veterinary practices, _____ _____ are the instruments primarily used for routine débridement and advanced periodontal therapy.

20. The portion of an ultrasonic scaler handpiece that converts electrical energy into mechanical energy is called the _____.

21. In general, dental hand instruments consist of three parts: (1) the _____, (2) the _____, and (3) the _____ _____.

22. Designed for subgingival scaling and root planing, a(n) _____ _____ has two cutting edges and can be adapted for all surfaces of the teeth.

435

23. Three benefits of nerve blocks in veterinary dentistry are _____ analgesia, _____ analgesia, and a decreased concentration of _____ _____ agents.

24. One should aspirate prior to injecting local analgesic when performing a dental nerve block to ensure that the needle is not in a(n) _____ _____.

25. A(n) _____-gauge needle is most commonly used for dental nerve blocks.

26. _____ materials are those that do not induce new bone, but act as a scaffold to allow existing bone cells to fill the defect.

27. _____ materials are those that will induce new bone growth by stimulating osteoblast precursors to form.

28. The three basic categories of home dental care intended to reduce oral bacteria are _____, _____, and use of _____.

29. Of the three basic categories of home dental care listed previously, _____ provides the most thorough method of plaque control for pets.

30. _____ is the facial morphology in which the upper jaw is wider than the lower jaw.

31. _____ _____ are small pieces of rubber that go around an endodontic file in order to mark a specific length in the canal.

32. The distance from the tip of the endodontic file and the rubber stop is known as the _____ _____.

33. Sodium hypochlorite is the most common irrigant in endodontic therapy because it has excellent _____ properties and the ability to break down _____ _____.

34. During endodontic therapy, _____ is defined as filling the canal with material that will seal it from the periapical area.

35. When sharpening hand instruments, the angle between the stone and the face should be approximately _____ degrees.

36. When performing endodontics, a(n) _____ is used to push the filling material apically and a(n) _____ is used to push the filling material laterally.

37. When significant periodontal disease exists, an iatrogenic jaw fracture more easily occurs when extracting the _____ mandibular molar and the mandibular _____ in cats and small-breed dogs.

38. When performing exodontia, the handle of the dental elevator should rest securely in the palm of the hand, and the _____ _____ is placed at the tip of the dental elevator to prevent inadvertent advancement of the tip into deeper structures.

39. _____ extraction is a type of tooth extraction that uses dental elevators placed in the periodontal space on the mesial or distal surface of the crown to fatigue the periodontal ligament.

40. _____ extraction is a type of tooth extraction in which a gingival flap is created, and then a window is created in the buccal bone over the tooth to be extracted.

41. A gingival flap with no releasing incision is called a(n) _____ flap, a gingival flap with one releasing incision is called a(n) _____ flap, and a gingival flap with two releasing incisions is called a(n) _____ flap.

42. The _____ is the animal species that is most commonly affected with tooth resorption.

43. There are _____ classes of malocclusion.

44. Class _____ malocclusion is the most common type receiving orthodontic correction in pets.

45. _____ _____ is a nonspecific term for a form of unilateral maxillary-mandibular asymmetry.

46. _____ _____ is the term used to describe the extraction of persistent deciduous or adult teeth that are problematic because of malocclusion.

47. Mandibular permanent canines erupt _____ in relationship to the persistent deciduous teeth, whereas maxillary permanent canines erupt _____ in relationship to the persistent deciduous teeth.

48. The best time to remove persistent deciduous teeth is before they cause _____ of their permanent counterparts.

49. The three typical types of dental trauma in dogs and cats are _____, a(n) _____ tooth fracture (in which there is no pulp exposure), and a(n) _____ tooth fracture (in which there is pulp exposure).

50. The most common oral tumor in the cat is _____ _____ _____.

51. The most common benign oral tumor in the dog is _____.

52. The four common malignant oral tumors in the dog are malignant _____, _____ _____ _____, _____, and _____.

53. A(n) _____ muzzle may be the treatment of choice in young animals with jaw fractures.

54. "Wolf teeth" is a term used to describe the permanent _____ _____ in the horse and are more commonly seen in the _____ arcade.

55. The premolars and molars in the horse are collectively known as _____ _____.

56. In the equine, intraoral dental radiographs are limited to evaluation of the incisors because of the large size of the _____, the small size of the _____, and limited _____ access.

57. Sinusitis and chronic unilateral nasal discharge related to dental disease in the horse usually affect the maxillary fourth _____; the first, second, and third _____ teeth; and the _____ sinus.

58. Extraoral exodontia is usually performed on the _____ teeth in the horse.

59. _____ _____ is the term for deviation of the incisive bone, maxilla, and nasal septum laterally from midline in the foal.

EXERCISE 36.12 CASE STUDY: PROFESSIONAL DENTAL CLEANING

You have just been hired as a veterinary technician in a small animal practice that emphasizes quality dental care. On your first day on the job, you are directed to the dental suite and asked to perform a professional dental cleaning on a 9-year-old, neutered male Toy Poodle. Wanting to make a good impression by providing excellent care to your patient, you mentally review the procedure. Respond to each of the following queries about the professional dental cleaning.

1. Power scaling instruments use a water-cooled vibrating tip to remove hard and soft deposits from the teeth and periodontal pockets.

   a. Explain how the vibrations of power scalers are measured.

   _____

   _____

   b. Briefly describe the two types of power scalers and how each operates.

   i. _____

   _____

   _____

   ii. _____

   _____

   _____

   c. Explain the disadvantage of using a sonic scaler.

   _____

   _____

2. The ultrasonic scaling unit contains an electronic generator inside plastic housing attached to a foot pedal by a cable. The handpiece is also attached by tubing to a water supply to provide a water stream from the ultrasonic scaler tip.

a. List the benefits of the water stream that comes from the ultrasonic scaler tip.

_____

_____

_____

_____

_____

_____

b. Identify the patient and human safety precautions that should be taken to reduce the amount of aerosolized bacteria caused by the ultrasonic scaler's water mist.

_____

_____

_____

_____

_____

c. How should the patient's eyes be protected during ultrasonic scaling?

_____

_____

d. Why is it important to intubate the patient and ensure that the endotracheal cuff is fully inflated prior to ultrasonic scaling?

_____

_____

3. The magnetostrictive scaler is the most common type of power scaler used in human and veterinary dentistry. Describe how the tip of a magnetostrictive scaler functions and how the tip should be properly used on tooth surfaces.

_____

_____

_____

_____

_____

_____

439

4. The power and water knobs of magnetostrictive units must be properly adjusted prior to the periodontal débridement procedure.

   a. What does the power knob do?

   _____

   _____

   _____

   b. When should the high-power versus low-power setting be used?

   _____

   _____

   _____

   c. Why is it necessary to have adequate water flow through the ultrasonic scaler handpiece?

   _____

   _____

   _____

5. Describe the proper technique required for removal of dental calculus using a supragingival hand scaler.

   _____

   _____

   _____

   _____

   _____

   _____

6. Angulation refers to the relationship of the face of a hand scaling instrument to the tooth. Explain proper curette angulation and the technique for removal of dental deposits from the gingival sulcus.

   _____

   _____

   _____

   _____

   _____

   _____

440

7. Polishing is the final but critical step performed on a dental patient as part of routine cleaning or advanced periodontal therapy.

   a. Explain the rationale for dental polishing.

   _____

   _____

   _____

   b. Describe proper polishing technique when using a motor-driven handpiece and rubber cup, including desired polishing paste, cup pressure, speed setting, and polishing time per tooth surface.

   _____

   _____

   _____

   _____

   _____

   _____

   _____

   _____

   _____

   c. After polishing, what is the final step that should be performed to finish the complete dental cleaning procedure?

   _____

   _____

   _____

37 Geriatric and Hospice Care: Supporting the Aged and Dying Patient

LEARNING OBJECTIVES

When you have completed this chapter, you will be able to:
1. Pronounce, define, and spell all of the key terms in this chapter.
2. List the life stages of dogs and cats, and describe the effects of aging on body systems, and describe how to integrate geriatric care.
3. Identify and explain the oral, cardiac, respiratory, neoplastic, renal, neurologic, orthopedic, and endocrine disorders commonly seen in geriatric dogs and cats.
4. Explain the changing nutritional needs of aging pets.
5. Discuss components of hospice nursing care for geriatric dogs and cats, including how to identify the appropriate time to discuss euthanasia with a pet's owner.
6. Discuss components of the physical examination of a geriatric horse.
7. List and describe disorders commonly seen in geriatric horses, including oral/nasal, vision, cardiac, respiratory, gastrointestinal, kidney, skin, neurologic, and orthopedic problems.
8. Identify and explain the chronic conditions that most commonly affect geriatric horses such as equine Cushing disease, heaves, laminitis, dental problems and sinusitis, equine recurrent uveitis (ERU), and neurologic and musculoskeletal defects.
9. Discuss the management, nutrition, and nursing care of geriatric horses, including end of life issues.

EXERCISE 37.1 DEFINITIONS: TERMS AND DEFINITIONS

Instructions: Define each term in your own words.

1. Laminitis: _____

   _____

2. Geriatric: _____

   _____

3. Hirsutism: _____

   _____

4. Hospice: _____

   _____

5. Incontinence: _____

   _____

6. Life stage: _____

_____

7. Wave mouth: _____

_____

EXERCISE 37.2 MATCHING: SIGNS OF EQUINE RECURRENT UVEITIS (ERU)

Instructions: Match each sign of ERU in column A with its corresponding description in column B by writing the appropriate letter in the space provided.

Column A

1. _____ Corneal edema
2. _____ Hyphema
3. _____ Photophobia
4. _____ Miosis
5. _____ Hypopyon
6. _____ Neovascularization
7. _____ Corneal ulceration
8. _____ Anterior uveitis

Column B

A. Constricted pupils.
B. Cellular debris in the eye.
C. Blood vessel growth on cornea.
D. Blue tint caused by increased fluid content.
E. Discomfort upon exposure to light.
F. Inflammation of the tissues in the forward chamber.
G. Loss of the epithelium on the front of the eye.
H. Hemorrhage in the eye.

EXERCISE 37.3 TRUE OR FALSE: COMPREHENSIVE

Instructions: Read the following statements and write "T" for true or "F" for false in the blanks provided. If a statement is false, correct the statement to make it true.

1. _____ The effects of aging in people are very different from the effects of aging in animals.

2. _____ The speed with which the aging process occurs in animals varies according to the species and breed.

3. _____ Geriatric animals that are ill most often have relatively specific symptoms that can be traced to a particular disease condition.

4. _____ At-home dental prophylaxis is not helpful in a geriatric patient with established dental disease.

5. _____ Signs of mild coughing and exercise intolerance in geriatric animals are most likely associated with muscle fatigue or arthritis that develops with age, and does not necessarily warrant further investigation.

6. _____ Chronic renal disease is very common in geriatric cats.

7. _____ Orthopedic disease is a common geriatric condition often successfully managed with appropriate care.

8. _____ Hypothyroidism is a common disease in middle-aged and geriatric cats that is characterized by increased appetite with weight loss, vomiting, and lack of grooming behavior.

9. _____ Life-threatening complications can develop with untreated hyperthyroidism in cats.

10. _____ Pain is more difficult to assess in animals than in humans because the signs of pain are subtler.

11. _____ An increased heart rate or an increased respiratory rate can be a sign that an animal is in pain.

12. _____ A feeding tube should be placed in any ill patient that is not eating to ensure adequate caloric intake.

13. _____ Slings are used in animals with functional forelimbs but little or no function of their hindlimbs.

14. _____ Heaves in horses is often related to a dust or mold allergy.

15. _____ Dyspnea, especially during inhalation, is a typical sign of heaves.

16. _____ In an aged horse, laminitis usually develops as a secondary condition to a preexisting problem.

17. _____ Eye pain and swelling in an aged horse requires treatment but is usually not serious.

18. _____ Geriatric horses often develop degenerative joint disease in the coxofemoral joints, stifles, and lumbar vertebrae.

19. _____ A horse may have gastrointestinal parasites even when the fecal examination is negative.

20. _____ A dog is no longer classified as pediatric after reaching 1 year of age.

21. _____ A large-breed dog ages more rapidly than a small-breed dog or a cat.

22. _____ In general, an animal needs more energy from food as it ages.

23. _____ Reduced dietary protein may decrease the risk of developing kidney disease and slow its progression in geriatric patients.

24. _____ All aging patients need the amount of fiber in their diet increased significantly.

25. _____ Home-cooked diets are a very acceptable alternative for senior pets.

26. _____ Dehydration may be seen in animals that are drinking less as well as in animals that are drinking more than normal.

EXERCISE 37.4 MULTIPLE CHOICE: COMPREHENSIVE

Instructions: Circle the one correct answer to each of the following questions.

1. A cat that is 8 years of age is considered to be a
   a. Young adult
   b. Mature adult
   c. Senior
   d. Geriatric

2. A Great Dane that is 8 years of age is considered to be a
   a. Young adult
   b. Mature adult
   c. Senior
   d. Geriatric

3. Which of the following is not a change you would expect to see in an aging patient?
   a. Decrease in caloric needs by 30% to 40%
   b. Decreased activity of the immune system
   c. Development of an immune-mediated disease
   d. Decreased susceptibility to infections

4. Which of the following is not a physical change you would expect to see in an aging patient?
   a. Decreased percentage of body fat
   b. Thickening and darkening of the skin
   c. Loss of muscle mass
   d. Thickened footpads

5. All geriatric animals are prone to heart disease, but the exact nature of cardiac disease varies among species and even among breeds. For instance, small-breed dogs are most prone to _____, although large-breed dogs and cats are not.
   a. Chronic valvular disease
   b. Hypertrophic cardiomyopathy
   c. Atrial fibrillation
   d. Dilated cardiomyopathy

6. Polyuria and polydipsia are commonly noted in animals with all of the following diseases but one. Which is it?
   a. Diabetes mellitus
   b. Hyperadrenocorticism
   c. Hypothyroidism
   d. Chronic renal disease

7. This endocrine disease is much more commonly seen in geriatric cats than in other species.
   a. Hyperadrenocorticism
   b. Diabetes mellitus
   c. Hypothyroidism
   d. Hyperthyroidism

8. Common signs of hyperthyroidism do *not* include
   a. Polyuria
   b. Increased appetite
   c. Heat seeking
   d. Weight loss

9. "Cushing disease" is an alternative name for
   a. Hyperadrenocorticism
   b. Diabetes mellitus
   c. Hypothyroidism
   d. Hyperthyroidism

10. The class of analgesic drugs that can cause significant side effects, especially with long-term use, and should only be used as a last resort is
    a. Nonsteroidal antiinflammatory drugs
    b. Glucocorticoids
    c. Opiates
    d. α_2-Agonists

11. A geriatric horse with a long, wavy hair coat that does not shed completely in the spring is likely to have
    a. Hypothyroidism
    b. Laminitis
    c. Cushing disease
    d. Heaves

12. The most common abnormal heart rhythm in geriatric horses is
    a. Ventricular tachycardia
    b. First-degree AV heart block
    c. Sinus arrhythmia
    d. Atrial fibrillation

13. The development of hypertrophied external abdominal oblique muscles as a result of increased effort on exhalation is typically seen in horses with
    a. Recurrent airway obstruction
    b. Sinusitis
    c. Pneumonia
    d. Laryngeal paralysis

14. Pituitary pars intermedia dysfunction (PPID) is an alternative name for
    a. Recurrent airway obstruction
    b. Equine recurrent uveitis
    c. Cushing disease
    d. Hirsutism

15. The reluctance of a horse to touch its nose to its shoulder is generally indicative of pain affecting the
    a. Nose
    b. Neck
    c. Jaw
    d. Shoulder

16. The signs of Cushing disease in horses include hirsutism, patchy sweating, polyuria, polydipsia, and
    a. Weight loss
    b. Laminitis
    c. Muscle hypertrophy
    d. Hyperactivity

17. The most important aspect of treatment for horses with heaves is
    a. Minimizing contact with allergens
    b. The bronchodilator clenbuterol
    c. Injections of steroids
    d. Regular use of an inhaler

18. Serial measurement of ACTH, insulin, and dextrose is used to diagnose
    a. Hyperthyroidism in cats
    b. Hypothyroidism in dogs
    c. PPID in horses
    d. Diabetes in dogs

19. An NSAID used to treat DJD in the horse that is less likely than other NSAIDs to cause adverse effects because it is a COX-2 inhibitor is
    a. Phenylbutazone
    b. Flunixin meglumine
    c. Dexamethasone
    d. Firocoxib

20. A geriatric horse that lives in a barn with poor air circulation, has a history of allergic reactions, and exhibits tachypnea and dyspnea may be exhibiting signs of
    a. Laminitis
    b. Heaves
    c. Sinusitis
    d. DJD

21. Pretreatment with a(n) _____ is recommended in horses with a history of vaccine reactions.
    a. Steroid
    b. Bronchodilator
    c. NSAID
    d. Antibiotic

446

EXERCISE 37.5 FILL-IN-THE-BLANK: COMPREHENSIVE

Instructions: Fill in each of the spaces provided with the missing word or words that complete the sentence.

1. Many veterinarians recommend that healthy geriatric small animals (those over _____ years of age) should be examined _____ time(s) a year.

2. Glucose is the necessary nutrient for the body's cells to perform their normal functions. For glucose to enter cells, the hormone _____ is required.

3. As a cat ages, it is prone to a(n) _____ in body weight, until approximately 11 to 12 years of age, when it is prone to a(n) _____ in body weight.

4. The most commonly used class of analgesics used to treat pain associated with degenerative joint disease and other forms of osteoarthritis is the _____.

5. To prevent formation of decubital ulcers, a recumbent patient should be turned from side to side every _____ hours.

6. A few hours after giving subcutaneous fluids between the shoulder blades, the fluids will usually shift to the _____ surface of the body because of the force of _____.

7. Position for bladder expression may vary patient to patient. For instance, the bladder can usually be expressed when a patient is in _____ recumbency, or when it is _____.

8. Geriatric horses are generally considered to be those older than _____ years of age.

9. A systolic murmur auscultated on the left side of the equine thorax suggests a common valvular disease of the geriatric horse known as _____ _____.

10. Common tumors in horses include squamous cell carcinomas, which often develop on the _____, and melanomas, which often develop around the _____ area.

11. Cushing disease in horses is caused by decreased production of the neurotransmitter _____ in the hypothalamus.

12. Cushing disease in horses is treated with the dopamine agonist _____.

13. To maintain health and keep the horse comfortable, a geriatric horse should have its hooves trimmed every _____ weeks and dental floating every _____ months.

14. Inflammation of the right dorsal colon and renal failure are potential adverse effects of _____ class drugs in the horse.

447

Instructions: Provide a short answer to each of the following questions in the space provided.

1. The need for hospice care for veterinary patients has increased in recent years. Describe some of the factors that has led to this increase.

   _____

   _____

   _____

2. As would be expected, difficulty chewing and dropping food from the mouth are signs of a deterioration of oral health (dental disease, gingivitis, a tumor, etc.). What are other signs of disease that may or may not be associated with oral disease, but should trigger an examination of the mouth?

   _____

   _____

3. What are some of the general signs that would indicate that a geriatric animal might have respiratory disease?

   _____

   _____

4. What is "cognitive dysfunction," and why does it sometimes strain the attachment between a pet and an owner?

   _____

   _____

   _____

5. Before giving any pain medication to a geriatric patient, and periodically while it is being given, blood work should be performed. Why is this necessary?

   _____

   _____

   _____

6. Decubital ulcers are a common complication in patients that cannot walk, such as those with spinal trauma or intervertebral disc disease.

   a. At what locations on the body do these ulcers most commonly form? What is it about these locations that predisposes them to ulcer formation?

   _____

   _____

   _____

   _____

b. What are some of the strategies that can be used to prevent decubital ulcers in recumbent patients? Include information about bedding, hygiene, and preventing undue pressure on the areas that are most at risk.

_____

_____

_____

_____

_____

_____

7. What conditions or factors predispose a patient to urine scalding?

_____

_____

_____

_____

_____

_____

8. Aging horses can develop one of a number of chronic diseases. For each of the following chronic diseases of the aged equine patient, indicate the part of the body that it effects and three common clinical signs associated with the condition. Because there are more than three clinical signs that may indicate each disease, pick three that you think are most important.

Disease Condition	Part of the Body Affected by this Condition	Three Important Signs of this Condition
Cushing disease		
Heaves		
Laminitis		
Wave mouth		
Chronic sinusitis		
Equine recurrent uveitis		
Neurologic deficits		
Osteoarthritis (DJD)		

9. Geriatric horses may have problems resulting from an overly long hair coat.

   a. What is the nature of the problems this can cause?

   _____

   _____

   _____

b. What can be done to keep these animals comfortable?

_____

_____

_____

10. Geriatric horses with a poor body condition as a consequence of inadequate caloric intake may require dietary changes or supplementation. What specific dietary changes can be employed to maintain body weight in these patients?

_____

_____

_____

38 The Human-Animal Bond and Euthanasia

LEARNING OBJECTIVES

When you have completed this chapter, you will be able to:
1. Pronounce, define, and spell all of the key terms in this chapter.
2. Discuss aspects of the human-animal bond.
3. List and describe the stages of grief and the role of veterinary professionals in grief counseling.
4. Do the following regarding euthanasia:
   - Discuss the impact of euthanasia and client grief on members of the veterinary health care team.
   - Discuss the legal and ethical issues related to euthanasia.
   - Discuss the role of the veterinary health care team in counseling owners considering euthanasia of their pet, and factors that owners need to consider when making decisions regarding euthanasia.
   - Describe considerations in scheduling euthanasia appointments and in preparing for unexpected events during euthanasia.
   - List signs and symptoms of staff burnout.
   - List and describe acceptable methods of euthanasia in animals.
   - Discuss special considerations related to euthanasia of large animals.

EXERCISE 38.1 MATCHING: TERMS AND DEFINITIONS

Instructions: Match each term in column A with its corresponding definition in column B by writing the appropriate letter in the space provided.

Column A

1. _____ Denial
2. _____ Catharsis
3. _____ Resolution
4. _____ Bargaining
5. _____ Validation
6. _____ Compassion
7. _____ Depression
8. _____ Anger

Column B

A. This manifestation of grief may be evident as irritability, sleep irregularity, restlessness, and an inability to concentrate.
B. This is the point in the grief process when the client's routines are reestablished and the pet is not forgotten but has been assigned to a special place in the bereaved individual's heart.
C. Guilt may be defined as this emotion turned inward.
D. Assuring a client that they made the right decision following euthanasia of a pet, and affirming that it is OK to grieve, are examples of this.
E. Focusing on a minor problem, such as a matted coat, after just having been given a poor prognosis for an animal with a terminal disease is a form of this.
F. Attempting to replace an animal that has died without grieving for the pet that was lost is a form of this.
G. This is the understanding of the suffering of others.
H. This is a release of emotion necessary to work through one's grief.

EXERCISE 38.2 DEFINITIONS: KEY TERMS

Instructions: Define each term in your own words.

1. Barbiturate: _____

_____

2. Bereavement: _____

_____

Chapter **38** **The Human-Animal Bond and Euthanasia**

3. Drug Enforcement Agency (DEA): _____

_____

4. Euthanasia: _____

_____

5. Grief: _____

_____

6. Grief process: _____

_____

EXERCISE 38.3 TRUE OR FALSE: COMPREHENSIVE

Instructions: Read the following statements and write "T" for true or "F" for false in the blanks provided. If a statement is false, correct the statement to make it true.

1. _____ People often view their pets as filling the role of partner, child, or best friend.

2. _____ Pet ownership can be good for human health, as it has been shown to be an important predictor of survival for people with coronary artery disease.

3. _____ The attachment of an owner to his or her guide dog is usually less strong than the attachment of an owner to his or her family pet.

4. _____ Family and friends who make up a person's support system often do not fully understand the importance of the bond between a pet and its owner.

5. _____ Most people in the United States are reasonably comfortable with talking about death.

6. _____ Veterinary professionals usually receive extensive training on how to counsel grieving clients in professional or technical school as a part of the regular curriculum.

7. _____ People usually experience the stages of grief in a specific order (first denial, then bargaining, anger, depression, and, finally, resolution).

8. _____ Clients experiencing denial will often never fully accept the reality of the situation they are experiencing.

9. _____ Clients going through the denial stage of the grief process can often get to a stage of acceptance only when they are forced to face the truth by a professional.

10. _____ When a client is going through the anger stage of grief, it is best that the veterinarian not allow the client to express his or her anger in front of the staff.

11. _____ Children usually are able to accept a loss more quickly than an adult.

12. _____ Once a client has made the decision to euthanize a pet, you are obligated to let the client know if you do not agree with the decision.

13. _____ In the event that a client does not want to be present during euthanasia, it is also best that he or she not be permitted to see the body after the animal is dead, as this tends to increase anxiety and grief.

14. _____ When performing euthanasia by injection of sodium pentobarbital, the animal may struggle or vocalize, even though it is not conscious.

15. _____ The Drug Enforcement Agency (DEA) of the U.S. Department of Justice requires that an accurate record be kept of the amount of barbiturate-class drug you use for each patient.

16. _____ Following euthanasia, once death has been confirmed by the vet, it is best to tell the client that the patient is dead.

17. _____ The use of dark humor by the staff to cope with the stress of euthanasia is an unfeeling action that has been shown to be ineffective.

EXERCISE 38.4 MULTIPLE CHOICE: COMPREHENSIVE

Instructions: Circle the one correct answer to each of the following questions.

1. The percentage of pet owners who classify their attachment to pets as "strong" is
   a. 25%
   b. 40%
   c. 50%
   d. 60%

2. During which stage of grief will a client often act in a way that makes him or her seem out of touch with reality?
   a. Anger
   b. Denial
   c. Depression
   d. Bargaining

3. A client comes into your practice to euthanize her pet. During the process, she says, "If only I had fed her a better quality food, maybe this would not be happening." This statement best characterizes which stage of the grief process?
   a. Denial
   b. Bargaining
   c. Anger
   d. Depression

4. In general, the best way to assist a client who is experiencing guilt is to say something like
   a. "I know how you feel."
   b. "We have a pet right here that is looking for a home and really needs you."
   c. "You did everything you could to help him."
   d. "Don't do this to yourself!"

5. A client comes into your practice to euthanize his pet. During the process, he says, "I'm thinking euthanasia may be a mistake. Rover seemed to be making a turn for the better this morning, and I think he can pull through." This statement best characterizes which stage of the grief process?
   a. Denial
   b. Bargaining
   c. Anger
   d. Depression

6. In general, the best way to assist a client who is expressing strong anger at the staff would be to
   a. Say, "If you're going to threaten me, you just need to leave now!"
   b. Say, "Please control yourself!"
   c. Say, "There's no need to be angry; you did everything you could to help him."
   d. Just listen attentively and do not say anything.

7. Clients most often may be reluctant to pay the bill when they are going through which stage of grief?
   a. Denial
   b. Bargaining
   c. Anger
   d. Depression

8. A client comes into your practice to euthanize his pet. During the process, he says, "Just last month I lost my wife; now I'm losing my dearest Buffy. I just don't know how I can go on without them." This statement best characterizes which stage of the grief process?
   a. Denial
   b. Depression
   c. Bargaining
   d. Anger

9. What is the best way to help a client make a decision whether or not to elect to euthanize a pet?
   a. Tell him or her what you would do if it were your pet
   b. Give him or her information about euthanasia and treatment alternatives
   c. Do not say anything; just listen
   d. Make the decision for him or her

10. A client comes into your practice to euthanize her pet. During the process, she says, "Isn't there any other treatment we can try? Just yesterday my neighbor was telling me about an herbal remedy that completely cured her cat's cancer." This statement best characterizes which stage of the grief process?
    a. Denial
    b. Bargaining
    c. Anger
    d. Depression
    e. Resolution

11. Identify the preferred route of sodium pentobarbital administration for euthanasia.
    a. Intravenous
    b. Intrahepatic
    c. Intracardiac
    d. Intraperitoneal

12. Which of the following is usually the most helpful in coping with the stress associated with euthanasia?
    a. Take time off
    b. Do something that you enjoy
    c. Talk with colleagues about it
    d. Make time for yourself

13. The most commonly used drug for euthanasia is
    a. Sodium pentothal
    b. Phenobarbital sodium
    c. Thiopental sodium
    d. Sodium pentobarbital

EXERCISE 38.5 FILL-IN-THE-BLANK: COMPREHENSIVE

Instructions: Fill in each of the spaces provided with the missing word or words that complete the sentence.

1. The person who first described the five stages of grieving (denial, bargaining, anger, depression, and resolution) was _____ _____.

2. A change in appetite, decreased energy level, withdrawal from others, irritability, sleep irregularity, restlessness, and inability to concentrate are signs of the stage of grief known as _____.

3. The grief process is quite variable in length and can last anywhere between a few _____ and many _____.

4. The word *euthanasia* is derived from the Greek root *eu*, meaning _____, and *thanatos*, meaning _____.

5. A factor that is much more important to consider when euthanizing large animals than when euthanizing small animals is _____.

EXERCISE 38.6 CASE STUDY #1: HELPING ADULTS THROUGH THE GRIEVING PROCESS

Mrs. Andreas came into your clinic today with her 12-year-old female Golden Retriever, Goldie. Goldie had not been feeling well for about a week, and Mrs. Andreas noticed a few large lumps under her jaw. A physical examination revealed generalized enlargement of the peripheral lymph nodes. A complete diagnostic workup was done, including a needle biopsy of the right submandibular lymph node. The tests revealed lymphoma (cancer of the lymph nodes). While the doctor was explaining the disease and the prognosis, Mrs. Andreas looked away and seemed preoccupied with other thoughts. The doctor then tried to discuss treatment options, but Mrs. Andreas cut him off and said she had to leave or Goldie would be late for an appointment at the groomers.

1. Which stage of grief do you think Mrs. Andreas is in?

   _____

2. Your initial feelings are irritation and frustration. Should you express these feelings to Mrs. Andreas? Why or why not?

   _____

   _____

   _____

   _____

   _____

   _____

3. What are some constructive steps you could take to help Mrs. Andreas come to terms with the diagnosis?

   _____

   _____

   _____

   _____

   _____

   _____

EXERCISE 38.7 CASE STUDY #2: HELPING CHILDREN THROUGH THE GRIEVING PROCESS

You have just returned home from the animal hospital. Bonnie, your 19-year-old Siamese cat, was euthanized as a result of complications related to chronic kidney failure. It has been a difficult few weeks, as Bonnie was failing for some time and required a lot of care. Her condition deteriorated very suddenly this morning, and so you had to make arrangements for euthanasia sooner than you had anticipated and did not have the opportunity to prepare your 6-year-old daughter, Lizzy. When you returned from the hospital, Lizzy had just come home from school. She noticed immediately how upset you were and started to cry. Even before today, she had been acting more clingy and quiet than usual.

1. What are some of the emotions that Lizzy may be feeling?

   _____

   _____

   _____

2. When explaining Bonnie's death, is it preferable to be honest or to make up a story that will "soften the blow"? Why?

   _____

   _____

   _____

3. In what way might Lizzy view Bonnie's death differently than an older child?

   _____

   _____

   _____

4. When talking with Lizzy about Bonnie's death, it is important that you avoid using euphemisms. What is a euphemism, and why is it best to not use them around children?

   _____

   _____

   _____

5. After telling Lizzy that Bonnie died, you are feeling unbelievably weary and tired from the whole ordeal, and tell her you do not really want to talk about it anymore. Why might this approach intensify Lizzy's feelings?

   _____

   _____

   _____

Chapter **38** **The Human-Animal Bond and Euthanasia**